Transfusion medicine: the French model

Transfusion medicine: the French model

Coordinated by
Alain Beauplet,
Rémi Courbil,
Jean-Marc Ouazan

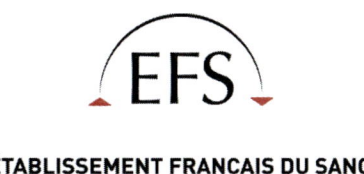

ÉTABLISSEMENT FRANÇAIS DU SANG

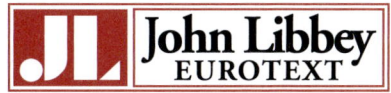

ISBN: 978-2-7420-1120-9

Éditions John Libbey Eurotext
127 Avenue de la République
92120 Montrouge, France
Tel: +33 (0)1 46 73 06 60
Email: contact@jle.com
http://www.jle.com

John Libbey Eurotext
42-46 High Street
Esher
KT10 9QY
United Kingdom

© 2013 John Libbey Eurotext. All rights reserved.

No part of this publication may be reproduced without the permission of the publisher or the Centre Français d'Exploitation du Droit de Copie, 20 Rue des Grands-Augustins, 75010 Paris.

Preface

Transfusion medicine

Blood transfusion is an essential, and irreplaceable, component of healthcare, underpinning modern medicine and surgery.

Over time, blood transfusion practice has evolved, leading to the emergence of **transfusion medicine** as we know it today – multidisciplinary and involving a series of complex processes.

Transfusion medicine now includes promoting donation, collecting blood from donors, and preparing and testing products. These activities are followed by distribution and delivery, which are closely associated with immunohaematology or possibly histocompatibility testing and transfusion support, to ensure the appropriate use of blood transfusion in patient management.

Safety is maintained through vigilance, monitoring and assessment processes targeting continual improvement in quality, which also entails training, research and development.

The French model

To optimize the provision of this aspect of healthcare, responsibility for blood transfusion services is clearly divided in France, with separation between:
– the producer of labile blood products (LBP): this role has been allocated to the French Blood Establishment (EFS), a central government agency (*établissement public de l'État*), which has had a monopoly over the collection, preparation, testing and distribution of LBP since 1 January 2000;
– the LBP user, *i.e.* health facilities (ES), whether public, private, semi-private or military, which transfuse the products to patients.

Three major features set **French transfusion medicine** apart from other international models:
- **in France, blood donation is underpinned by four founding principles: altruism, voluntarism, anonymity and absence of profit**, which are upheld by the EFS. These principles contribute to increased safety levels for donors and recipients.
  "Ethical blood donation" is the basis for the non-ownership and non-commercialization of the human body and products derived therefrom, principles that are now enshrined in bioethics law.
  It is also the unshakeable foundation of French society through the related concepts of generosity, solidarity and selflessness;
- French lawmakers opted to give **the EFS a monopoly over the distribution of LBP** to guarantee across the country:
– homogeneous distribution of LBP to all types of ES (public, private, etc.) and areas of activity (medicine, surgery, obstetrics, etc.),
– optimal access to LBP meeting the individual needs of each recipient (specific processing or testing) and avoiding the dispersion of stocks of these rare, precious and perishable products,

— records of recipients enabling permanent traceability of the donor-donation-product-patient chain,
— self-sufficiency in LBP at all times, for which a single government agency is clearly and solely accountable;
- **the strong link between immunohaematology, delivery and transfusion support**, which is essential for health safety and is the core of the French blood transfusion model. Immunohaematology is inseparable from the selection of blood components and its sole purpose is to ensure appropriate delivery: the right product to the right patient. The EFS also provides transfusion support to guide prescribers towards the "right prescription", *i.e.* consistent with current professional guidelines, the medical condition in question and patient characteristics. Transfusion support is an essential component of optimal LBP management for optimal recipient safety.

And because the EFS is financed by the State, **efficiency** is a major strategic objective alongside **self-sufficiency** and **safety**.

The French Blood Establishment

The EFS, which was founded under the authority of the Ministry of Health on 1 January 2000 by the Act of 1 July 1998 and was ISO 9001 certified in 2008, is the **sole public provider of national blood transfusion services in France**. Its role is to maintain the country's self-sufficiency in LBP, whilst meeting the highest quality and safety standards. Formed by 17 regional establishments (14 on the mainland and 3 in overseas *départements*), the EFS is a **major contributor to public health in France**, managing the collection (in 2011: 3.2 million donations were made in its 151 permanent sites and 50,000 annual mobile sessions), preparation, testing (with its 17 technical platforms) and distribution of LBP (in 2011: 2.4 million packed red blood cells, 380,000 therapeutic plasmas and 29,000 platelet concentrates) and delivery, for each patient, from its 156 sites (in 2011: over 560,000 recipients transfused in more than 1,900 ES).

The EFS is also France's largest medical testing laboratory with recognized expertise in immunohaematology (in 2011: 376 million tests conducted) and histocompatibility (in 2011: 106 million tests conducted). Finally, in addition to its core purpose, the EFS provides treatments and conducts research in innovative areas such as engineering and cell and tissue therapy.

The mapping of EFS processes (Figure 1) shows the extent and complexity of its activities.

Every day, continuity in public transfusion services is ensured through the commitment and professionalism of nearly 10,000 EFS employees.

François Toujas
Chairman of the EFS

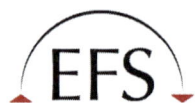

Preface

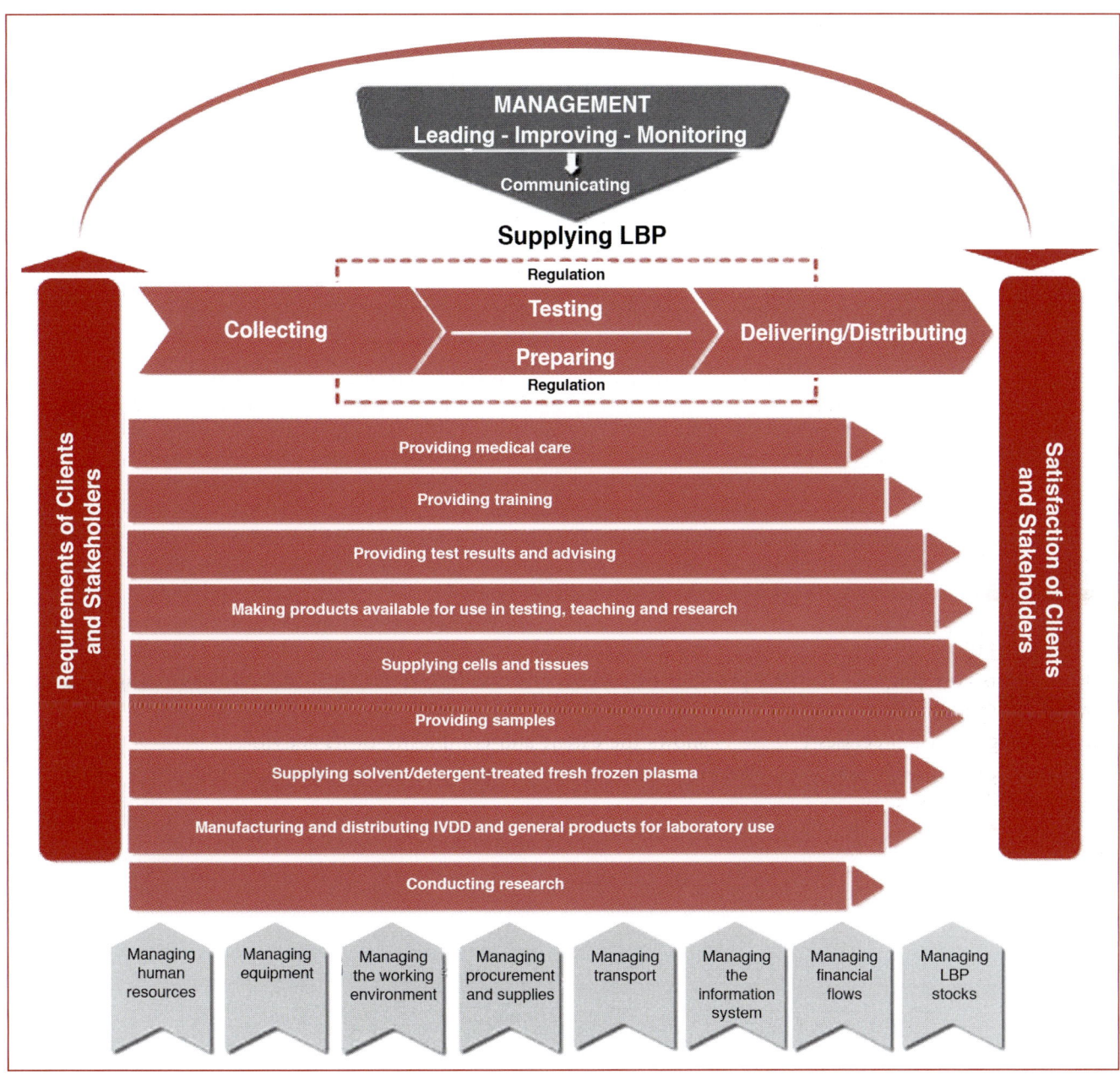

Figure 1. Mapping of EFS processes.
LBP: labile blood products; IVDD: *in vitro* diagnostic medical devices.

Contents

Preface V
F. Toujas

List of the authors XI

Part I. Organisation of blood transfusion services

1. Organisation of blood transfusion services in France 3
J.-M. Ouazan, S. Valcke

2. Other organisational models for blood transfusion services 13
O. Nasr

3. The Council of Europe: Pioneering Blood Safety since the 1950's 19
G. Rautmann

Part II. French transfusion medicine

4. Communication 25
F. Le Failler

5. Blood collection 32
F. Chenus, B. Danic, G. Woimant

6. Preparation 45
P. Chavarin, D. Dernis, C. Vignoli

7. Donation testing 61
A. Assal, C. Corbi, P. Gallian

8. Patient testing 73
F. Hau, C. Krause, F. Roubinet

9. Distribution, delivery and transfusion support 83
S. Assari, A. François, F. Roubinet

10. Transfusion 94
J. Chiaroni, R. Courbil, S. Mathieu-Nafissi, J.-F. Quaranta

Part III. Transfusion safety in France

11. Assessment	109
S. Begue, A. Chabanel, M. Sillam	
12. Monitoring	123
R. Courbil, A. Fialaire-Legendre, S. Jbilou, F. Maire, D. Narbey, N. Ribon, E. Terme	
13. Improvement	138
E. Bizot-Touzard, É. Hergon, W. Sghaier	

Part IV. Research within the EFS and the future of transfusion medicine

14. Research within the EFS and the future of transfusion medicine	155
P. Tiberghien	
15. The cell and tissue therapy within the EFS	163
A. Fialaire-Legendre	

Part V. The EFS's European and international activities

16. The EFS, a European stakeholder in blood transfusion	169
Y. Charpak, N. Prunier	
17. The EFS's international activities	172
L. Sobaga	

Conclusion	181
A. Beauplet, R. Courbil, J.-M. Ouazan	
Regulatory references	183
J. Debeir	

Annexes

The EFS staff	191
Table showing selling price before tax for labile blood products in France	192
Glossary	193

List of the authors

Assal Azzedine, Director of EFS Aquitaine-Limousin

Assari Suzanne, Clinical Trial Manager within the Medical Division

Beauplet Alain, Director of International Affairs of the EFS

Bégué Stéphane, Head of Quality Control and Assessment of LBP within the Medical Division

Bizot-Touzard Emeline, Project Manager within the Regulatory Affairs and Quality Division

Chabanel Anne, "Quality Control and Assessment of LBP" expert within the Medical Division

Charpak Yves, Director of Surveys and Prospective of the EFS

Chavarin Patricia, Deputy Director of EFS Auvergne-Loire

Chenus Florence, Collection Manager of EFS Aquitaine-Limousin

Chiaroni Jacques, Director of EFS Alpes-Méditerranée

Corbi Cécile, Donation Testing Laboratory Manager of EFS Centre-Atlantique

Courbil Rémi, Medical Director of the EFS

Danic Bruno, Deputy Director of EFS Bretagne

Debeir Joëlle, Head of the "Authorization, Inspection and Regulation" Unit within the Regulatory Affairs and Quality Division

Dernis Dominique, "Preparation" expert within the Medical Division

Fialaire-Legendre Anne, "Cell and tissue therapy" expert within the Medical Division

François Anne, "Distribution/delivery" expert within the Medical Division

Gallian Pierre, "Donation Testing" expert within the Medical Division

Hau Françoise, "Histocompatibility" expert within the Medical Division

Hergon Eric, Director of Regulatory Affairs and Quality of the EFS

Jbilou Saadia, Project Manager within the Medical Division

Krause Claire, "Immunohaematology" expert within the Medical Division

Le Failler Françoise, Director of Communication of the EFS

Maire Françoise, Deputy Director of the Medical Division

Mathieu-Nafissi Suzanne, "Health centres" expert within the Medical Division

Narbey David, "Haemovigilance, medical devices and pharmacovigilance expert" within the Medical Division

Nasr Olivier, Project Manager within the International Affairs Division
Ouazan Jean-Marc, Director of the Office of the Chairman of the EFS
Prunier Nina, Project Manager Europe
Quaranta Jean-François, Risk and Quality Manager within Nice University Hospital
Rautmann Guy, Scientific Officer, European Directorate for the Quality of Medicines & HealthCare, Council of Europe
Ribon Nicolas, Project Manager within the Medical Division
Roubinet Francis, Director of EFS Pyrénées-Méditerranée
Sghaier Wided, "Risk Management" Project Manager within the Regulatory Affairs and Quality Division
Sillam Magali, Database Manager within the Medical Division
Sobaga Leslie, Deputy Director of the International Affairs Division
Terme Emmanuel, "Reagent vigilance" expert within the Medical Division
Tiberghien Pierre, Responsible Person of the EFS
Toujas François, Chairman of the EFS
Valcke Samuel, Director of Legal Affairs of the EFS
Vignoli Catherine, Head of Labile Blood Product Preparation of EFS Alpes-Méditerranée
Woimant Geneviève, "Collection" expert within the Medical Division

Part I
Organisation of blood transfusion services

1. Organisation of blood transfusion services in France

Jean-Marc Ouazan
Samuel Valcke

The French Blood Establishment (EFS), a central government agency (*établissement public de l'État*), is now responsible in law for managing national blood transfusion services in France. Since it was founded on 1 January 2000, it has ensured that the country remains self-sufficient in blood products whilst meeting the highest safety and ethical standards.

Yet since Karl Landsteiner distinguished the main blood groups in 1900 and World War I established the place of blood transfusion in modern medicine – the first transfusion with known blood groups was performed in 1918 – the organisation of blood transfusion services has undergone several major changes.

The move towards nationalization: the three periods of change in blood transfusion services

In the interwar period, led by a number of visionary figures, France developed a network of blood establishments (ETS), most of which were opened with public hospitals. The first such establishment was founded by Arnaud Tzanck at Paris's Saint-Antoine Hospital in 1928.

It was only after the Second World War, however, that France's ruling class, still strongly influenced by the ideals of the *Résistance*, began to supervise and coordinate these individual initiatives and organize universal blood transfusion services for the first time. In the Act of 21 July 1952 on the use of human blood, plasma and derived products in medicine, French lawmakers laid **"the foundation stone" of national blood transfusion services**. This Act outlines the ethical principles underpinning the services: voluntary, anonymous donations and the absence of profit. Supported by the Decree of 16 January 1954, it brought the services under State

Jean-Marc Ouazan, jean-marc.ouazan@efs.sante.fr
Samuel Valcke, samuel.valcke@efs.sante.fr

control, setting out the type of legal structure that blood establishments can adopt (which must be non-profit-making rather than commercial companies), requiring them to obtain prior government authorization, with the appointment of their director subject to the approval of the Public Health Minister, and determining the geographical areas they cover and type of service they provide.

It was in this legislative and regulatory framework that the 150 or so national structures, regional establishments and some local facilities authorized to provide blood transfusion services were to develop over 4 decades. Amongst these different organisations and geographical disparities, the type of services provided by the structures also varied. Whilst they all provided essential blood transfusion services, from taking blood from the donor's arm to preparing labile blood products for direct transfusion to patients (packed red blood cells, platelets and plasma), a very small number also carried out fractionation, which involves extracting stable products, also known as medicinal products derived from human blood or human plasma (coagulation factors intended primarily for haemophiliacs, albumins and immunoglobulins), for injection into patients.

The **second major period of change** was sparked by the health crisis that marked French society in the early 1990s. To benefit from what is now seen as the first modern health crisis, the authorities made a number of sweeping changes to the organisation of blood transfusion services in the Act of 4 January 1993 on blood transfusion and medicinal product safety.

As well as transposing the European directive of 14 June 1989, which aligned certain measures on medicinal products derived from human blood or human plasma throughout Europe for the first time, the primary aim of this Act was to ensure the safety of blood transfusions and outline a series of organisational and operational principles that are still in use today.

- *First principle:* the Act reduced the number of service providers significantly, from 150 or so to 43, and required them to form public-interest groups (PIGs) with standard bylaws. Alongside these newly formed groups of blood establishments, the 6 structures that carried out fractionation remained unchanged, as did the subsidiary budget of public hospitals in Paris and Ile-de-France (AP-HP).

- *Second principle:* it separated the production of labile and stable blood products. The former remained the responsibility of blood establishments, now in the form of PIGs, whilst the latter was entrusted to a new, specially created structure: the French Fractionation Laboratory (LFB). The LFB, which was initially formed by PIGs, would be transformed into a corporation with public capital (*société anonyme à capital public*) by the Order of 28 July 2005. This move reinforced the separation between transfusion and fractionation service providers because it prevented the LFB and its affiliates from holding a direct or indirect stake in a structure that collects blood or blood components, and vice versa.

- *Third principle:* it increased State control over transfusion service providers by creating a government-funded health watchdog: the French Blood Agency (AFS). Its role was to approve blood establishments and their directors, prepare area plans for the organisation of blood transfusion services (STOTS) for the Health Minister's approval and determine the geographical area covered by each establishment. It also drew up *Good Transfusion Practice* for the Health Minister's approval and inspected blood establishments to ensure that their services complied with this good practice.

The 1993 Act had barely come into effect – the newly formed PIGs would only be introduced in spring 1995 – when it was replaced by new legislation with a broader scope than blood transfusion services. The Act of 1 July 1998 on increased health monitoring and greater control over medicinal products for human use marked the start of the **third major period of change** in the organisation of blood transfusion services in France.

Leaving the ethical principles underpinning the services unchanged, the Act confirmed the separation of blood transfusion services from approval, supervision and monitoring. The latter were transferred to a new government agency with a larger remit: the French Health Products Safety Agency (Afssaps[1]), which merged the roles of the French Blood Agency (AFS) and the French Medicines Agency. The former, meanwhile, now formally recognized as public services, were entrusted to a single agency with sole power in the area: the EFS.

Blood transfusion in France: an "ethical" public service

All of France's public services are governed by standard legal principles. Citizens must be treated equally and not encounter any discrimination. All patients, irrespective of their personal circumstances, are therefore entitled to receive appropriate labile blood products in sufficient quantities. This **principle of equality** in public services also implies neutrality. The **principle of**

---

1. The Act of 29 December 2011 on increasing medicines and health products safety transformed the Afssaps into the French National Agency for the Safety of Medicines and Health Products (ANSM).

continuity demands continuous public services, with no interruption other than those which are prescribed by law. This principle is particularly relevant to blood transfusion as the services may be needed at any time day or night and on any day of the week, month or year. Finally, the **principle of mutability** requires public services to adapt to the needs of the population and act in the general interest. In relation to transfusion, this involves adapting the means of collecting and issuing blood products to demographic and social changes, as well as constantly increasing the scientific, medical and technological research needed to maintain the highest standards of product quality and safety.

In addition to these principles, which apply uniformly to all public services, blood transfusion services are also subject to the **ethical principles** laid down in Article L. 1221-1 of the French Public Health Code. This crucially important article is the basis on which all regulations governing the donation of blood and the use of elements isolated or otherwise produced from the human body must be determined: "Blood transfusion services are provided to benefit the recipient and underpinned by the ethical principles of voluntary, anonymous donations and the absence of profit [...]."

The first of these principles is, therefore, **voluntary** donations. Donors may not receive any form of payment, whether direct or indirect. This principle is absolute:

> "The donation of blood or blood components may not lead to any form of direct or indirect payment. Therefore, no cash payments, gift vouchers, discount vouchers or other documents making it possible to obtain a benefit from a third party may be provided, nor any items of value, services or benefits." (Article D. 1221-1 of the French Public Health Code).

This principle is not, however, universal across Europe. Germany, the UK and Austria still provide payment for certain types of donations. The debates surrounding the proposed European directive on blood donation in 2001 demonstrate this, as Council members agreed only to "encourage voluntary and unpaid donations".

Yet this principle must not penalize donors financially. The regulations allow employers in particular to give their employees paid leave for blood donation in certain circumstances, provided that the leave is no longer than the time needed for travel to, and possibly from, the workplace and donation centre, the personal interview, medical tests, the donation itself and the period of rest and refreshment deemed medically necessary. It also allows the EFS to reimburse the transport costs incurred by donors, albeit on an individual rather than a flat-rate basis.

The second principle, **anonymous donations**, was laid down as early as 1952 and later extended to all products derived from the human body by the Act of 29 July 1994. It means that the recipient may not know the identity of the donor, nor the donor that of the recipient. No information making it possible to identify either the person donating blood or the person receiving it may be disclosed. This naturally **prohibits directed donations**, except where judged necessary by the attending physician (patients with a rare blood group or transfusion between mother and baby).

This principle emphasizes the altruistic and selfless nature of blood donation. It is consistent with the French republican value of *fraternité*: blood donation is the first link in the national solidarity chain benefitting transfused patients, irrespective of the identity, social background, ethnic origin or religious beliefs of donors and recipients. It highlights the principle of equality and ensures that it applies to all patients, neither excluding nor privileging anyone. In the process, it contributes to national self-sufficiency in blood products. It also promotes health safety, taking away any pressure from donors, who can speak freely, openly and honestly during the personal interview prior to the donation. Finally, it makes it impossible for the recipient to hold the donor liable if a pathogenic agent is transmitted by the blood, which would almost certainly dissuade others from donating.

The third principle, **absence of profit**, does not, of course, mean that blood products are provided free of charge. Providing quality public services has a cost: collecting donations in mobile units or permanent sites – the donation centres designed to accommodate appropriately and safely the millions of donors who give a little of their time and themselves to benefit others every year, preparing the products, conducting the screening tests that all donations must undergo to ensure the safety of the products, distributing and issuing the products where they are needed by patients, providing transfusion support services as well as analyzing the compatibility of the product and recipient. Therefore, blood products are sold to public or private hospitals on the basis of a price per product category, with this price reflecting only the costs and charges incurred by the establishment and generating no profit. Moreover, these prices are not freely decided by the establishment but set by a decree from the Ministers in charge of Health and Social Security.

Although not an ethical principle in the strict sense, the **freely given consent of donors** is a legal requirement for blood collection. On that basis, no donation of blood or blood components for therapeutic use in others may be taken from a minor or vulnerable adult who is under legal protection (guardianship, trusteeship or court order). Nonetheless, a donation may be taken from minors on an exceptional basis, *i.e.* in a medical emergency or when an immunologically compatible adult donor cannot be found. The donation may only be taken if both parents/guardians provide their express written consent, although the minor's refusal is final.

In order to be freely given, the donor's consent must be informed. In the pre-donation interview, therefore, prospective donors are given comprehensive information by a physician on the donation method that will be used and the risks incurred, however negligible. In this respect, the Act clearly states that the EFS is liable, even without fault, for the risks donors incur when giving blood and must take out insurance covering its liability for these risks. Prospective donors are also told how their donation may be used, *i.e.* for therapeutic or other purposes.

At the end of the personal interview, which makes it possible to collect information on their health and medical history, prospective donors acknowledge that they have read and understood the detailed information provided, have had an opportunity to ask questions and obtain answers, and have given their informed consent to the next stage in the donation process. Finally, they confirm that all the information they have provided is, to the best of their knowledge, correct.

The **honesty of donors** is an essential aspect contributing to the safety of the blood transfusion process. As blood transfusion services are provided to benefit the recipient, without harming the donor, donor selection criteria have been developed to screen out people who should not give blood, either because donating could be detrimental to their health or because their donations could present a risk to others. These restrictions are determined by the Health Minister and updated periodically to reflect advances in scientific and medical knowledge as well as the introduction of new techniques for screening for and reducing pathogenic agents.

A public service managed by a single agency: the EFS

It was therefore the Act of 1 July 1998 that gave a single government agency sole control over the management of all blood transfusion services in France, replacing the blood establishments that had largely been brought together in public-interest groups (PIGs) following the Act of 4 January 1993 and taking over powers from the French Blood Agency (AFS) which had not already been moved to the Afssaps.

The Act made provision for the **transfer** of the rights, obligations, assets, liabilities and property, both movable and immovable, pertaining to the blood transfusion services provided by the previous structures to the EFS. For immovable property in particular, the EFS was granted either full ownership or, in the public hospital sector, right of possession. Finally, the EFS became the new employer of the staff working in the previous structures, whether they were employed by the public or private sector, with a major merger of the statutes, bylaws and legal requirements leading to the adoption of a single collective agreement.

The first wave of transfers was followed by two further waves, triggered by the 2000 Amending Finance Act and the Order of 1 September 2005, which would enable the EFS to absorb almost all the structures that were not included in the initial 1998 transfer.

Under the terms of the Act, the EFS is a **central government agency** operating under the auspices of the Health Minister. As such, it is governed by the principle of speciality, which requires it to allocate all its resources to the roles specifically designated to it by the Act, prohibiting all other activities.

Pursuant to the Act, it ensures that the needs for blood products are met and that transfusion services adapt to medical, scientific and technological advances, in line with the ethical principles. In the framework of plans for the organisation of blood transfusion services (SOTS), it organizes blood collection, donation screening, and the preparation, distribution and delivery of blood products throughout the country. In this framework, its **roles** are to:

– manage the national blood transfusion services over which it has a monopoly in France, as well as related services. Note that the French Armed Forces Blood Transfusion Centre (CTSA) provides these services within the armed forces;
– promote blood donation, encourage the correct and proper use of donated blood, and ensure that all parties adhere strictly to the ethical principles;
– guarantee high quality standards within blood establishments and implement good practice in compliance with the laws and regulations on blood transfusion services;
– within the haemovigilance network, share data on the health safety of blood products with the French National Agency for the Safety of Medicines and Health Products (ANSM) and epidemiological data with the French Institute for Public Health Surveillance (InVS);
– devise, update and implement the SOTS;
– with research and testing bodies, encourage, undertake or participate in research in areas relating to blood transfusion and related or ancillary services, and promote the dissemination of scientific and technical knowledge in these areas;
– maintain a national database of donors and recipients of rare blood groups and a bank of rare blood groups,

1. Organisation of blood transfusion services in France

and coordinate the work of laboratories involved in these activities;
– participate in providing emergency aid in the event of a national or international disaster requiring the use of blood transfusion resources;
– participate in scientific and technical cooperation between France and the European and international community.

The **organisation and structure** of the EFS reflect the unique nature of its roles.

Like all government agencies, the EFS is led by a **Board of Directors** which determines the main thrusts of its policy and broadly how it should be implemented. In addition to the State representatives that supervise its activities, which include the Directorate-General for Health (DGS), the Directorate-General for Care Provision (DGOS), the Social Security Directorate (DSS) and the Budget Directorate representing the Finance Minister, the Board of Directors also comprises representatives of organisations promoting voluntary blood donations, patients' associations, health insurance funds, public and private hospitals, EFS staff members and qualified figures in the field.

Following the directions set by the Board of Directors, whose decisions he/she prepares and implements, the **Chairman** of the Board of Directors, who is appointed by Presidential decree effectively manages the EFS. Acting as an Executive Chairman, he/she performs all the duties that are not reserved for the Board of Directors. He/she recruits, appoints and manages the staff of establishments over which he/she has authority. He/she represents the EFS in all civil matters and may instigate legal proceedings in its name. He/she enters into contracts, agreements and arrangements as well as deeds of purchase and sale. He/she also monitors income and expenditure. Based on the opinions of the Board of Directors, the Chairman appoints the directors of blood establishments for a four-year term and delegates powers to them, the type and extent of which are determined for the management of the establishment in question.

Alongside the Chairman and appointed by him/her, a **responsible person** is accountable for blood transfusion safety. This major new position in the blood transfusion system, born from the dual ambition to harmonize the regulations applicable to various health products at European level and make all parties in the health system responsible for product quality and safety, was created by the Directive of 27 January 2003 setting standards of quality and safety for the collection, testing, processing, storage and distribution of human blood and blood components, which was transposed into French law by the Order of 1 September 2005 and its implementing decree of 1 February 2006. The "responsible person" ensures compliance with laws and regulations on the quality and safety of blood products in blood establishments. For this purpose, he/she has authority over the directors of blood establishments. He/she oversees the implementation, evaluation and update of the quality assurance system in line with good practice and takes the necessary steps to ensure the complete traceability of blood products, irrespective of their destination. Finally, he/she is responsible for implementing the haemovigilance system within the EFS.

The EFS also has a **Scientific Committee**, whose members are appointed by the Health Minister and whose purpose is to give opinions or make observations on all medical, scientific and technical issues affecting fulfilment of the EFS's roles or the quality and safety of blood transfusions. It is also involved in determining research policy and assessing EFS programmes.

In addition to the statutory bodies provided for by the French Public Health Code, the EFS has chosen to form an **Ethics Committee**. The role of this committee, which was created by decision of the Board of Directors in 2012, is to assist, in its areas of expertise, the Chairman, responsible person and Board of Directors, to which it submits wholly independent and objective opinions and recommendations on the ethical issues raised by the activities of the EFS, whether they relate to national blood transfusion services, research or the activities described by the French Public Health Code as "linked to blood transfusion" (immunohaematological tests) or "auxiliary" (advanced therapy medicinal products, cell and tissue engineering, blood products for laboratory use, teaching and research, laboratory reagents, provision of care, laboratory testing, etc.). Furthermore, pursuant to the Act of 29 December 2011 on increasing medicines and health products safety, the committee has a role in preventing and managing conflicts of interest. In this role, it assesses the policy implemented within the EFS and may be called on in the event of a specific set of circumstances producing a new, difficult or complex conflict of interest.

A public health stakeholder present throughout and heavily involved in the medical sector

The EFS provides **blood transfusion services** throughout the country *via* its 17 blood establishments, which are regional centres without corporate status (Figure 2):

Transfusion medicine: the French model

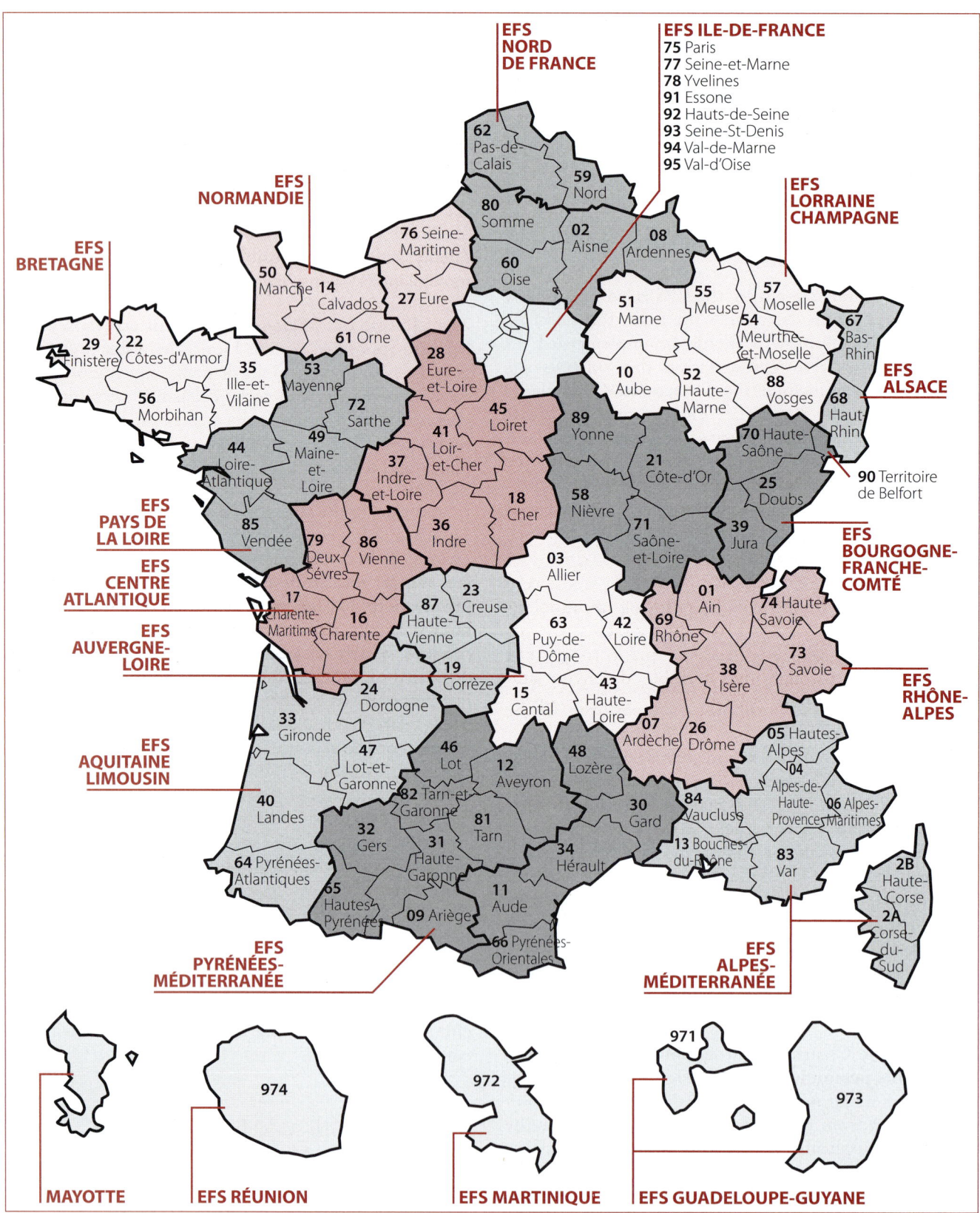

Figure 2. The EFS, a decentralised public establishment, with 17 regional establishment.
Source: EFS.

1. Organisation of blood transfusion services in France

- blood collection, which is taken after prospective donors have been found to meet the medical requirements and selection criteria set by the Health Minister. This is linked to promoting blood donation with organisations that work to increase the number of voluntary donations;
- donation screening, which involves conducting a series of laboratory tests and screenings on every donation;
- the preparation of blood products, which is an industrial process undertaken on specialized platforms and which transforms the "raw material" taken from the donor's arm to the "end product" used for medical purposes;
- distribution, which involves the "wholesale" supply of labile blood products (LBP) to a hospital operating a blood bank or to another blood establishment;
- delivery which is providing LBP to a hospital on medical prescription with a view to administration to a given patient and which requires the EFS's delivery sites to be located as close as possible to the health facility.

Linked to these primary roles, over which the EFS has a monopoly, is the **conduct of immunohaematological tests** on blood product recipients. This helps secure very high safety levels for patients by ensuring immunological compatibility between LBP and recipients. Immunohaematology provides analyses prior to patient transfusion and, through links with blood delivery sites and transfusion support services, makes a major contribution to the safety of the French transfusion system. It is a round-the-clock, locally available service ensuring continuous national blood transfusion services.

In addition, the EFS develops several **activities linked to or resulting from its primary role**, each of which are carried out within a specific legal framework supervised by the ANSM and/or regional health agencies (ARS), including:
- the preparation, storage, and distribution of human tissue (corneas, amniotic membranes, bone grafts, heart valves, blood vessels, skin, etc.) and cells other than blood cells, as well as gene and cell therapy preparations (haematopoietic stem cells, for which the EFS meets nearly 60% of national requirements) as well as the preparation and distribution of advanced therapy medicinal products for which the EFS will acquire drug establishment status;
- the provision of care in the specific framework of its health centres (bloodletting, outpatient transfusion, plasma exchange, erythrocyte exchange, extracorporeal photochemotherapy, collection of haematopoietic stem cells, etc.);
- the production of blood components or blood products for non-therapeutic purposes (teaching, research, production of reagents, etc.) as well as the production and distribution of laboratory reagents for testing within a specialized production unit and, occasionally, in partnership with industrial groups.

To provide quality services throughout the transfusion chain, blood establishments must be approved by the ANSM, an independent health watchdog. This **approval**, which is granted for 5 years, is renewable and subject to strict administrative, technical, medical and sanitary conditions. The ANSM inspects blood establishments at least biennially to ensure that the transfusion services they provide meet good transfusion practice, as determined by the Director-General of the ANSM, as well as the relevant operation and equipment standards. For this purpose, the Director-General of the agency may request all necessary information from blood establishments and has appropriate powers of sanction, which can lead to the withdrawal of approval.

As a **key partner in healthcare**, the EFS maintains close relationships with the 1,900 or so **health facilities**, which are strictly regulated. In addition to close physical proximity to healthcare facilities – half of the EFS's facilities are located on a hospital site – every public or private hospital chooses a single blood establishment, known as the referent blood establishment ensuring product safety and traceability, which distributes and delivers the blood products that the health facility needs. Furthermore, when a health facility is authorized by the ARS to operate a blood bank, an agreement is reached between that health facility and its referent blood establishment to maintain the bank and monitor the products stored therein.

To ensure consistent dealings with health stakeholders throughout the country, the EFS organizes its activities in the framework of **SOTS**, which determine the geographical area and resources allocated to each blood establishment. These plans, which are prepared by the EFS, are adopted by the Health Minister for 5 years based on the opinions of the Director-Generals of ARS. For each blood establishment, they include permanent collection sites, specialized platforms preparing LBP, specialized interregional platforms screening donations, sites distributing LBP to health facilities operating a blood bank, sites delivering LBP and the list of health facilities authorized to deliver labile blood products.

Through its activity and involvement in health facilities, the EFS makes it possible to transfuse over 560,000 patients each year. In addition, through the plasma it supplies to the **LFB**, its sole partner in this field, the EFS also contributes to treating the 500,000 patients to whom medicinal products derived from human blood are administered.

Transfusion medicine: the French model

Finally, as a natural extension of its roles and to facilitate continuous improvement and anticipate future advances, the EFS develops an active **research policy** in all the fields covered by its activities in liaison with academic partners such as universities, the French National Institute of Health and Medical Research (INSERM), the French National Centre for Scientific Research (CNRS), and industrial partners.

The EFS, the product of several successive periods of change and sole provider of national blood transfusion services, is now a vital scientific, technical and medical participant in public health policy (Figure 3).

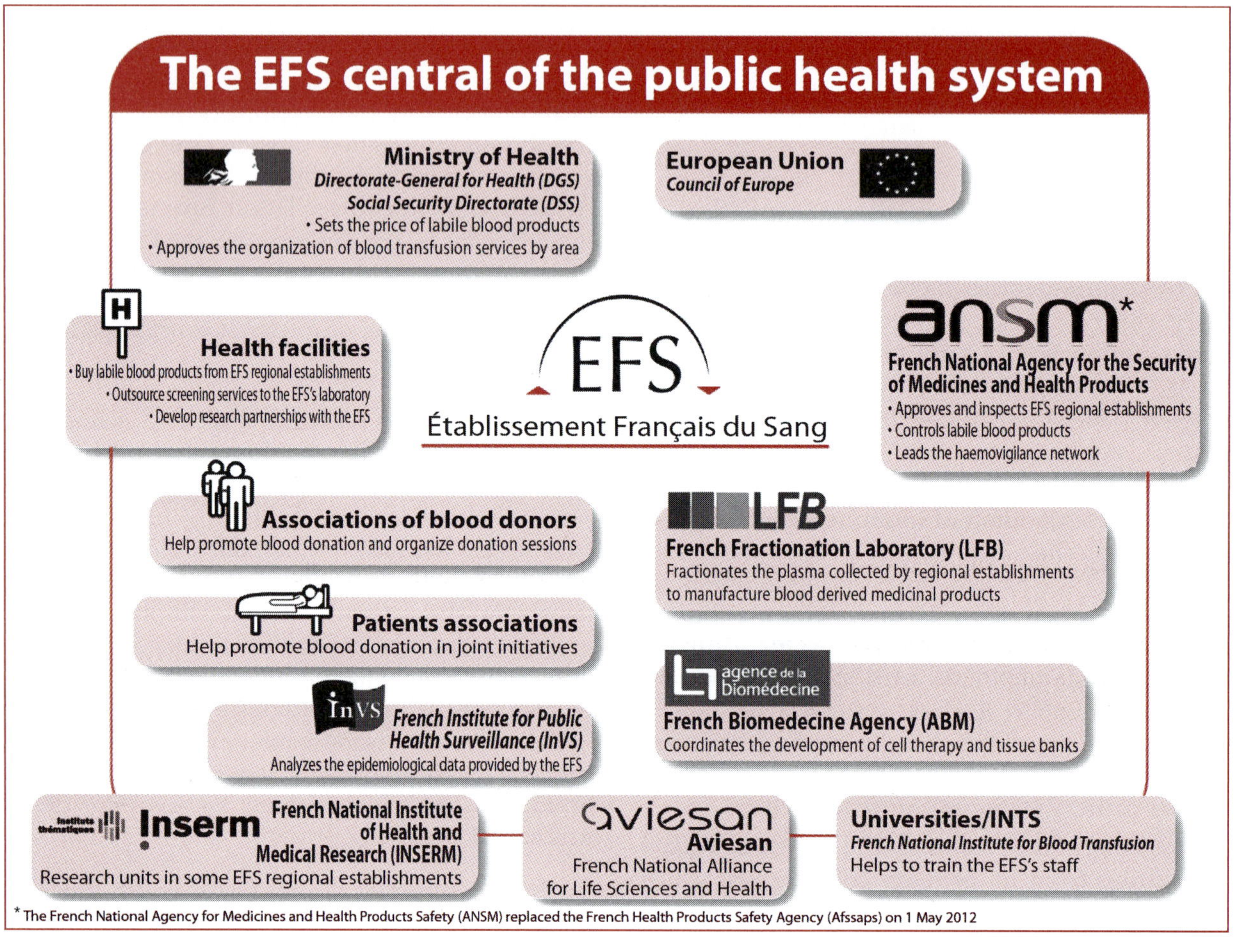

Figure 3. The EFS central to the public health system.

The partnership policy of the EFS

Another unique feature of the French transfusion model is the partnership policy of the EFS. As a result of its history, values and growing patient needs for blood products, the national blood transfusion service has formed several partnerships that enter into a specific model combining management and development. This model positions the EFS at the crossroads of 3 economic and institutional areas: the service sector, the public health sector and the commercial sector (Figure 4).

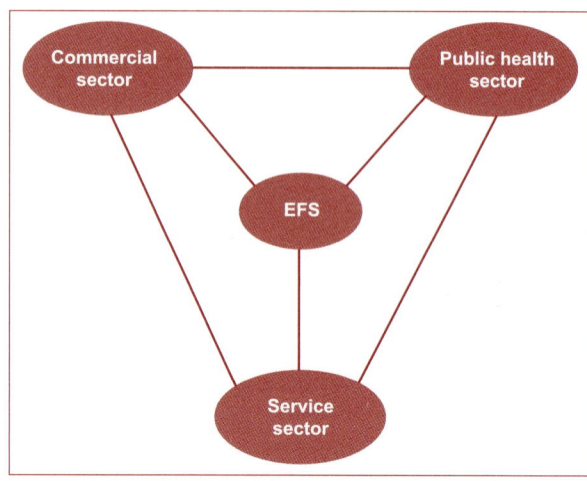

Figure 4. The three economic and constitutional spheres.

1. Organisation of blood transfusion services in France

At the base of this model is the **service sector**, or third sector as it has been described by Jacques Delors, which is also known as the social and solidary economy. What defines it as such is the way in which the EFS's main resource, blood donation, the raw material involved in transfusions, is used, which is guided by strong values (altruism, voluntarism, anonymity and absence of profit). By extension, these ethical principles apply to the public services. In this social and solidary sphere, the EFS's partnership policy aims to inform and mobilize blood donors and their representatives whilst making it easier to donate.

The public health sector is the establishment's second sphere of influence. It is formed by the administrative authorities that approve the budgets, set product prices and ensure high safety standards. It is therefore with the support of agencies (primarily the ANSM) and the use of surveillance and haemovigilance procedures that high safety standards are met, for the benefit of patients.

The partnerships aim to highlight requirements for blood products, by making the link between the generosity of donors and the needs of patients. The transfusion chain can then provide experiences and endorsements to promote blood donation.

The third sphere is the **commercial sector**. Although the establishment's employees are subject to private law, its procurement (which accounts for nearly one third of its revenue) is subject to market forces. Some activities linked to medicinal products, meanwhile, fall in the competitive sector. In this sphere, the involvement of private organisations is another aspect of the partnership policy.

To explore the components of this policy in more detail, we will distinguish between 2 major types of cooperation.

Institutional partnerships

These are required by France's laws and regulations, which changed following the health crises at the end of the twentieth century.

These traumatic health crises forced the authorities to reform the legislative framework of blood transfusion. The major aim of the 1993 and 1998 laws was to guarantee transfusion safety by laying down a number of organisational and operational principles:
- the drastic reduction in the number of service providers, initially from 150 to 43 and later to a single establishment on 1 January 2000;
- the separation of the production of labile and stable blood products, with the former provided by the EFS and the latter by the LFB;
- the institutionalization of the participation of donors and patients in the EFS's Board of Directors.

The participation of the French Federation for Voluntary Blood Donation

This is building on past foundations as blood donors and their associations, with the help of physicians, created many structures in the 1960s to keep pace with growing needs for blood products. The State's wish to move away from the balkanization of transfusion led to the involvement of the French Federation for Voluntary Blood Donation (FFDSB) in the EFS Board of Directors.

It does not affect the special relationships that the EFS profits from with the FFDSB and other partner associations in any way.

National and local agreements structure this partnership. Associations participate in promoting donation and organizing donation sessions, notably providing hospitality for donors. Their work also contributes to retaining donors and conveying the values of blood donation: citizenship, solidarity, generosity and altruism. The EFS also provides funding for these associations to help them fulfil their role.

Patients associations

On the legislator's decision, a representative of the French Association of Haemophiliacs (AFH) sits on the EFS's Board of Directors. It is important and right that haemophiliacs, who have suffered greatly from the effects of the health crisis, help prevent history repeating itself *via* monitoring.

Other patients associations have formed partnerships with the EFS. They raise awareness of blood donation by highlighting the need for labile blood products.

Partnerships resulting from voluntary schemes

Voluntary schemes result from efforts by the EFS's Communication Office to meet ever-growing demand for blood products, which has been prompted by the renewed quality of the products, the ageing of the population and ever-more complex therapeutic practices, although it is impossible to measure the extent to which each factor is involved precisely.

From 2004 to 2012, donations of packed red blood cells increased by over 25%, which led the EFS to refine its communication policy and diversify its partnerships. Throughout the year, and particularly at the time of events like World Blood Donor Day, this makes it possible to increase the mobilization of donors and boost donation levels.

Transfusion medicine: the French model

Awareness-raising partnerships

Promoting blood donation requires investment. Raising awareness is one aspect. **Educational campaigns** bring information to pupils from the final year of primary school, as well as teachers and parents, in cooperation with MGEN, a leading authority in education circles.

In the framework of Citizen Action Days and with the support of the **Ministry of Defence**, it involves raising awareness of the notion of citizenship amongst young people who have reached the age of legal responsibility, giving them information and encouraging them to give blood, which is often seen as the first act of good citizenship.

By providing specific materials, the EFS makes such a scheme possible.

Collection partnerships

Collection partnerships are a major aim of the EFS's partnership policy. It makes its resources, influence and organisation available to the EFS to improve the services provided in donation sessions and to encourage people to donate, often for the first time. With the help of the French Round Table and top chefs, better refreshments are now provided. J.-F. Piège from Hotel de Crillon (at that time), Eric Frachon from the Ritz and Anne-Sophie Pic have, with their high profile and high-quality services, attracted many donors.

Rotary Clubs also help boost the appeal of donation sessions across the country. In Toulouse, for example, they are able to access the prestigious Salle des Illustres in City Hall and have for many years organized the largest donation session in Europe, with over 3,000 donors attending.

Public sector partnerships

These partnerships are formed between the EFS and other public organisations. With the Association of French Mayors (AMF), local elected representatives and town/city services provide locations and advertising for donation sessions.

Similar schemes are in operation in the academic world [the National Centre for Pupil and Student Welfare (CNOUS), Conference of University Presidents (CPU) and Conference of Grandes Écoles (CGE)], but involve student initiatives only.

Corporate partnerships

In many companies, blood donation is promoted as a good cause and teambuilding exercise. Several big businesses support donation sessions and organize them on their premises or nearby. Arcelor, Peugeot, Legrand, La Poste and France Télécom, for example, are active throughout the year.

"General public" partnerships aim to raise the EFS's profile amongst both the customers and staff of such companies, particularly on World Blood Donor Day. They include partnerships with France Télévisions and Allo Ciné, which offer the EFS banners on their website and/or advertising slots whenever possible.

"Sector" partnerships aim to raise the EFS's profile amongst a specific audience. Only one section of the public is targeted, reflecting the partner's area of activity. Adecco Medical, for example, builds awareness amongst its employees and temporary workers; Banque Populaire does the same amongst its clients.

With its diverse partnerships and multifaceted relationships working to promote blood donation, the cooperation established by the EFS reopens and enriches the debate on the participation of users in public health services. **In mobilizing its partners to increase self-sufficiency, the EFS makes them into health system stakeholders supporting a noble and ethical cause.**

2. Other organisational models for blood transfusion services

Olivier Nasr

Although blood donation sessions were first organized using a list of voluntary donors, by the British Red Cross in London as early as 1921, it was only after the end of World War II that the first national structures were put in place.

Blood transfusion, an essential component of healthcare in wartime, was then extended to surgical and medical practice in peacetime.

Health authorities were immediately faced with problems linked to the collection of blood, the equipment available to the structures and staff training.

Over time, they developed national organisations that often reflected the country's level of development, social equality, culture, history, political regime and health system.

Ethical principles based on voluntary, unpaid donations were adopted by the League of Red Cross Societies at its seventeenth international conference in Stockholm in August 1948. These principles were taken up by the Council of Europe as early as 1956 and defended by the World Health Organisation (WHO) in May 1975, at the 28th World Health Assembly.

However, Edwin Cohn's development of human blood plasma fractionation using ethanol at Harvard in 1941 had already created an opportunity at the end of World War II that commercial companies would later exploit: a huge demand for plasma-derived products made most countries reliant on the American market, which was based on paid plasma donations.

The health crises of the 1990s prompted the political authorities to implement new organisations to ensure the quality and safety of blood products.

The introduction of a quality assurance system and the consolidation of labile blood product preparation and screening activities on modern, specialized platforms

Olivier Nasr, olivier.nasr@efs.sante.fr

with automated machinery and integrated IT solutions were the result of these moves.

In 2013, the transfusion sector is characterized by huge institutional, economic and ethical diversity, making comparisons difficult, particularly as it is constantly changing and sources of information can be sparse or nonexistent.

We can, however, identify 5 major forms of organisation, which may sometimes coexist in the same country:
- **countries whose blood transfusion system is placed strictly and directly under the responsibility of public health centres with organisation that is, to some extent, centralized:** this is the case in France, the UK, the Republic of Ireland, Poland and China;
- **countries whose organisation is fully delegated to the blood services of the national Red Cross:** this is the case in Belgium, Switzerland, Luxembourg, Finland, Japan, New Zealand and Australia;
- **countries whose blood transfusion system is fully managed by hospitals:** this is the case in Denmark, Sweden and Italy;
- **countries whose blood transfusion system is fully managed by non-profit-making organisations:** this is the case in the Netherlands and Canada, following the withdrawal of both their national Red Crosses;
- **countries whose blood transfusion system is mixed:** this is the case in Germany, Austria and the United States, where different organisations coexist: the national Red Cross, non-profit-making community organisations, hospitals and commercial companies (essentially for paid plasma donations).

We will give a brief overview of the transfusion system in 5 countries representing these major forms of organisation.

The UK

The UK is a parliamentary constitutional monarchy.

It comprises England, Scotland, Wales and Northern Ireland. These 4 constituent nations cannot be compared to the administrative subdivisions of other countries and, since devolution in 1999, the UK can be considered as a unitary state with certain characteristics of a federal state.

This explains the unique organisation of public transfusion services, which are divided into 4 separate entities, each reporting to its local government:
– National Health Service Blood and Transplant (NHSBT) for England and North Wales;
– Scottish National Blood Transfusion Service (SNBTS) for Scotland;
– Welsh Blood Service (WBS) for the rest of Wales;
– Northern Ireland Blood Transfusion Service (NIBTS) for Northern Ireland.

Since 2005, following the transposition of European directives into British law, a government agency, the Medicines and Healthcare Products Regulatory Agency (MHRA) is responsible for regulating, inspecting and granting authorizations to all blood establishments.

Donors of whole blood and blood components are volunteers.

England and North Wales: 51 million inhabitants

NHS Blood and Transplant brings together several operational units:
– Blood Donation (previously the National Blood Service) is responsible for organizing and managing the fifteen blood establishments in England and distributing labile blood products to 300 health facilities.

Since the centre was opened in Filton, near Bristol, in June 2008, which is thought to be the biggest in the world with the ability to process 600,000 donations every year, the preparation of labile blood products has been consolidated on 5 specialized platforms and screening on 3 specialized platforms. There is talk in 2013 of retaining only 2 platforms for screening (Filton and Manchester);
– UK Transplant is responsible for organizing organ donations for the entire UK and maintaining the national organ donor register;
– Tissues: the Liverpool Tissue Bank is responsible for collecting, preparing, processing and distributing tissue to health facilities;
– Stem Cell Services: the UK's biggest supplier of haematopoietic stem cells (bone marrow and cord blood);
– Specialist Therapeutic Services: services responsible for collecting stem cells and plasma exchanges;
– Diagnostic Services: immunology, immunogenetic and immunohaematology laboratories, including the famous International Blood Group Reference Laboratory in Bristol.

Scotland: 5 million inhabitants

Scotland has legislative power and general competence over administrative matters (health, justice, policing, agriculture, etc.).

SNBTS collected 244,850 whole blood donations in 2012: 25% on permanent sites (Edinburgh, Glasgow, Dundee, Aberdeen and Inverness) and 75% in mobile units.

The preparation and screening of labile blood products are consolidated at the Edinburgh and Glasgow sites.

The Scottish Fractionation Centre in Edinburgh was definitively closed in 2007.

Wales (Centre, West and South): 2.2 million inhabitants

WBS collects approximately 100,000 donations per annum, primarily in mobile units.

The preparation and screening of labile blood products are consolidated at the Talbot Green site near Cardiff.

Discussions are ongoing between the health authorities and NHSBT on making WBS the sole provider of blood transfusion services in Wales by 2016.

Northern Ireland: 1.7 million inhabitants

In 2012, NIBTS collected approximately 58,000 donations with its 3 mobile units (250 collections per annum) and carried out 4,700 cytapheresis procedures at its permanent site in Belfast City Hospital, where the preparation and screening of labile blood products are consolidated.

Bio Products Laboratory Limited (BPL)

Bio Products Laboratory Limited (BPL) based in Elstree, north London, is the sole pharmaceutical structure responsible for producing plasma-derived medicinal products and biotechnologies.

As a precautionary measure against the new variant prion (nvMCJ), British plasma has not been fractionated since 1998.

In 2000, the British Government paid £50 million to buy a private American company, Life Resources Incorporated, specializing in the paid collection of plasma.

The company was renamed DCI Biologicals Limited in 2002. Its head office is in Gallup, New Mexico, and it operates 32 plasmapheresis centres throughout the United States. The British Government now wishes to sell it.

The plasma collected in the United States is transferred to Elstree for fractionation and some is stored in the form of methylene blue virally inactivated fresh frozen plasma for patients born after 1996 only.

Japan

Japan is a parliamentary constitutional monarchy.

It is formed by 4 main islands (Hokkaido, Honshu, Shikoku and Kyushu) and a vast number of smaller islands covering an area of approximately 2,500 km.

It is subdivided into 8 regions and 47 prefectures. This administrative organisation was devised in 1871, based on the French model.

In 1990, the State delegated the blood transfusion system to the Japanese Red Cross Society, which is the only national provider of transfusion services. Donors of whole blood and blood components are volunteers. Two hundred milliliters or 400 mL of whole blood may be donated, depending on the donor's weight.

Table I. The UK in figures.	
OECD 2009	
Surface area	244,820 sq km
Population	60,930,000 inhabitants
	< 15 years = 17.7%
	> 65 years = 15.8%
GDP per capita	35,151 USD
Health expenditure	9.8% of GDP
Infant mortality	4.6/1,000 live births
Life expectancy at birth M/F	78.3/82.5
Collection 2010	
Whole blood	2,235,400 units
Platelets	293,343 procedures
Plasma	350,426 procedures
Distribution 2010	
PRBCs	2,175,905 units
Platelets	285,768 units
	– 80% from aphaeresis
	– 20% from whole blood
Plasma	366,466 units
	– standard: 292,884 units
	– MB: 17,113 units
	– SD: 57,487 units (Octapharma)

OECD: Organisation for Economic Co-operation and Development; GDP: gross domestic product; PRBCs: packed red blood cells; MB: pathogen reduced by methylene blue; SD: virus inactivated by solvent/detergent.

Since 2006, platelet concentrates have been collected solely by aphaeresis.

The system is organized in line with the country's administrative structure, with 47 Blood Centres responsible for collecting, preparing and distributing labile blood products and plasma-derived medicinal products.

In April 2012, an administrative consolidation led to the creation of 7 superstructures known as Block Blood Centres.

Standard donation screening tests (immunohaematology, viral serology, haematology and biochemistry) are consolidated on 10 specialized platforms and NAT testing [hepatitis B virus (HBV), hepatitis C virus (HCV) and human immunodeficiency virus (HIV) pooled] on 4 specialized platforms.

In June 2012, the national fractionation industry was restructured, leading to the creation of a single non-profit-making structure, the *Japan Blood Products Organisation* (JBPO) in Chitose (Hokkaido), which is able to fractionate 800,000 litres per annum.

Table II. Japan in figures.	
OECD 2009	
Surface area	377,000 sq km
Population	127,510,000 inhabitants
	< 15 years = 13.3%
	> 65 years = 22.7%
GDP per capita	32,018 USD
Health expenditure	8.5% of GDP (2008)
Infant mortality	2.4/1,000 live births
Life expectancy at birth M/F	79.6/86.4
Collection 2011	
Whole blood	3,731,003 units
	– 3,301,605 of 400 mL
	– 429,398 of 200 mL
Aphaeresis (plasma + platelets):	1,521,179 procedures
Distribution 2011	
Whole blood	378 units
	– 40 of 200 mL
	– 338 of 400 mL
PRBCs	3,468,431 units
	– 399,708 from 200 mL of WB
	– 3,068,723 from 400 mL of WB
APC	8,756,916 units
	– 1 unit = 0.2×10^{11} platelets
FFP	992,867 units
	– 54,656 from 200 mL of WB
	– 751,837 from 400 mL of WB
	– 186,374 by aphaeresis
FFP for fractionation	956,582 litres

OECD: Organisation for Economic Co-operation and Development; GDP: gross domestic product; PRBCs: packed red blood cells; WB: whole blood; APC: aphaeresis platelet concentrate; FFP: fresh-frozen plasma.

Italy

Italy is a parliamentary republic.

The country is divided into 20 regions, including fifteen with "ordinary statute" and 5 with "special statute", which are autonomous. The 1999 institutional reform significantly increased the powers of the regions, which choose their form of government and enjoy a high level of financial and fiscal autonomy.

The transfusion system is a public hospital system based on voluntary donations of whole blood and blood components.

The transfusion structures are hospital services organized in accordance with the healthcare provision in the region or province to which they belong.

In total, Italy has 322 hospital transfusion services (*servizio transfusionale*) and 4 managed by the armed forces (Rome, Florence, La Spezia and Taranto).

The main particularity of the system is the vital role played by Associations of Voluntary Blood Donors (AVIS, the oldest and largest, FIDAS and FRATRES) and, to a lesser extent, the Italian Red Cross.

These associations manage not only donor recruitment but also donation sessions in 1,340 collection sites (*unita di raccolta*) throughout the country.

They operate under the responsibility of the referent hospital transfusion services and are authorized by the regional and national health authorities.

They receive funding, on the basis of the number of donations, from specific programmes supported by the regions and the State.

Plasma for fractionation is sold, for custom processing, to the private Italian company Kedrion, which has 2 fractionation units in Bologna and Naples.

This company also fractionates the unethical plasma collected in the United States, Germany and Austria.

European Directives have been transposed into Italian law by Act 219 of 21 October 2005, which reorganized the national and regional governance of the system.

- **At national level:**
- creation, within the National Institute of Health, of the National Blood Centre (*Centro Nazionale Sangue*), which has been in operation since August 2007. Its roles include the coordination and scientific and technical supervision of regional coordination centres (*Centro Regionale di Coordinamento*);
- creation of a national consultative commission comprised of the directors of regional centres, representatives of associations of voluntary blood donors, representatives of associations of leukaemia and thalassemia patients, and representatives of learned societies in transfusion medicine and cell therapy. It is chaired by the Health Minister or his/her representative.

- **At regional level:**
- creation of 20 regional hospital centres whose role is to facilitate coordination and exchanges between the various transfusion centres in the regions.

2. Other organisational models for blood transfusion services

Table III. Italy in figures.	
OECD 2009	
Surface area	310,226 sq km
Population	60,193,000 inhabitants
	< 15 years = 14%
	> 65 years = 20.2%
GDP per capita	32,413 USD
Health expenditure	9.5% of GDP
Infant mortality	3.3/1,000 live births
Life expectancy at birth M/F	79.1/84.5
Collection	
Whole blood (2011)	2,653,136 units
Aphaeresis (2009)	477,215 procedures (including military centres):
	– 371,049 simple plasmapheresis
	– 60,072 combined aphaeresis (plasma-platelets)
	– 24,216 combined aphaeresis (plasma-erythrocytes)
	– 8,626 combined aphaeresis (erythrocytes-platelets)
	– 9,194 single cytapheresis
	– 3,079 double cytapheresis
	– 979 double erythropheresis
Distribution	
PRBCs (2011)	2,668,134 units
Plasma for fractionation (Kedrion 2012)	768,435 kg
	– 194,751 kg from plasmapheresis and freezing < 6 hours (category A)
	– 503,824 kg from whole blood and freezing < 7 hours (category B)
	– 69,242 kg from whole blood and freezing > 7 hours and < 72 hours (category C)
	– 618 kg specific anti-HBs plasma

OECD: Organisation for Economic Co-operation and Development; GDP: gross domestic product; PRBCs: packed red blood cells.

Netherlands

The Netherlands is a parliamentary constitutional monarchy.

It is a decentralized unitary state divided into 12 provinces, which do not have very extensive powers although each one has a local assembly.

Each province is governed by a commissioner appointed by the monarch and an elected legislative body.

The municipalities are led by an elected council and mayor (burgomaster) appointed by the monarch.

Most power is held by the central government.

Until 1998, the Dutch Red Cross was responsible for the transfusion system.

It had 22 regional transfusion centres and a plasma fractionation unit in Amsterdam, the Central Laboratory of Blood Transfusion (CLB), created under the aegis of the central government, Red Cross and municipality of Amsterdam.

With the 1998 Blood Supply Act, and following the merger of the 22 regional centres and CLB, a new organisation was put in place with the creation of Sanquin, a non-profit-making foundation that became the sole national provider of blood transfusion and plasma fractionation services on the basis of voluntary, unpaid donations.

In 2001, Sanquin consolidated the preparation of labile blood products at 4 regional centres (Amsterdam, Groningen, Rotterdam and Nijmegen) and centralized donation screening on the specialized platform in Amsterdam.

Eighty per cent of whole blood and 100% of aphaeresis donations are made on 56 permanent sites.

For plasma fractionation, Sanquin and the Central Fractionation Unit of the Belgian Red Cross (CAF-DCF) merged in 1998, leading to the creation of a limited liability cooperative company: Sanquin-CAF-DCF.

In February 2008, an industrial agreement with a 24.99% minority interest was reached with the French Fractionation Laboratory (LFB).

Note that Sanquin has been responsible for the Council of Europe's European Bank of Frozen Blood of Rare Groups, based in Amsterdam, since 1969.

Table IV. The Netherlands in figures.	
OECD 2009	
Surface area	41,500 sq km
Population	16,530,000 inhabitants
	< 15 years = 17.7%
	> 65 years = 15.2%
GDP per capita	40,804 USD
Health expenditure	11.2% of GDP
Infant mortality	3.8/1,000 live births
Life expectancy at birth M/F	78.5/82.7
Collection (2011)	
Whole blood	538,282 units
Plasma aphaeresis	347,554 procedures
Distribution (2011)	
PRBCs	544,324 units
Platelets from whole blood	290,623 pools
Therapeutic plasma	89,631 units
Plasma for fractionation	347,044 kg

OECD: Organisation for Economic Co-operation and Development; GDP: gross domestic product; PRBCs: packed red blood cells.

Germany

Germany is a federal republic.

Powers are divided between the federal state (the *Bund*) and 16 federated states (the *Länder*) in line with the principle of subsidiarity.

The federated states each have their own constitution, parliament and government, but most legislative power is held by the federal state.

Three *Länder* are city-states: Hamburg, Bremen and Berlin.

The German blood transfusion system is a mixed system with both paid and unpaid donations, even in some non-profit-making establishments.

The 1998 Transfusion Act added to existing regulations on the collection and use of whole blood and blood components.

In the Federal Health Ministry, the Paul Ehrlich Institute (PEI) became the body responsible for monitoring the country's supply of whole blood and blood products and the Robert Koch Institute (RKI) was given responsibility for the epidemiological follow up of donors.

The non-profit-making sector is formed by:
– the blood services of the German Red Cross (DRK BTS), which collect 75% of whole blood donations (10% on permanent sites and 90% in mobile units, with approximately 50,000 mobile collections per annum) and 12% of plasma donations. The DRK has 12 blood establishments and 36 collection sites;
– 59 transfusion centres managed by municipalities and hospitals, which collect 19% of whole blood donations and 4% of plasma donations;
– the armed forces blood transfusion centre in Coblence.

The profit-making sector is represented by:
– 16 private collection centres, which collect approximately 6% of whole blood donations and 44% of plasma donations;
– the 17 plasmapheresis centres of the pharmaceutical fractionation industry, which collect 40% of plasma donations.

In private centres and municipal and hospital centres, donors receive, on average, a €25 payment for donating whole blood and €20 for donating plasma.

Note that 3 plasma fractionation sites belong to private companies:
– CSL Behring;
– Biotest;
– Octapharma, which acquired the Red Cross fractionation unit in Sprige/Hanover in 2008.

Table V. Germany in figures.	
OECD 2009	
Surface area	357,027 sq km
Population	81,902,000 inhabitants
	< 15 years = 13.5%
	> 65 years = 20.5%
GDP per capita	36,332 USD
Health expenditure	11.6% of GDP
Infant mortality	3.5/1,000 live births
Life expectancy at birth M/F	77.8/82.8
Collection 2011	
Whole blood	4,925,540 units
Aphaeresis	2,645,681 procedures
	– 2,406,874 plasmapheresis
	– 191,743 cytapheresis
	– 15,691 erythropheresis
	– 31,373 combined aphaeresis
Distribution 2011	
PRBCs	4,311,110 units
Platelets	493,472 units
	– 40% from whole blood
	– 60% by aphaeresis
Therapeutic FFP	1,100,663 units
	– 1,045,809 plasma extraction from 270 mL
	– 54,854 SD aphaeresis plasma from 250 mL
FFP for fractionation	2,998,386 litres
	– 1,820,781 litres by aphaeresis
	– 1,177,605 litres from whole blood

OECD: Organisation for Economic Co-operation and Development; GDP: gross domestic product; PRBCs: packed red blood cells; FFP: fresh frozen plasma.

3. The Council of Europe: Pioneering Blood Safety since the 1950's

Guy Rautmann

The History

Founded in 1949, the Council of Europe (CoE)[1] is the oldest and largest of all European institutions and now numbers 47 Member States. One of the founding principles of the CoE is increasing co-operation between Member States to improve the quality of life for all Europeans.

Since the CoE was established in 1949, the key to its success has been its collaborative work process. The CoE co-ordinates inter-governmental co-operation, involving experts from European states and the contributions of other international organisations like the World Health Organisation (WHO) and the European Union (EU).

In the field of health, the CoE has consistently selected ethical problems for study in all Member states. The most important ethical issues relate to the non-commercialisation of human substances, *i.e.* blood and its components, organs, tissues and cells.

Co-operation among Member States in the field of blood transfusion began in the 1950s. From the outset, these activities were inspired by the following guiding principles: promotion of voluntary, non-remunerated blood donation, self-sufficiency, optimal use of blood and blood products, mutual assistance and protection of the donor and the recipient.

1953 North Sea Flood Disaster

It was this event, which took place in 1953 and mainly affected the Netherlands, which mobilised the CoE and its Member States in the field of blood safety.

---

[1]. A political organisation set up in 1949, the Council of Europe works to promote democracy and human rights continent-wide. It also develops common responses to social, cultural and legal challenges in its 47 Member States.

Guy Rautmann, guy.rautmann@edqm.eu

The Dutch province of Zeeland and the neighboring regions of Belgium were hardest hit, with 133 towns and villages flooded and over 1,800 casualties. At the time, there was no transparency or common good practices for blood transfusion in Europe, and no real understanding of the need for safe storage of blood products. Indeed, the disaster demonstrated a need for safety guidelines on the collection, storage and use of blood products in Europe.

This prompted the CoE to initiate the collaborative elaboration of a series of Recommendations for the safe preparation and use of quality blood components within Member States; an inter-governmental working process that has been successful throughout the history of the CoE.

Milestones

The first result of this co-operation was the adoption of the *European Agreement on the Exchange of Therapeutic Substances of Human Origin* (*European Treaty Series, No. 26*) in 1958. It was followed by the *European Agreement on the Exchange of Blood Grouping Reagents* (*European Treaty Series, No. 39*) in 1962 and the *European Agreement on the Exchange of Tissue-Typing Reagents* (*European Treaty Series, No. 84*) in 1976.

Based on these 3 agreements, the CoE has established a blood transfusion programme, the aim of which is to ensure the safe supply of good quality blood and blood products.

Since then, the CoE has adopted a number of recommendations covering ethical, social, scientific and training aspects of blood transfusion. Whereas agreements are binding on the States that ratify them, recommendations are policy statements to governments proposing a common course of action to be followed. *Recommendation No. R (88) 4* on the responsibilities of Health Authorities in the field of blood transfusion is one such influential recommendation.

In 1986, a Select Committee of Experts on Quality Assurance in Blood Transfusion Services published proposals on quality assurance in blood transfusion services. Based on these proposals, the Select Committee produced a more comprehensive guide on blood components in 1995. The immediate success and widespread acceptance of this document was such that the Committee of Ministers adopted it as a technical appendix to what then became known as *Recommendation No. R (95) 15*.

Recommendation No. R (95) 15 states that its technical appendix will be regularly up-dated to keep it in line with scientific progress and, to this end, the Committee was charged with producing annual up-dates in the form of a guide. During the elaboration of the 4th Edition, a public consultation procedure was introduced for the first time with great success. The publication of subsequent editions was based on this procedure.

The European Committee on Blood Transfusion (CD-P-TS) today

In 2007, the secretariat responsible for blood transfusion activities was transferred to the European Directorate for the Quality of Medicines and Healthcare (EDQM[2]). The CD-P-TS, a Steering Committee of the CoE, has since been in charge of co-ordinating the actions of the CoE in this area. This group is charged with updating *Recommendation No. R (95) 15* in the form of the *"Guide to the preparation, use and quality assurance of blood components"*, which is published by the EDQM and is, currently, in its 17th Edition. (17th edition to be published in 2013. See *The Guide* below.)

Thirty-five countries, including CoE Member States, parties to the *Convention on the Elaboration of a European Pharmacopoeia* and observers are represented on the CD-P-TS and its groups of experts. The European Commission, the World Health Organisation (WHO) and the CoE Committee on Bioethics are special observers to the CD-P-TS.

The objectives of the European Committee on Blood Transfusion

- Examine questions related to blood transfusion, notably on quality and safety standards and their implementation.
- Assist Member States in improving blood transfusion services and, if needed, in restructuring them to promote the principle of voluntary non-remunerated donations.
- Assist Member States in elaborating common European standards for quality management systems to be implemented in blood establishments involved in the collection, production and distribution of blood components.
- Define and promote the implementation of quality and safety standards in the collection, storage, distribution and use of blood components.
- Propose ethical, safety and quality standards for professional practices and product specifications.
- Ensure the transfer and development of knowledge and expertise through training and networking.
- Establish good practices in transfusion medicine and monitor their use in Europe.

---

2. The European Directorate for the Quality of Medicines & HealthCare (EDQM) contributes to protecting and promoting public and animal health in Europe by establishing high quality standards for human and veterinary medicinal products, blood transfusion and transplantation of organs tissues and cells and the safe and appropriate use of medicines.

3. The Council of Europe: Pioneering Blood Safety since the 1950's

- Assess epidemiological risks linked to blood transfusion and, in particular, for new transmissible diseases.
- Ensure the availability of rare blood components by providing suitable tools such as the European Bank of Frozen Blood of Rare Groups and, in the future, a centralised European database.

The European Committee on Blood Transfusion attains its objectives by:

- setting standards and preparing guidance on professional practices (*e.g.* the "*Guide to the preparation, use and quality assurance of blood components*");
- organising international surveys (*e.g.* enquiries on the collection, testing and use of blood components in Europe). The data are evaluated in reports, which are published on the EDQM's website;
- elaborating tools for professionals to promote continuous improvement of an ethical, organisational and regulatory approach to blood transfusion by means of resolutions (*e.g.* the *Resolution on donor responsibility and on the limitation of the donation of blood and its components CM/Res(2008)5*);
- providing practical, external quality assurance tools for blood establishments such as proficiency testing scheme studies and audits of blood establishments by peers;
- participating in World Blood Donor Day to thank blood donors for their life-saving generosity and to promote blood donation.

The Guide (17th Edition)

For a number of years the CoE has been publishing the "*Guide to the Preparation, Use and Quality Assurance of Blood Components*". This guide acts as the technical annex to *Recommendation No. R (95) 15*, which states that the guide must be continually updated to include the latest developments and state-of-the-art scientific processes identified by the experts of the CD-P-TS.

This guide is specifically designed for use by blood transfusion professionals working in transfusion services and establishments, hospitals and regulatory authorities.

The *Guide* is updated through an on-going collaborative and consultative process, whereby a group of experts is given access to updated texts and can suggest changes, make comments and also view existing comments made by their international colleagues.

The EDQM produces the *Guide* in the two official languages of the CoE (English and French), while translations into other languages (*e.g.* Greek, Polish and Turkish) are carried out under the responsibility of external parties. It is made available in both printed and electronic formats.

World Blood Donor Day (WBDD) helps to raise public awareness of the need for blood donations and promotes the principle of voluntary, non-remunerated donations. This year is the 10th anniversary of the global event, which will be hosted in Paris, France. The CoE/EDQM has been promoting WBDD for a number of years and provides practical support to some Member States in the preparation and production of campaign materials. The message of WBDD is not only a noteworthy cause in itself, but also provides a platform for the CoE to contribute and highlight on a global stage its expertise in the area of blood transfusion.

The CoE/EDQM is very pleased to be collaborating on WBDD 2013 with all of the partner organisations, including the WHO and the Etablissement Français du Sang.

The Future

There are a number of factors that may detrimentally influence and impact the supply, quality and safety of blood components and their derivatives in our changing world:

- ageing populations in developed countries;
- increasing instances of pandemics and natural disasters;
- new and emerging pathogens disseminated through geographical changes in populations (movement of labour) or forecasted climate change;
- levels of geopolitical and economic support for safe practices.

For these reasons, the activities of the CD-P-TS and the CoE/EDQM will continue to be of the utmost importance for the public health of European citizens in the future.

For more information, visit the website:
www.edqm.eu

To access the *Guide*:
http://tots.edqm.eu/entry.htm

To register the *Guide*:
www.edqm.eu/register

EDQM – Council of Europe
7 allée Kastner, CS 30026
F-67081 Strasbourg
France
Tel: +33 (0) 388 413 030
Fax: +33 (0) 388 412 771

Part II
French transfusion medicine

4. Communication

Françoise Le Failler

As well as its primary objective, self-sufficiency is a major and ongoing concern for the French Blood Establishment (EFS). Meeting patient needs is a constant challenge, and one that is overcome each year through the actions and efforts of collection teams, donor relations and communication campaigns.

Between 1988 and 2001, the use of labile blood products (LBP) fell by 30% following a series of damaging health crises: sales declined whilst autologous donations remained at high levels (close to 100,880 in 2000, a sign of deep distrust over the quality of LBP).

The communication policy was, until 2003, deliberately restrained and centred on blood donation rather than the EFS. As an institution, the EFS maintained a very low profile at that time.

From 2001 onwards, and particularly after 2004, the use of LBP increased very significantly. Over the same period, in a sign of renewed confidence, the number of autologous donations plummeted to just 1,800 in 2011.

The communication policy has helped the EFS address the upturn in demand for blood products. At no time in France have patients ever not received the LBP they need.

Context

Statistics

In France, there were approximately 1,700,000 voluntary blood donors in 2011, with an average of 1.8 blood donations per annum, per person. Sales are relatively consistent and experience few dips across the year. To meet these needs, approximately 10,000 blood donations are required every day.

In gender terms, the vast majority of new donors are women. They account for just over half of known donors. Yet most donations continue, quite noticeably, to be made by men. This gap is widening year on year.

Françoise Le Failler, francoise.lefailler@efs.sante.fr

Transfusion medicine: the French model

Between 2002 and 2011, sales of packed red blood cells rose by 25.5%, giving an increase of nearly 500,000 bags (2002: 1,938,501 and 2011: 2,432,076 or +493,575). The number of donors also rose in the same period, by 26.5% or 360,000 (2002: 1,364,124, 2011: 1,725,495 or +361,371).

Awareness of donors and non-donors: an essential prerequisite to action

To develop an effective communication policy, it is essential to identify current and potential donors, to understand their motivations and expectations, and to anticipate behavioural changes affecting their relationship with blood donation.

All studies report that blood donation is perceived very positively, a view shared by active donors and non-donors. Two extremes can be found amongst them: "super-donors" and "super non-donors", *i.e.* vocal supporters of the two camps. "Super-donors" say, "Of course we have to give blood, it's no bother. What's the problem? Anyway, it should be compulsory."

"Super non-donors", meanwhile, say, "No way, don't even talk to me about it." This position can be explained by physical reasons: "I'd faint straight away. I can't even give a blood sample." These people represent a very small section of the population.

As part of the *Living Standards and Aspirations in France* study conducted by the French Research Centre for the Study and Monitoring of Living Standards (CREDOC), the EFS commissioned a study on French attitudes to blood donation in June 2007. Donors and non-donors have similar views. Both say that donating blood is worthwhile, essential, and a good and necessary thing to do. 98% think that it can save lives and is, therefore, beneficial. 90% think that it is a good deed and 88% even think that giving blood is easy, at least whole blood. The figures suggest that approximately 4% of the eligible population gives blood. However, 34% of respondents say that they plan to give blood in the next 6 months.

We can note a discrepancy between the need to give blood and the need for greater resonance with the public. Although the benefits of blood donation are recognized, many donors and non-donors alike believe that it is not sufficiently publicized.

One of the barriers cited is lack of information. Sixty-five per cent of French people say, "You don't hear enough about giving blood in this country". Another barrier: giving blood is not an automatic habit and has to be instilled. Most people never consider it. There is, then, a contradiction between awareness of the importance of giving blood and the feeling that there is insufficient information about it. The other reasons given include lack of time and not knowing where blood donation sites are located. Mobile units and extended opening hours are strong incentives for people who work.

Finally, blood-related fears are still reported: 17% of French people are scared of needles, 12% cannot stand the sight of blood and 8% are afraid of feeling unwell after donating. The factors that would encourage French people to give more relate to the lifesaving potential of donated blood. They would be more motivated to donate if their donation could save a close friend or relative, if there was a national health emergency, if rare blood was needed and if there was a guarantee that lives would be saved.

Donors and socio-economic categories
Lifestyle and Blood Donation study
(Bernard Cuneo, Priscilla Duboz, Research Unit 6578 – Aix-Marseille University)

This study, which was conducted in 2008, identified four lifestyle groups relevant to blood donation.

- The first group comprises young people who give blood once and never again. It includes many students who are childless, not yet in employment and frequent travellers.
- The second group comprises people aged 26–35. It includes many socio-economic categories in intermediate occupations as defined by the French National Institute for Statistics and Economic Studies (INSEE), such as office workers, health workers (not doctors or pharmacists), and education workers (not teachers in higher education). This group includes the most regular donors.
- The third, more mature group comprises people aged 36–55. Here blood donation is less frequent. It includes members of associations. In this group, which is most likely to be in stable employment, there is strong demand for donation sessions in the workplace and direct invitations.
- The fourth group is more removed from blood donation. It is the oldest group, comprising over 55s. Since the age limit on blood donation was raised to 70, these donors no longer see themselves as too old to give blood and are starting to donate once more.

All the studies conducted on donors in recent years have the same aim: greater knowledge of the community of current and potential donors in order to develop an ever-more effective communication policy, encourage people to donate for the first time and increase repeat donations.

4. Communication

How does communication help the EFS achieve self-sufficiency?

The stock levels in each blood establishment are displayed on the EFS's computer screens each morning. This daily update, which one journalist called "the *Wall Street* of blood", demonstrates the difficulty of achieving self-sufficiency. Stock levels are monitored day by day. This means that communication on blood donation is a constant challenge, due in particular to various external factors that may affect donations and donors (bad weather, epidemics, etc.). Communication must, therefore, take a humble stance as it seeks to fulfil its aims. In national campaigns, there are never any guarantees that the expected results will be achieved. Nothing is ever certain. There is always an element of doubt in communication initiatives, which may lessen their impact.

The challenges

The need to balance short-term results and long-term strategies

Communication has two stages: the short and long term. These two stages are reflected in how communication is organized.

In the short term, the aim is to contribute to current blood collection efforts. This is an issue that cannot wait. Urgency has long been a hallmark of communication and collection by the EFS. The EFS has seen huge surges when it was heavily publicized in the media. The collection teams managed donors' waiting times. This situation caused real problems. In recent years, there has been a shift away from the emphasis on urgency, even though the EFS's teams coped with it well. They reacted quickly but the situation was far from ideal, both for staff working conditions and the image conveyed to donors. There was also a risk of losing media credibility. For that reason, the focus has been moved to publicizing blood donation throughout the year.

The service is dominated by variations across the year: whilst demand for LBP is constant, donations fluctuate widely due to school term dates (fewer donors during the holidays) and seasonal variations: bad weather, epidemics (influenza, gastroenteritis, etc.), strikes, student demonstrations, disruptions to public transport, and so on.

To implement a long-term communication policy, an annual programme of seasonal campaigns has been developed.

Some campaigns are said to have a "slow burn" effect. This involves anticipating a foreseeable drop in donation numbers. This is the aim of the November campaign in particular, which prepares for Christmas and New Year, a difficult period when there are fewer donors (Figure 5).

Other campaigns are described as "quick burn", where the aim is to build up blood stocks very quickly. These actions have to be short, timely and achieve results fast. In a saturated media environment, blood donation is not a subject that should be trivialized. The messages must be honest and pertinent.

The need to balance internal and external stakeholders

The glasshouse that is the Internet, the most powerful of all the media, means that targeted communication (donors, EFS staff members, physicians, associations, etc.) has lost all meaning. Today, information is

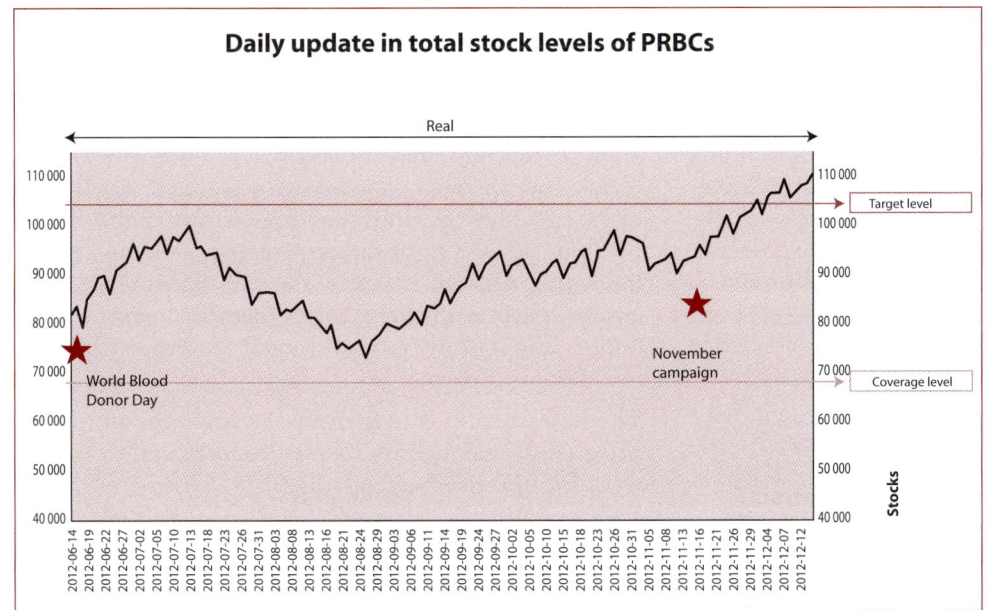

Figure 5. Changes in national stock levels of PRBCs (2012).
PRBCs: packed red blood cells.

accessible to everyone. The information the EFS provides to each party must be consistent.

Internal communication, which has too often been overlooked, plays a key role.

The aim is to go further than small, individual initiatives and deliver a comprehensive programme giving stakeholders the resources they need to better understand the institution, its role, its aims and the results it expects.

The aim is also to garner support. Support cannot be assumed. It is won through information and explanations of the policies implemented. Senior managers have a decisive role to play in this communication, notably in educating teams so that they understand and adopt the strategic decisions taken by the establishment.

This remark applies to all the EFS's activities but is particularly relevant to blood donation and collection, which bring its staff into constant contact with civil society (donors, media, associations, etc.). They are the best ambassadors for the service. Their expertise and dedication are regularly highlighted by donors in studies. It is vital, then, that actions and messages involving internal and external stakeholders are complementary.

The communication policy boosting self-sufficiency
Its aims

To contribute to self-sufficiency, communication must not only inform but also inspire to act and create committed, long-term donors.

Its work to achieve self-sufficiency has four aims, which are to:
– clearly situate the EFS and its role;
– convey an identity that all audiences recognize;
– raise awareness;
– ensure that messages are consistent.

Communication has been shaped by the ethical values underpinning blood donation: altruism, volunteerism and absence of profit. On this basis, moralizing, patronizing and reprehending messages are rejected. For national blood transfusion services, it involves building a community of donors with three aims: professionalism, proximity and modernity. Over the years, the discourse has evolved, with messages on the purpose and use of donations (diseases treated with blood products, daily needs, etc.) and donation sites gradually replacing previous campaigns that praised donors.

Communication stakeholders

Within the EFS, various stakeholders are involved at different levels:

- **At head office: the National Communication Department (DIRCOM)**

Based on the EFS's strategic objectives, DIRCOM devises the national communication policy (external and internal) and oversees its implementation. It manages the EFS's image, raising its profile and improving its reputation. It implements tools, partnerships and national awareness-raising and recruitment campaigns aimed at donors and non-donors.

- **In regional establishments (ETS)**
  – Communication teams implement the national policy through local initiatives that boost donor numbers. They work with various partners: associations, companies and local authorities. They coordinate these networks of partners.
  – The teams in charge of scheduling blood collection: donation sessions and communication initiatives must be coordinated. A major blood donation drive implies a major publicity drive. However, there is little point in widespread communication if there are insufficient facilities to accommodate donors.
  – Finally, teams from the Donor Relations and Marketing Departments add to the initiatives by creating and developing personalized relationships with donors.

Work within the communication network makes it possible to review the initiatives put in place and share good practice.

All blood collection personnel have a role to play because they are in contact with donors. They provide information to parties outside the EFS.

Types of initiatives
- **Campaigns**

The campaigns developed include initiatives for use by the EFS's regional establishments, which implement them at grassroots level with their partners.

As a minimum, a national campaign includes posters, radio commercials and web advertising.

Depending on the donation targets, a campaign may be supplemented and strengthened by other tools: press releases, advertisements (radio, web, billboards, television, etc.) and promotional items.

Some campaigns may undergo a pre-implementation review, which involves assessing a planned visual with different audiences: understanding, consistency with the EFS's image or aim of the campaign, and so on. Working with a research institute, the EFS forms three focus groups, each with eight to 10 members: non-donors, donors and a third group bringing together EFS staff members and partner associations.

The ultimate aim is to identify the strengths and weaknesses of the campaign's creative concept and to suggest areas for improvement.

- **Events**

The aims of blood donation events are to:
– recruit new donors,

4. Communication

– raise the profile and reputation of the EFS,
– increase blood donation numbers significantly.
These events are highlights in the calendar of the EFS and its establishments.

14 June is a key date for the EFS each year, with 350 collection sites in France marking World Blood Donor Day.

Events and press relations are closely linked: every year, journalists give significant coverage to World Blood Donor Day. This event aims to become bigger and better known in the media year after year.

• **Press relations**

Press relations have a very important place in communication relating to self-sufficiency.

Blood donation is an area that interests the media and receives widespread coverage.

The media are a good way to promote the cause of blood donation and to mobilize donors and non-donors.

Blood donation and "supply issues" interest journalists. All communication with the media must be developed in advance so as to manage the discourse, avoid any scaremongering and deliver the right messages in line with the establishment's strategy.

Any person who comes into contact with the media must therefore be aware of the journalist's agenda ("angle" of the article) and prepare for the interview with the communication teams. They will provide the information needed for this purpose (press packs, key figures, etc.).

• **Digital communication**

The verdict is in: it is impossible to escape the ubiquity of the Internet.

The dominance of social networks, the strong emergence of mobile tools and the growth in the tablets market are central to the digital communication strategy.

Dialogue with the public must be shaped around these technologies, with users made central to the strategy and discourse once more. These two requirements have led the EFS to implement a strategy based on producing content that is specifically designed for digital formats.

Note that users are fickle, the pace of change is ever-quickening, and support for a brand and its values is won or lost in the first few seconds. Opportunities for the audience to see the messages must therefore be increased.

It is important that the content created is multilayered, and that the visual and graphic elements convey the values and identity just as much as the discourse.

The aim is to deliver continuous services and messages, irrespective of the users, their needs and their personal circumstances.

The EFS is available on the following media:
– website: www.dondusang.net;
– mobile tools: iPhone app, mobile site (android or tablet);
– social networks *via* Facebook (around 30,000 people have consulted the EFS's page), Twitter and YouTube.

• **Institutional communication**

The EFS's institutional communication aims to meet several objectives, which are to:
– provide information on the institution and its role in providing national blood transfusion services;
– increase the EFS's profile and associate it with blood donation;
– act as an institution and implement government decisions on relevant topics (ethics of blood donation, monopoly, health safety, etc.);
– improve the EFS's attractiveness as an employer.

The EFS is a public health stakeholder. But although everyone is aware of the product (blood), who really knows what the EFS is and what its roles are? How can we raise awareness of the EFS as an institutional partner in the public health system?

Alongside conventional communication campaigns (posters, leaflets, etc.), this involves working more closely with opinion leaders. At grassroots level, the EFS has already developed close ties with local media.

The aim now is to develop stronger relationships with local elected representatives. Opportunities to increase their understanding of the EFS must be created so that they can then publicize the EFS and its work with donors and patients. This type of initiative adopts a long-term approach.

• **Review of communication initiatives**

Reviewing communication initiatives is a particularly important step for a public service. It is important to review what initiatives achieve as well as what they cost (example of the review of World Blood Donor Day 2012 within the EFS in the text box below).

Conclusion

To communicate with donors on a daily basis and anticipate the changes brought about by social and technological advances, it is necessary to:
– implement communication initiatives, which are essential and urgently needed;
– consider tomorrow's communication.

One of the objectives of the communication policy is clear: mobilizing donors to meet patients' needs. The EFS has therefore moved away from short-term campaigns, which even led to urgent national appeals for donors, and towards a long-term mobilization policy.

Transfusion medicine: the French model

Review of World Blood Donor Day 2012

A quantitative response

- *The donation numbers, donors and new donors*

Date	Known donors	New donors	Donations	% donors who were able to donate	% new donors
14/06/2012	17,542	6,363	21,117	88%	26.6%

On 14 June 2012, 21,117 donors gave blood, whilst in the week of 14 June a total of 75,705 bags were donated.

- *The number of press mentions*

There were 976 press mentions of World Blood Donor Day 2012 (*versus* 2011: 970, 2010: 649, 2009: 397, 2008: 248 and 2007: 147).

Most major national channels covered World Blood Donor Day in their news bulletins: TF1, France 2, France 3, i>Télé, LCI, M6, etc. It was also widely covered in the written press, with a 30% increase in the number of mentions (excluding websites) *versus* 2011. Note significant coverage in the regional press too, with 70% of mentions.

- *Visitor numbers to the website*

	2011			2012			Difference
	Event website	Site dondusang.net	Total	Event website	Site dondusang.net	Total	%
Visits	5,757	28,426	34,183	27,357	16,971	44,328	29.7%
Pages seen	15,489	79,665	95,154	44,046	66,306	110,352	16.0%
Visitors	5,452	26,773	32,225	26,600	15,891	42,491	31.9%

Qualitative responses: post-event reviews

Every year, the communication initiatives on World Blood Donor Day are reviewed by an independent panel. Several aspects are examined: is the EFS seen as the instigator of the initiative? Have the messages been understood? Did they encourage blood donations? These are just some of the questions that will make it possible to choose stronger messages and communication mechanisms in future initiatives.

Mobilization is staggered throughout the year. One annual highlight is World Blood Donor Day on 14 June.

It is also tailored to the target donor. One example is the student campaign, which is run twice in the year, in February and November (Figure 6). A specific tool has also been designed for young people turning 18. It is publicized by the French Ministry of Defence as part of Citizen Action Days (Figure 7).

This mobilization is also organized by collection type. Communication on permanent sites has been developed across the country.

Similarly, to support the EFS's communication in businesses that host donation sessions, specific tools have been created to raise awareness of blood donation and encourage people to give.

We have come far since the propaganda of the 1950s. Within the EFS, in communication and many other areas, significant advances have been made. Yet communication on blood transfusion services still faces many challenges.

We are particularly mindful of the precautions needed when publicizing advances in research on universal blood. Cultured red blood cells may indeed make it possible to better manage patients with a rare blood group, who receive repeated transfusions and present complex transfusion problems, but no product is yet able to replace human blood. Communication on this subject must therefore be extremely cautious as there is a major risk of discouraging donors, who may wrongly think that it is possible to manufacture blood in huge amounts *in vitro*. There is also a question mark over launching campaigns to recruit donors of certain blood groups. This would involve developing national communication focused on the O-negative group in

4. Communication

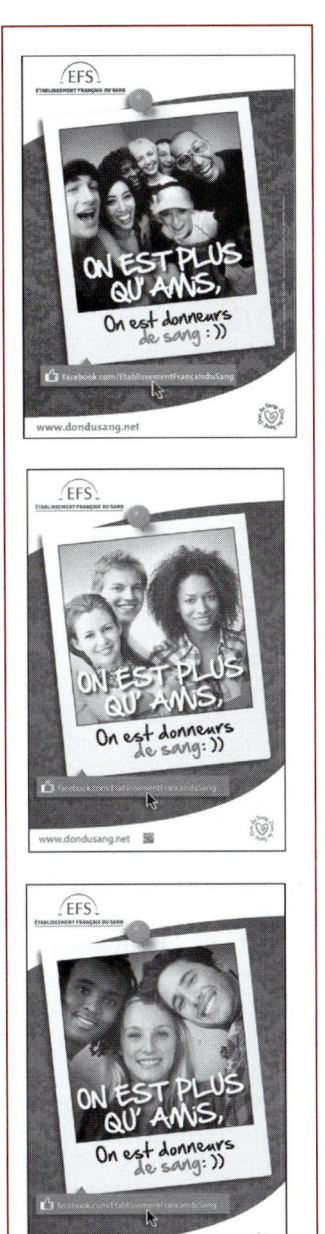

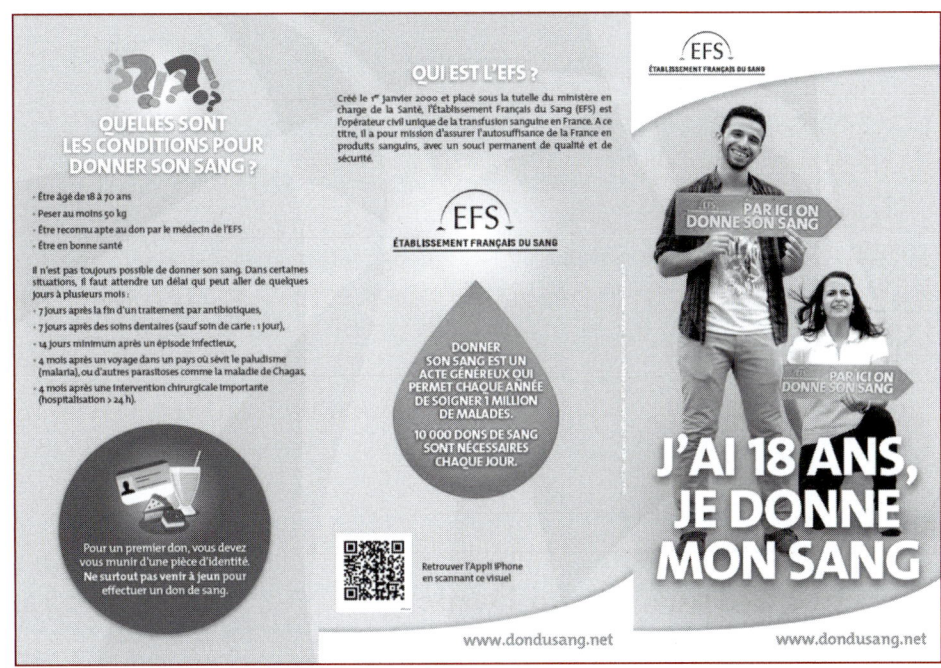

Figure 7. Leaflet for Citizen Action Day 2012.
© EFS.

Figure 6. Posters of the 2013 student campaign.
© EFS.

particular. These donors are identified in the EFS's databases and contacted individually at local level. A major, nationwide initiative aimed at these donors is being considered.

Tomorrow's communication will stand at the crossroads of three requirements: efficiency, quality and self-sufficiency. These 3 requirements will be met on 2 conditions:

– excellent synergies between the communication and communication teams; and
– greater internal communication to increase the impact and consistency of the messages conveyed by EFS staff members.

Awareness of present realities and future challenges is the line of communication that should generate action and promote an essential public service: blood donation.

5. Blood collection

Florence Chenus, Bruno Danic, Geneviève Woimant

Since 2000, blood collection has been managed by a single government agency, the French Blood Establishment (EFS).

In 2011, as a result of the staff's work, who numbers over 3,000 full-time equivalents, the EFS collected 3,190,226 donations in its 151 permanent sites and donation centres, as well as through the 50,000 donation sessions organized across the country, including:
– 2,588,716 of homologous, autologous and non-therapeutic whole blood;
– 466,474 of plasmapheresis,
– 134,398 of platelet aphaeresis, single or combined.

These donations supplied 914,750 litres of raw plasma material intended for fractionation and provided to the French Fractionation Laboratory (LFB) for the preparation of medicinal products derived from human blood and plasma: immunoglobulins, albumin and coagulation factors. The medicinal products prepared by the LFB from the plasma collected by the EFS are used solely by health centres in France.

The "communication" phase is located upstream of "collection" services. These services have two essential components: firstly, organizing the donation collection system and managing the donor database and, secondly, collecting the raw material, *i.e.* blood, and samples for the specialized platforms preparing blood products and testing donations. Downstream are the "preparation" and "testing" phases. The two activities combine to transform the raw material into a distributable or issuable end product.

Medico-technical description of "collection" services

The absolute necessity to guarantee the safety of donors and recipients is an essential part of the EFS's culture. It is underpinned by the regulatory framework and

Florence Chenus, florence.chenus@efs.sante.fr.
Bruno Danic, bruno.danic@efs.sante.fr.
Geneviève Woimant, genevieve.woimant@efs.sante.fr.

5. Blood collection

monitored by the French National Agency for Medicines and Health Products Safety (ANSM). The EFS draws on quality management to achieve the targets set by the State. Internally, it has developed various tools to ensure the safety of "collection" services across the country.

The EFS has chosen to use the preliminary risk analysis method for its comprehensive risk management programme. This method of identifying, assessing and reducing risk covers all potential hazards (strategy, management, information technology, medical issues, etc.).

Each transfusion site must obtain internal authorization to provide "collection" services, whether on permanent sites and/or in mobile units. This authorization is granted for 4 years, once the Establishment Authorization Technical Committee has approved a self-assessment completed by the director of the regional blood establishment (ETS) for all sites involved in the services. This self-assessment is designed in accordance with national guidelines. Between each authorization, the collection services provided by the ETS are audited, on the basis of at least one site each year, to verify compliance with current regulations and progress in the action plans undertaken. After 4 years, a further self-assessment is carried out to review the authorization (Figure 8).

Donation collection system

The EFS's role is to ensure the availability of labile blood products (LBP) across the country. The anticipation of transfusion needs and the regulation of stock levels are managed at national and regional level. Every year, the EFS sets each ETS production targets reflecting their forecast level of activity. The ETS then organizes the collection of blood in its vicinity in accordance with its targets.

In the geographical area allocated to the site, local managers, site managers and/or collection managers organize, provide and adapt the collection services. They ensure that the targets are met, as required by law and the establishment's internal regulations.

To do this, with the help of volunteers brought together under the term "Logistics Unit", they plan the collections, manage the availability of staff, venues, equipment, supplies and vehicles, and assess the need to publicize the donation session. Analysis of the results using indicators and dashboards makes it possible, if necessary, to adapt the facilities to the targets and/or changing situations.

The year-long planning of permanent and mobile collections

An initial plan is developed in spring for the following year. Mobile collections are scheduled in each area over the weeks and months ahead to ensure the regular supply of LBP, in both quality and quantity, in the region. Difficult periods are the school holidays and public

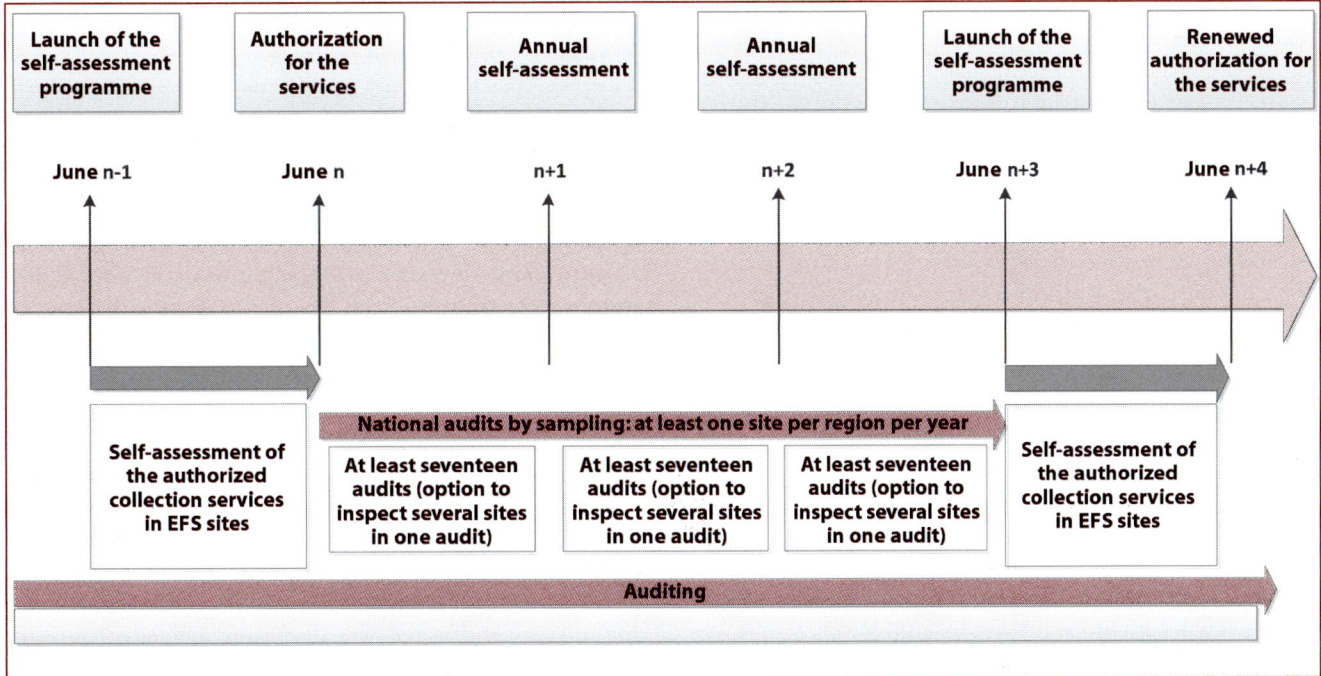

Figure 8. Cycle of initial authorization (2011–2015) and renewal.
EFS: French Blood Establishment.

holidays that fall close together or to the weekend. The scheduling must also take into account local particularities, such as the availability of venues, trading hours and possibly the availability of partners to help to organize the collection.

Rooms may be booked in town halls by the EFS or donors associations depending on the partnerships formed. The plan becomes definitive in or around June. It is then supplemented by donation sessions in businesses. Finally, after the long summer holidays, the plan is finalized with the addition of sessions in colleges and universities, which are scheduled in accordance with the availability of the premises and students. Several parties are involved. In addition to the usual partners brought together in associations, partnerships are established with service clubs (International Rotary, French Round Table, Lions Clubs, etc.), local authorities, municipalities, public transport networks, educational institutions, major companies, and so on. The links in the blood collection chain rely on volunteers in town halls, work councils, occupational health departments, preventive medicine services in colleges and universities…

Throughout the year, plans may be adapted to unforeseeable circumstances: the temporary unavailability of venues or donors, participation in an event or additional donation sessions to cover a fall in blood stocks, for any reason: a sudden increase in requirements or fall in donor numbers due, for example, to bad weather, seasonal epidemics, strikes, etc.

> Predictions of the donation numbers expected from each session are based on analysis of previous figures from the same period in the last 3 years. This analysis reflects occasional variations caused by efforts to promote the session or any other unforeseeable event that might affect the numbers attained. It makes it possible to determine, with a very small margin of error, the session's contribution to maintaining sufficient stocks of packed red blood cells to cover 12 to 14 days of sales and the staffing levels required to provide optimal services.

The times of the sessions are determined by the availability of the target group of donors and the logistical constraints of processing blood products.

Planning the staffing levels of donation sessions

Staffing levels are decided based on the predicted number of possible donors and blood donations. The organisation must provide the best possible balance between the optimal use of the allocated resources, the quality of service provided to donors and the time needed to complete each stage in the donation process: registration, pre-donation interview, collection, rest and refreshments. Maximum ratios determining the number of interviews per physician are set at national level, as are the donation numbers taken by state-registered nurses. These ratios are adapted to the donor profile: whole blood/aphaeresis and new/regular donors. A secretary, driver and refreshments supervisor usually complete the team. Associations promoting voluntary blood donation often contribute to the refreshments provided, helping to create a relaxing and enjoyable experience after donating.

Assessment of donation sites

This involves producing records that demonstrate compliance with regulatory standards and detail the equipment available onsite. A site plan shows the entrances and exits, power points, nearest available parking and a suggested layout of the donation collection facilities. The arrangements may be finalized by the completion of a room hire agreement for the specified day. Finally, one or more journey plans are created, and the team's travelling time is calculated.

The availability of equipment, supplies and vehicles

Appropriate equipment, in sufficient quantities to meet requirements (mechanical agitators, portable sealers, cell separators, donation chairs, etc.), is essential for the conduct of the session. Other necessities include the barcodes used to identify donations, single-use medical devices (SUDs), sample tubes, medical supplies (antiseptics, dressings, first-aid kits, etc.), donation guides and refreshments.

Managing the donor database

In France, 4.3% of the eligible population contributes to maintaining LBP stock levels every year. Yet needs are increasing by approximately 2 to 3% year on year. For that reason, it is important that the EFS ensures the availability of a growing number of blood products at all times and devises a sustainable donation collection system reflecting the lifestyles of the groups it hopes to attract, increasing the number of donors and securing repeat donations.

The blood donor database is refreshed and expanded by communication campaigns orchestrated at national level and implemented in the regions by the ETS. At local level, the EFS provides the donors associations with all the tools they need to promote blood donation and so raise awareness amongst local people. The role of the EFS's communication services is to increase knowledge and understanding of the donation collection system. Studies conducted by the EFS show that posters, leaflets and direct invitations from another donor are the triggers most frequently cited by new donors.

The personalized relationship with donors borrows an organisational style and tools from social marketing. It aims to ensure the successful solicitation of donors, maintaining constant links between them and the EFS without veering into harassment. All methods of communication are used: social networks, emails, SMS, letters, newsletters, etc.

Regular surveys are used to review the effectiveness of the campaigns and tools, measure donor satisfaction and adapt the organisational style.

Quality indicators of blood donation collection

Analysis of completed donation sessions is used to update all the sources of information that will be used when planning future collections. This is undertaken on a daily basis by examining reports on the conduct of donation sessions, including the results generated and any notable incidents. It may be supplemented by analysis of the donations that were declined and the results of blood donation testing, particularly if a transmissible disease marker is found.

In addition to the ongoing review of services, quality indicators make it possible to monitor, analyze, react and anticipate in order to ensure continuous improvement in performance.

The quality levels of donated products, including managing in-process losses, the quality of service provided to donors and reports of nonconformities are analyzed daily, weekly, monthly and even annually if necessary. Internal audits are conducted at regional and national level. The entire system is detailed in preventive and/or corrective action plans whose effectiveness is assessed.

The main activity indicators are:
– number of bags collected per collection type;
– number and characteristics of the donation sessions, in total and per collection type;
– number of donors who attended, and how many were able to give blood;
– number of first donations;
– number of attendees who were unable to give blood.

The main quality indicators used to assess the performance of the services include:
– analysis of in-process losses: insufficient volumes, blood seals, defective sealers, incorrectly labelled products or tubes;
– quality control of the donated products;
– complaints made by internal and external parties: specialized platforms, donors, partners, etc.,
– adverse reactions, serious adverse reactions and serious incidents occurring in the transfusion chain as a result of blood donation.

The various donation sites

A donation session can be defined as a particular moment in time when a volunteer can go to a designated place and give blood. The characteristics of this place are used to define the two types of donation site currently in use: permanent and mobile.

The permanent site or donation centre

The EFS has 151 permanent sites and donation centres, primarily located in large and medium-sized cities. These sites offer donation facilities with long opening hours, which the EFS tries to adapt to the lifestyles of urban populations. In particular, the EFS is developing donation by appointment on its permanent sites to save donors time. These sites collect all forms of donation in the best possible conditions: whole blood, apheresis and voluntary donors for bone marrow donations. All apheresis donations are made on these sites and the EFS has the target of collecting at least 20% of the whole blood donations needed every year here.

Frequently, donation centres form part of the collection service, with the other part entailing the organisation and preparation of mobile donation sessions.

The space provided for homologous donations is formed by a series of areas laid out in the same logical order as the donation process:
- *a reception area*, with an IT system (computer and printer) giving access to donor's records database in the medico-technical software. This area has all the administrative documents needed to inform and register prospective donors;
- *one or more health screening areas*, which also have the facilities to view and update donors' records, as well as the equipment needed to measure the clinical and biological parameters required by law: a stethoscope, tensiometer, photometer to determine haemoglobin levels before the donation, and possibly weighing scales. This area has the documents needed to evaluate the suitability of the prospective donor: list of malaria-endemic countries, medicinal product monographs and current guidelines;
- *one or more collection rooms*, which are provided in areas with ergonomic donation chairs, cell separators and whole blood collection monitors, as well as all the equipment and supplies needed for the different types of donation (*e.g.* a photometer to determine the haemoglobin in capillary blood and perhaps an automated blood count analyzer, etc.);
- *a rest area*, which is separate but situated immediately alongside the team, particularly the physician, for individual monitoring should the donor feel unwell;
- *a refreshments area* serving food and drinks that meet food safety standards.

Transfusion medicine: the French model

All the premises meet the regulatory standards governing public buildings in terms of safety, cleanliness, ventilation, lighting, temperature and accessibility, particularly disabled access. Some areas may need to be temperature controlled to provide the storage conditions required by both donated products (storage of whole blood, plasma, platelet concentrates and packed red blood cells from aphaeresis prior to transport, which are kept between +20 °C and +24 °C), and some collection devices and solutions, generally between 0 °C and +25 °C.

Mobile blood collection

The EFS often sends a donation collection team to areas closest to the population being served. This team holds donation sessions in the venue provided, often at no cost, or in one of its specially equipped blood donation vehicles known as "mobile collection units".

Because mobile blood collection covers the entire country, it enables the maximum number of prospective donors to give blood. Over 80% of whole blood donations are made in 50,000 mobile collections every year. It is essential that these facilities are well advertised, clearly signposted and easily accessible to the public, with sufficient parking in the vicinity.

Irrespective of the type of mobile blood collection, the facilities are laid out in the same logical order as permanent sites, reflecting the different stages in the donation process. The venues provided meet minimum health and safety standards applicable to public buildings in terms of hygiene (toilets and washroom facilities), accessibility (special provisions for disabled people), ventilation, lighting, temperature and security (stairs, emergency exits, etc.). They provide sufficient space to create the different areas within a coherent layout, including areas that ensure donor confidentiality.

The same equipment is used in these donation sessions as in permanent sites. The team must in particular have practical means of communication. The donation chairs must be portable, foldaway and suitable for use in different venues. However, they must also balance practical requirements with the comfort of the donor.

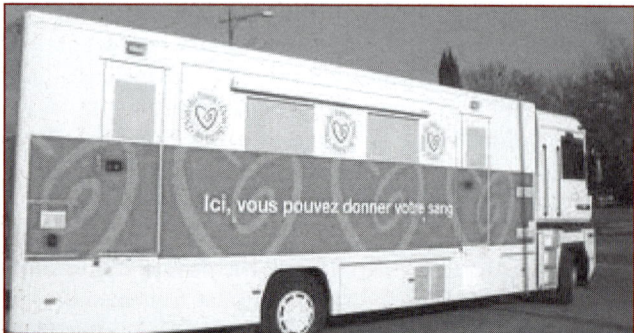
© EFS.

The various donation stages

The four-stage "donation process" is the same in permanent sites and mobile units.

Registration

On arrival, prospective donors are met by a member of the collection team. This stage makes it possible to create the donor's records in the computer system using a series of open-ended questions and proof of identity. Registering these details in the system generates a donor number. The type of information that is recorded and used to locate existing records is outlined in a national procedure preventing the creation of duplicates and ensuring the traceability of previous attendances. The donor's records, which are confirmed at each attendance and updated if necessary, are used to print the donation collection form. A unique, non-reusable donation number is allocated to this form. Shown as a series of figures and a barcode, the number has 11 digits: the first 2 correspond to the ETS, the next 2 to the year, the following 6 to the serial numbers allocated to the collection site, and finally a check digit is used for error detection. The donation collection form is handed to the prospective donor, who reads it and confirms that the details are correct. At this stage, donors are also given documents on blood donation safety: pre-donation information, whose content is determined by the Director-General of the ANSM, additional pre-donation information on aphaeresis if necessary, and the questionnaire to complete before the pre-donation interview, whose style and content are defined in law. Prospective donors read the information and complete the questionnaire in a private, confidential area.

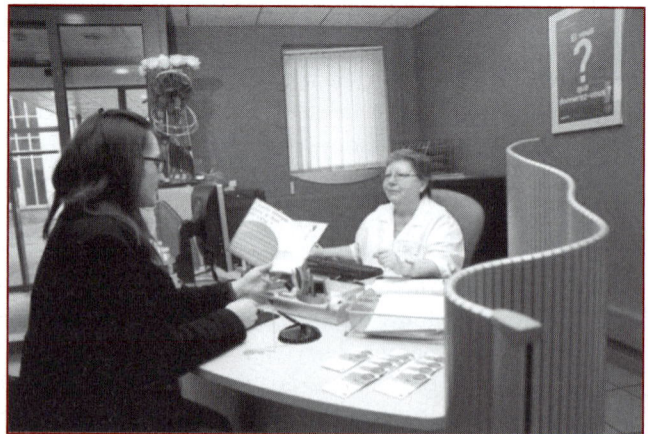
© EFS.

Pre-donation interview

The pre-donation interview is conducted one-to-one by an authorized and trained medical doctor. No third parties are present to maintain donor confidentiality. He/she checks the prospective donor's suitability to give blood in line with criteria designed to protect the health of the donor and limit the risks of transmitting a pathogen to the recipient. The physician must ensure that the issues surrounding blood donation safety have been understood by the donor, which requires a sufficient command of French to read and understand the information documents, as well as to maintain a high level of conversation in the pre-donation interview.

After confirming the prospective donor's identity, the doctor goes over all the items on the questionnaire, asking any additional questions that may be required. The donation contraindications ensuring donor safety are based on identifying a cardiovascular irregularity, blood anomaly and any condition that could be worsened by giving 500 mL of blood. The contraindications ensuring recipient safety are based on identifying any ongoing or recent infection, as well as activities that may expose, or have exposed, donors to an infection that could be transmitted to the recipient by transfusion. Blood donor selection criteria are defined in a Ministerial Order, itself based on a European directive. This remains an essential stage in blood donation because the tests conducted on donations may not always detect very recent contamination.

The doctor carries out a clinical examination limited to measuring the donor's blood pressure, heart rate and looking for signs of anaemia. He/she measures, or orders tests on, capillary and venous haemoglobin levels and other laboratory values depending on the requirements of the session. He/she examines the medical and family histories and details of previous donations, if any, advises the donor to stay hydrated and provides recommendations for the hours following the donation. He/she reminds the donor of the importance of reporting adverse reactions at any time, as well as new or forgotten information that may undermine the safety of the donated products, particularly any signs of infection in the fortnight after donating.

Because donors may feel unwell after giving blood, they are given a series of written recommendations: to avoid

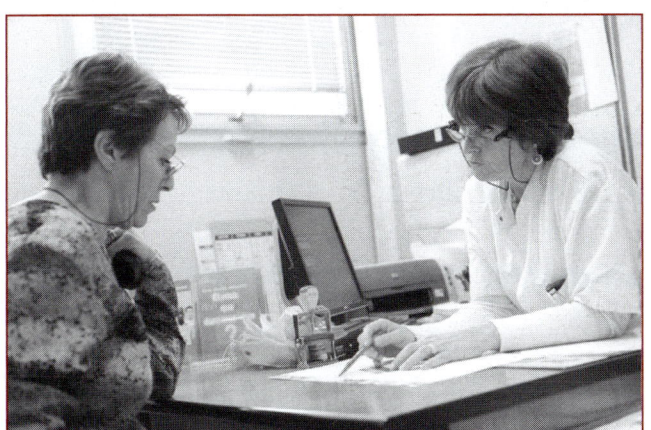
© EFS.

vigorous exercise for 12 hours after the donation, as well as any hazardous occupation or hobby that could put them or others at the risk of harm, such as working at height or driving a bus.

After answering the prospective donor's questions, the physician signs the donation collection form to confirm that the pre-donation interview is satisfactory. The donor signs to confirm that he/she has been made aware of all the safety issues and wishes to continue the donation process (informed consent).

Collection of the donation and samples

Blood is taken by an authorized and trained nurse. After checking that the donation collection form corresponds to the right donor, he/she reads the doctor's recommendations and ensures that all the previous stages have been completed correctly.

Based on the information provided, he/she selects the type of SUDs and any solutions required by the donation. He/she positions the SUDs on the blood collection monitor or cell separator and enters the parameters that will determine the characteristics of the donated product: volume for whole blood, clinical and biological parameters for aphaeresis. To do this, he/she provides details of the donor's weight, height, sex, haematocrit and platelet levels, and haemoglobin concentration. Finally, he/she prepares the tubes needed to test the donation and a tube for the sample bank.

- **Selecting the venipuncture site**

The creases of both elbows are inspected to locate the most suitable venipuncture site. Following friction (hydroalcoholic disinfection of the nurse's bare hands), the area is made aseptic using an iodine- or chlorhexidine-based disinfectant solution applied in 2 to 4 circular motions. The contact time of the disinfectant solution is that recommended by the supplier. Further palpation of the venipuncture site requires to repeat the disinfection procedure. The opening and use-by dates of the disinfectant solutions are marked on the bottles.

- **Collection**

The clamps of the collection line and sample pouch are closed before the cap is removed from the needle. The venisection of the basilic vein should be clean, rapid and immediate to avoid activating the tissue factors causing coagulation. The length of catheterization is determined by the type of donation: short for whole blood, medium for aphaeresis. The venipuncture site is then protected by a compress or drape, which may be used only once in some cases. The first 40 millilitres of whole blood are diverted to the sample pouch. By removing the skin tissue that may have been detached by the bevel of the needle, this practice reduces the risk of bacterial

Transfusion medicine: the French model

contamination in the donated product. When full, its line is permanently closed, often by heat sealing. The collection line is then unclamped and the donation begins in earnest. The following stage involves filling the sample tubes for testing and linking the donor/bags/tubes. To do this, the nurse asks the donor to confirm his/her full name and date of birth. He/she then identifies the bags and tubes using the donation number. From this moment on, the link is consolidated, anonymity is protected and traceability is assured.

The collection is constantly monitored. This includes signs of adverse reactions in donors, the flow rate, volume collected, operation of the monitors, volumes of solutions used and progress in hydration.

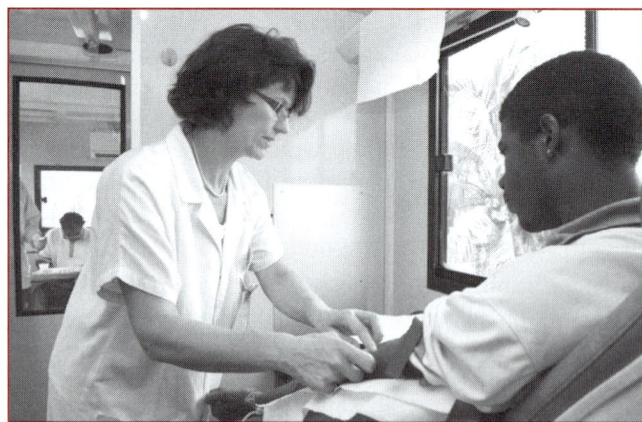
© EFS.

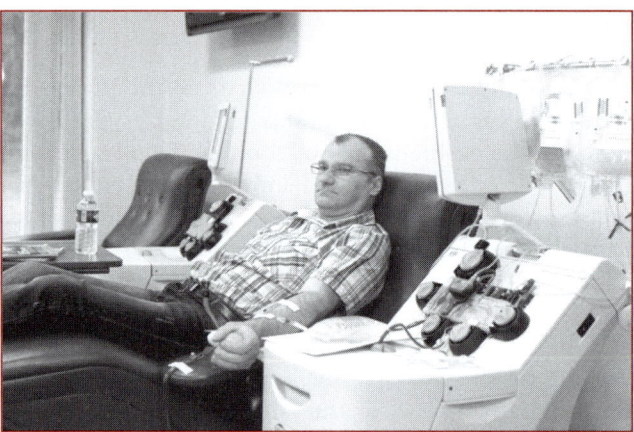
© EFS.

• **The end of the collection**

This is managed by the monitor as soon as the specified volume has been taken. The line is irreversibly closed by heat sealing. The needle is removed using a needle cover to limit the risk of accidental blood exposure. Donors are monitored for a few more moments; in aphaeresis, blood pressure is measured. They are then directed towards the refreshments area. The donation and tubes are packaged for transport, and information on the procedure is recorded. Used supplies are placed in the containers provided for infectious waste disposal.

Two stages are critical in preventing accidental blood exposure due to the risk of transcutaneous inoculation: the venipuncture and, more importantly, the removal of the needle. It is highly recommended that gloves are worn for these stages.

Refreshments and post-donation monitoring

Refreshments conclude the donation process. This is an opportunity to rehydrate and monitor donors. They are offered unlimited amounts of water and various sweet, non-alcoholic drinks, confectionary, charcuterie and hot or cold meals. The refreshments are transported and stored in suitable containers and appropriate temperatures. The persons providing refreshments, whether they are professionals or volunteers, must meet current hygiene standards to protect the health of donors. They are authorized and trained in preventing accidental blood exposure, detecting the first signs of ill health, recognizing information that is relevant to blood donation safety, and answering basic questions on the different types of donation. They ensure that donors are given sufficient fluids (at least 300 mL) and rest. Pre-prepared refreshments are stored in refrigerated containers and provided to donors as and when required. They are disposed of after the session. The refrigerated containers are regularly cleaned (and these actions are recorded) and their temperature controls are checked periodically in accordance with storage standards.

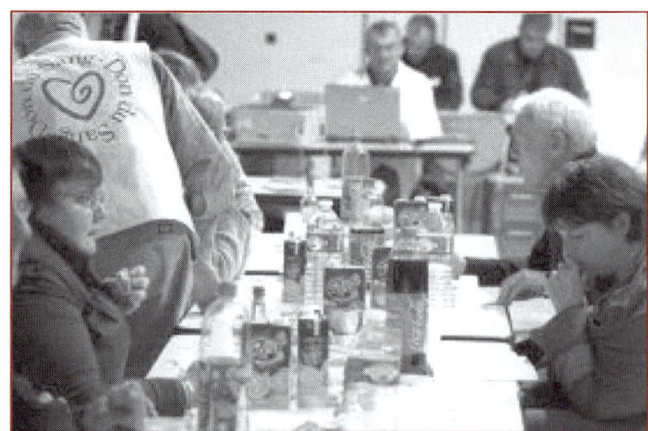
© EFS.

The different types of donation and collection techniques

Irrespective of the type of homologous donation, collections are made in line with the ethical principles that are volunteerism, anonymity and the absence of profit.

5. Blood collection

Whole blood donation

This remains almost the sole source of the packed red blood cells that patients need. Over 80% of donations are made in mobile blood collections.

Regulations limit the volume collected to 500 mL (excluding blood samples) and 13% of the circulating blood volume. This type of donation requires a minimum weight of 50 kg and height of 1.36 metre.

Just before the donation, haemoglobin levels are ascertained by photometric measurement in new donors, donors who have not given blood for at least 2 years, if haemoglobin levels were < 12.5 g/dL in women and < 13.5 g/dL in men at the time of the previous donation or if ordered by the doctor, particularly if he/she considers that there is a possibility of anaemia. If there is no measuring equipment available, donations cannot be made.

The volume, annual frequency and intervals between each type of donation are defined in law. The donation volume is calculated based on the weight, height and sex of the donor. Three standard volumes that meet this requirement, and corpulence in particular, have been defined in prescription charts (Table VI).

Table VI. Chart showing the total volumes to prescribe and plan in whole blood donation.

Estimation of total blood volumes that can be collected in accordance with Gilcher's Rule of Five		Men/Women 136 cm ≤ Height ≤ 144 cm Weight ≥ 50 kg			
		420 mL			
		Women		Men	
		145 cm ≤ Height ≤ 164 cm	Height ≥ 165 cm	145 cm ≤ Height ≤ 164 cm	Height ≥ 165 cm
WEIGHT	50 kg	450 mL	420 mL	480 mL	450 mL
	51 kg				
	52 kg				
	53 kg				
		145 cm ≤ Height ≤ 170 cm	Height ≥ 171 cm	Height ≥ 145 cm	
	54 kg	480 mL	450 mL	480 mL	
	55 kg				
	56 kg				
	≥ 57 kg	Men / Women Height ≥ 145 cm			
		480 mL			

Donations are made in permanent sites and mobile units alike, with or without an appointment. The whole process takes approximately 1 hour. The donation itself takes 5 to 10 minutes on average, the time needed to collect by gravity a sufficient volume of whole blood to prepare an adult unit of leucocyte-depleted packed red blood cells and nearly 300 mL of plasma. The preparation platform can also extract a buffy coat to form a standard pool of platelet concentrates. If the donation period exceeds 12 minutes, it is thought that the slow blood flow may have activated haemostasis and the buffy coat will not be used; after 15 minutes, the plasma will be downgraded to category 2, which cannot be used to prepare coagulation factors.

The **single-use device** is authorized by the ANSM, closed, sterile and apyrogenic. According to current guidelines, it comprises 4 siamese bags and a filter to leucodeplete whole blood or 5 bags, a filter to leucodeplete packed red blood cells and a filter to leucodeplete plasma. The first bag contains 66.5 mL of anticoagulant citrate-phosphate-dextrose (CPD). The volume of saline-adenine-glucose-mannitol (SAGM) is 105 mL. The label placed on the bottom of the bag by the manufacturer marks the location of the "donation barcode number".

The mechanical **agitator** has an automatic shutoff used once the target volume has been reached and, in some cases, a barcode scanner and data capture unit transferring the information collected during the donation to blood management software by radiofrequency. The automated system measures the volume collected, flow rate and time spent at every stage in the donation, whilst constantly agitating the product to mix the blood/anticoagulant.

Donation by aphaeresis

Donations by aphaeresis are made by appointment, solely in permanent sites.

Five types of homologous aphaeresis are regularly practiced in France: plasmapheresis, packed red blood cells/plasma combined aphaeresis, aphaeresis platelet concentrate/packed red blood cells, aphaeresis platelet concentrate/packed red blood cells/plasma, and the donation of granulocytes. The connectable extremities of solutions enabling their use (anticoagulant and NaCl 0.9‰ solution) are secured using a specific male-female system that is different for each solution type. Each type of separator is configured in the same way in all regions. The only anticoagulant is acid-citrate-dextrose-A. All these precautions aim to prevent solution inversion, particularly citrate intoxication.

Clinical and biological selection follows the same guidelines as whole blood, with any additional requirements depending on the type of aphaeresis donation: the volume collected may not exceed 16% of total blood volume or 750 mL in the case of plasmapheresis, and 13% of total blood volume or 650 mL in the case of cell aphaeresis.

A minimum height of 1.50 metre is required, and the EFS tends not to recruit donors who weigh less than 55 kg. The volume collected is calculated in accordance with the donor's sex, weight and height, so as not to exceed 20% of their total blood volume.

Particular attention is paid to previous histories of blackouts, faints or collapse and their contributing factors, particularly cardiovascular risk factors after the age of 60.

Fluids are always provided (500 mL to be drunk during the donation process).

Donors are required to rest for at least 20 minutes after donating.

To ensure their safety, blood protein levels are measured at the time of the first donation and then controlled once annually. When they are below 60 g/L or above 80 g/L, electrophoresis is carried out.

- **Plasmapheresis**

Over time, women are no longer being allowed to make donations that will be used to prepare therapeutic plasma (whose safety is ensured by quarantine, solvent/detergent viral inactivation or amotosalen). This simple measure, which is compatible with supply targets, makes it possible to avoid the anti-HLA or anti-granulocyte antibody, which is synthesized in pregnancy and could cause a TRALI (Transfusion-Related Acute Lung Injury) in the recipient.

The donation requires donors to be available for approximately 1‰ hours, with an average donating time of 60 minutes. The volume is determined by weight, height and gender charts and the type of separator.

- **Combined platelet aphaeresis**

Women can continue to make these donations if they are childless or screen negative for anti-HLA antibodies.

The donation requires donors to be available for approximately 2‰ hours, with an average donating time of 90 minutes. A minimum platelets level of 150 G/L is required to make a donation in order to guarantee a sufficient quantity of active principle.

Leukapheresis is indicated on a case-by-case basis for the specific needs of a patient presenting with an antibiotherapy-resistant infection in the context of severe neutropenia. These donations are subject to specific criteria for the authorization of premises and staff. The selection criteria of prospective donors are defined in law. The donation is made by bi-puncture.

Special cases

Donations of rare blood groups for laboratory use, research or teaching are subject to inclusion and exclusion criteria that are defined in law. For non-therapeutic donations, which all donors are able to make, the doctor provides specific information, detailing if necessary the specific tests that may be conducted. The donor's specific written consent to non-therapeutic use is recorded.

Patients treated with bloodletting for iron overload of genetic or metabolic origin can give blood if they meet the regulatory selection criteria. However, these donations can only be made under special conditions in order to ensure compliance with ethical guidelines, and particularly the absence of secondary benefit. Donations are only authorized if they are made on a permanent ETS site with a health centre in which the patient can be monitored.

Autotransfusion

Also known as autologous transfusion, its practice is falling sharply. It can be made in the form of whole blood donations or erythrapheresis. Protocol indications should now be limited to rare blood groups, whose frequency is less than 4/1,000, or complex poly-immunizations with phenotype compatibility < 4/100,000.

The transport of raw materials and samples

It meets the regulatory requirements governing such transport, from the collection site to the specialized platform. From the collection site to the referral site, transport containers are often managed by the collection team. Donations and sample tubes are packaged at the collection site. From 6 hours after the collection, the sample tubes are stored in containers refrigerated to between +2 °C and +10 °C. They are supplied with transport documents making it possible to check compliance upon reception by the specialized platform. At the referral site, they are transferred to specific storage areas, where they are kept in the temperatures required by law. They may then be repackaged, depending on the temperature-control equipment in the vehicle providing the transfer. The containers, which are of standardized size and shape and either reusable or single-use, are identified in accordance with regulations and adapted to each transport method and product type. When they are not single-use, the containers are cleaned and disinfected in accordance with established procedures. From the referral site to the specialized platform, the containers are managed by authorized carriers.

The close interrelation between collection and distribution services

Distribution services are responsible for providing the LBP patients need to health centres, either by direct issue or through blood banks. These products must be supplied with the immunohaematological characteristics and in the urgent timescales required. Constant communication between the collection services and preparation platforms is necessary to ensure the permanent availability of products with short shelf lives, such as platelet concentrates, without running the risk of an unwarranted appeal for donors, which would lead to the non-use of donated products.

Conclusion

Although subject to the same monitoring as the entire transfusion chain, the "collection" phase is particularly concerned by the regulatory framework surrounding health protection and safety: the epidemiological monitoring of blood donors is underpinned by the information collected during the discovery of a transmissible infection marker whilst all adverse reactions experienced by donors, post-donation information and nonconformities in the process must be reported. Some may even be treated as serious incidents and lead to a 5 M-type causal analysis (Man-Machine-Medium-Mission-Management) to prevent reoccurrence. As a process with significant human involvement, both professionals and donors, the safety of blood collection can only be ensured through the personal commitment of all parties. With its numerous organisational constraints, both internal and external, it is also a process in direct and constant contact with the "outside world": the general public, local elected representatives, the media... and so it shapes public opinion of transfusion medicine professionals.

Key points
1. The main types of donation and regulatory restrictions

REQUIREMENTS PERTAINING TO VARIOUS TYPES OF HOMOLOGOUS DONATIONS

TYPE OF DONATION / Selection criteria	WHOLE BLOOD DONATION	COMBINED APHAERESIS DONATION — PLATELETS–PLASMA	COMBINED APHAERESIS DONATION — PLATELETS–RED CELLS	COMBINED APHAERESIS DONATION — PLATELETS–PLASMA–RED CELLS	SINGLE APHAERESIS DONATION — PLASMA	SINGLE APHAERESIS DONATION — GRANULOCYTES	SINGLE APHAERESIS DONATION — MONONUCLEAR HAEMATOPOIETIC CELLS
Age limit	18–70; first donation after 60 or donation after 65: decided on medical grounds	18–65; first donation after 60 decided on medical grounds	18–65; first donation after 60 decided on medical grounds	18–65; first donation after 60 decided on medical grounds	18–65; first donation after 60 decided on medical grounds	18–50	18–50
Interval between two donations	8 weeks with any other donation of red blood cells; 4 weeks with a donation of platelets/plasma; 2 weeks with a donation of plasma	4 weeks with any other donation of cells; 2 weeks with a donation of plasma	8 weeks with any other donation of red blood cells; 4 weeks with a donation of platelets/plasma; 2 weeks with a donation of plasma	8 weeks with any other donation of red blood cells; 4 weeks with a donation of platelets/plasma; 2 weeks with a donation of plasma	2 weeks with any other type of donation	4 weeks with any other donation of cells	4 weeks with any other donation of cells; 2 weeks with a donation of plasma
Maximum frequency over 12 months	♂ 6 donations / ♀ 4 donations (exemption possible, subject to conditions, if genetic or metabolic iron overload)	♂-♀ 12 donations	♂ 6 donations / ♀ 4 donations	♂ 6 donations / ♀ 4 donations	♂-♀ 24 donations	♂-♀ 2 donations, 4 decided on medical grounds	♂-♀ 1 donation decided on medical grounds
	Total: packed red blood cells from whole blood and/or aphaeresis: ♂ ≤ 6 donations – ♀ ≤ 4 donations; platelet donations ≤ 12 donations; plasma donations ≤ 24 donations. Total all types of donations combined ≤ 24 over 12 rolling months (tolerance of 15 days)						
Volume collected, excluding the sample bag (40 mL) and anticoagulant	≤ 13% of the estimated total blood volume; maximum 500 mL	≤ 13% of the estimated total blood volume; maximum 650 mL	≤ 13% of the estimated total blood volume; maximum 650 mL	≤ 13% of the estimated total blood volume; maximum 650 mL	≤ 16% of the estimated total blood volume; minimum 500 mL maximum 750 mL	≤ 13% of the estimated total blood volume; maximum 650 mL	≤ 13% of the estimated total blood volume; maximum 650 mL
Minimum weight	50 kg	50 kg	50 kg	50 kg	50 kg	50 kg	50 kg
Minimum height	1.36 metre	1.50 metre	1.50 metre	1.50 metre	1.50 metre	1.50 metre	1.50 metre
Haemoglobin level	♂ ≥ 13 g/dL ♀ ≥ 12 g/dL. Must be checked immediately before donating if new donor; last donation > 2 years; last rate ♂ < 13.5 g/dL ♀ < 12.5 g/dL; history or signs of anaemia (clinical, biological)	♂ ≥ 13 g/dL ♀ ≥ 12 g/dL	♂ ≥ 13 g/dL ♀ ≥ 12 g/dL	♂ ≥ 13 g/dL ♀ ≥ 12 g/dL	♂ ≥ 13 g/dL, up to 12 g/dL decided on medical grounds; ♀ ≥ 12 g/dL, up to 11 g/dL decided on medical grounds	♂ ≥ 13 g/dL ♀ ≥ 12 g/dL	♂ ≥ 13 g/dL ♀ ≥ 12 g/dL

Platelet level		≥ **150 x 10⁹/L** exemption for HLA or HPA compatible			
Anti-HLA antibodies		Negative for ♀			
Hemostasis				Platelet, prothrombine and activated cephalin time normal	
Protein level		≥ **60 g/L**			
COLLECTION OF RARE BLOOD					
Indications	Therapeutic emergency requiring tissue compatibility – Donors selected to ensure transfusion coverage in the event of complex immunization or rare phenotype – rare phenotype and requested by the French National Bank of Rare Phenotype Blood (BNSPR)				
Exemptions	Age < 18: prospective donor willing and consent of the parents/guardians Weight < 50 kg, if collection of whole blood: maximum volume ≤ 13% of the estimated total blood volume Timeframe < 4 weeks: donation of HLA-compatible platelets and/or granulocytes Annual frequency ↗: donation of granulocytes 4 instead of 2 Risk of transmissible disease Any other contre-indication on a case-by-case basis except transfusion risk to the donor				
Decision-making	Jointly: physician in charge of the collection and physician responsible for collections in the ETS On assessment of the prospective donor's clinical and biological suitability (safety of donating) If there is a risk of transmissible disease: jointly physician responsible for collections in the ETS, physician responsible for distribution and delivery and, where appropriate, the local BNSPR representative, supplemented by increased post donation biological or clinical monitoring				
NON-THERAPEUTIC COLLECTION					
Indications	Laboratory research – Manufacturing *in vitro* diagnostic medical devices – Conducting tests and medical analysis – Teaching				
Exemptions	Weight < 50 kg, if collection of whole blood: maximum volume ≤ 13% of the estimated total blood volume Contre-indication related to transfusion risk to the recipient; contre-indication with donor risk possible, depending on the volume, type and frequency of collections In the event of positive HIV, HCV, HBsAg marker; collection in accordance with a specific procedure and agreement, scientific purpose or manufacture of reagents (exceptional)				
IRON OVERLOAD OF GENETIC OR METABOLIC ORIGIN					
Indications	Patient requiring blood depletion whose condition is compatible with the selection criteria for whole blood donation laid down in the Order Depletion protocol outlining the monthly frequency, rate, volume, eligibility and initial consent				
Exemptions	Inter-donation interval and annual frequency				
Decision-making	Initial collection of the patient's informed consent for inclusion in the donor process; during the visit to the health centre On the day of the donation, assessment of suitability in view of the selection criteria for blood donors Verification of consistency between the depletions protocol (medical prescription) and the requirements of homologous collections				

PRBCs: packed red blood cells; TBV: total blood volume; BNSPR: French National Bank of Rare Blood Phenotypes; PL: prothrombine level; ACT: activatedcephalin time; ETS: blood establishment.

2. Donation type depending on patient needs: the right product to the right patient

Donor orientation table.				
Donor's blood group		Phenotype	First-line donation (ideal donation)	Alternative
A (45%)	CcDee K-NEG ccdee K-NEG CcDEe K-NEG ccDEe K-NEG CCDee K-NEG	14% 7% 5% 5% 8%	Whole blood	Plateletpheresis
	All others (including K-POS)	6%	Plateletpheresis	Whole blood
O (43%)	CcDee K-NEG ccdee K-NEG CcDEe K-NEG ccDEe K-NEG CCDee K-NEG	13% 6% 5% 5% 8%	Whole blood	Plateletpheresis
	All others (including K-POS)	6%	Plateletpheresis	Whole blood
B (9%)	ccdee K-NEG CCDee K-NEG	1% 2%	Whole blood	Plasmapheresi
	All others	6%	Plasmapheresis	Plateletpheresis
AB (3%)	All	3%	Plasmapheresis	None

6. Preparation

**Patricia Chavarin,
Dominique Dernis,
Catherine Vignoli**

Introduction

History of the activity

It was only with the widespread availability of plastic blood bags in the early 1970s that the preparation of labile blood products (LBP) was able to develop fully.

The "preparation" phase covers all the steps involved in obtaining LBP from the raw or processed materials that are blood and blood components, including primary and secondary preparation, labelling, storage and quality control. The preparation, packaging and release of plasma for fractionation [French Fractionation Laboratory (LFB)] are also included in this process, as is supplying LBP to distribution sites.

Division of the activity across France

Currently there are 14 blood establishments (ETS) in mainland France and 3 in overseas *départements*, each with its own specialized platform preparing LBP. The target of one platform per ETS is still active. Therefore, the logistics of transporting blood products – bringing raw materials to the preparation platform and taking end products to various sites – continue to develop.

In total the preparation platforms represent near 500 full-time equivalents, which are organized to process over 3,200,000 donations every year.

The design of the preparation services must meet regulatory requirements, organizing the activity into logical flows, with no reverse movements or mixing of the bags. The same blood management software is used by all the ETS to ensure the traceability of each operation.

Mapping of the process

The "preparation" phase is the link in the transfusion chain that, along with the "testing" phase, starts with

Patricia Chavarin, patricia.chavarin@efs.sante.fr,
Dominique Dernis, dominique.dernis@efs.sante.fr,
Catherine Vignoli, catherine.vignoli@efs.sante.fr

the receipt of raw material from the "collection" phase and ends with the availability of end products, LBP, for the "distribution/issue" phase.

All these steps form part of the macro-process "provision of LBP".

Upstream: the "collection" link

This involves collecting blood and blood components. Donations are collected using sterile, closed, single-use devices (SUDs). The SUDs meet strict specifications and result from calls for tender, pursuant to the regulations of the French Public Procurement Code.

Tubes for the donation testing laboratory and sample bank are taken at the same time.

At this stage, the bags and tubes are identified using a unique donation number, in the form of a barcode, which was generated by the collection. A red line on the tubes for testing marks products that require urgent results.

Downstream: the "distribution/issue" link

This involves the receipt, storage and sharing out of end products pending their issue to transfusion sites, other ETS or even the hospital blood banks.

Medico-technical description of "preparation" services

The various operations

• **Leucodepleting the products**

The raw materials are received, recorded, weighed, centrifuged and separated. Leucocytes are also removed from the products during the preparation phase.

• **Quarantining processed products**

Processed products are quarantined pending the results of the donation testing laboratory. Their labelling is then used to move them to the next stage, depending on their compliance:
– compliant products: storage and availability for the "distribution/issue" phase;
– noncompliant products: destruction or if possible, depending on the reason for noncompliance, reassignment to non-therapeutic use.

• **Destroying noncompliant products**

As well as positive results identified by the donation testing laboratory, there are other reasons why LBP may be noncompliant: unacceptable leucodepletion, breakdown in the sterile transfer system, plasma contaminated with red blood cells, etc. These products will be destroyed. The nonconformities are recorded, graded and used to produce indicators measuring the effectiveness of preventive and corrective action.

Source and use of the various types of raw material

• **The collection of whole blood**

Whole blood is no longer used without a preparation stage. It must be leucocyte-depleted, centrifuged and separated to obtain transfusable end products: packed red blood cells (PRBCs), plasma and platelet concentrate (PC).

Whole blood is transported to the preparation site:
– if it is prepared within 24 hours, it will be transported between +18 °C and +24 °C;
– if it is prepared between 24 hours and 72 hours, it should be transported between +2 °C and +10 °C;
– after 72 hours, it can no longer be separated.

• **Collection by aphaeresis**

This type of collection provides semi-finished products directly: erythrapheresis (red blood cells), plasmapheresis (plasma), cytapheresis (platelets or granulocytes) or the combination of several products through combined aphaeresis. Leucocytes are removed during the donation process or later in the preparation phase.

There are 2 separate physical flows and timescales: one for homologous blood donation and another for autologous blood donation.

Selecting the device

• **Selection criteria**

Several single-use devices (SUDs) can be used to collect whole blood. They are all sterile, closed and provided with filters removing leucocytes from LBP. Selecting the devices through calls for tender has reduced variation within the French Blood Establishment (EFS).

The device is chosen in accordance with the LBP required:
– SUDs with an integrated filter for whole blood: preparing PRBCs and plasma. As the whole blood filter removes platelets, they cannot be obtained (Figure 9);
– SUDs with integrated filters for PRBCs and plasma: preparing PRBCs, plasma and buffy coats (Figure 10).

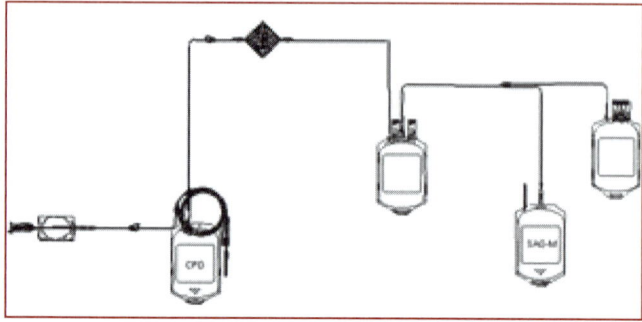

Figure 9. Integrated filtration of whole blood.

6. Preparation

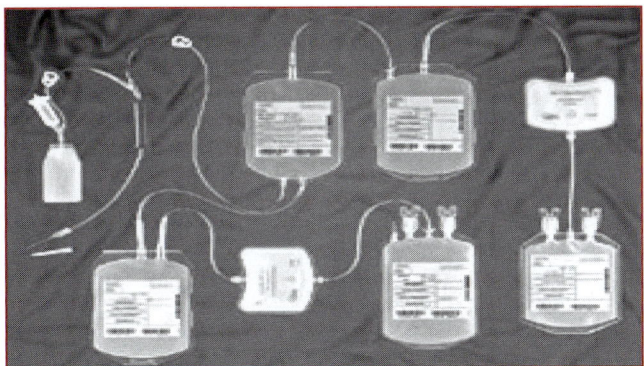

Figure 10. Integrated filtration of packed red blood cells and plasma.
© EFS.

Receiving the raw material

Upon receiving the raw material, it is essential to make the following checks:

- **Conformity of the transport**
  - Verification that the number of packages actually received is consistent with the number expected (transport documents)
  - Conformity of the transport temperatures, in view of good transport practice

- **Control of the specifications**

This control involves checking the appearance of the product (colour, volume, etc.), the identification number (consistent, not duplicated, etc.) and the condition of the SUDs (intact, no leaks), etc.

The unique identification number and batch number of the collection device are entered into the blood management software to record each donation.

All products are weighed and the volumes that are unsuitable for LBP, *i.e.* too much or too little, are removed.

By regulations, the type and number of donated products must be checked against the type and number of products received.

Leucodepletion

- **Principle**

Filtering removes most of the leucocytes found in a blood product. It is mandatory in France for all LBP, except autologous LBP.

- **Benefits**

Leucodepletion aims to:
- reduce the risk of transmitting intraleukocytic pathogens: viruses (CMV, EBV, HTLV), bacteria (*Yersinia enterocolitica*) and possibly prions;
- prevent anti-HLA immunization, which has been associated with chills/hyperthermia-type reactions.

For whole blood, there are 2 possibilities:
- either the donation was collected using an SUD with a whole blood filter, in which case leucocytes will already have been removed from all LBP resulting from the separation of the filtered whole blood;
- or the donation was collected using an SUD with PRBC and plasma filters, in which case leucocytes will be removed from each LBP in the separation stage.

Sealing

The tubing of the SUDs is sealed at several stages in the process to separate the 2 compartments of the device. The regulation requires systematic checks of the airtightness of seals to ensure that there is no breakdown in the sterile system.

Centrifugation

- **Folding the devices**

This operation makes it possible to separate the various cells and plasma depending on their respective density. The devices must first be folded in exactly the right place (Figure 11).

- **Weighing and placing in centrifuge cups**

The folded devices are then placed in centrifuge cups, with equal weight in opposing cups (Figures 12 and 13). The centrifugation programme is tailored to each device and confirmed (acceleration, maximum speed, temperature, duration, braking, etc.). This ensures optimal and reproducible separation of the various blood components (Figures 14 and 15).

Separation

The cups are carefully removed from the centrifuge to prevent any resuspension of the cells in the plasma and to maintain a clear separation between the various phases.

A blood separation machine uses pressure to direct the various blood components to their respective transfer bag (Figure 16).

Labelling

- **Affixing the label**

The bag of LBP can be permanently labelled as soon as the donation testing is complete and the results have been transferred to the blood management software.

The label is affixed manually. Checking the donation label placed at the time of the collection against the label affixed by the preparation technician ensures the safety of this critical stage (Figure 17).

Transfusion medicine: the French model

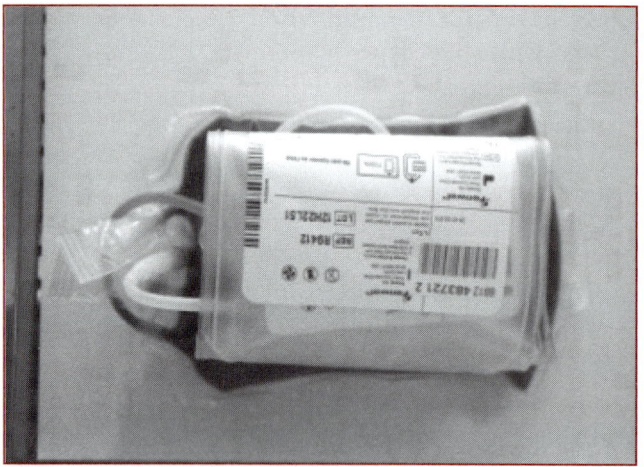

Figure 11. Folding.
© EFS.

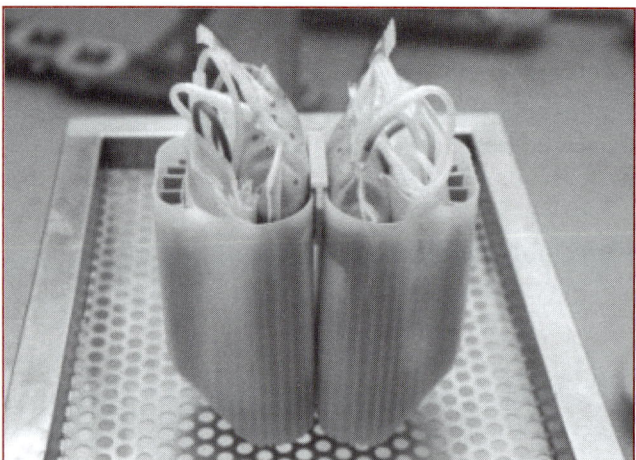

Figure 12. Placing in centrifuge cups.
© EFS.

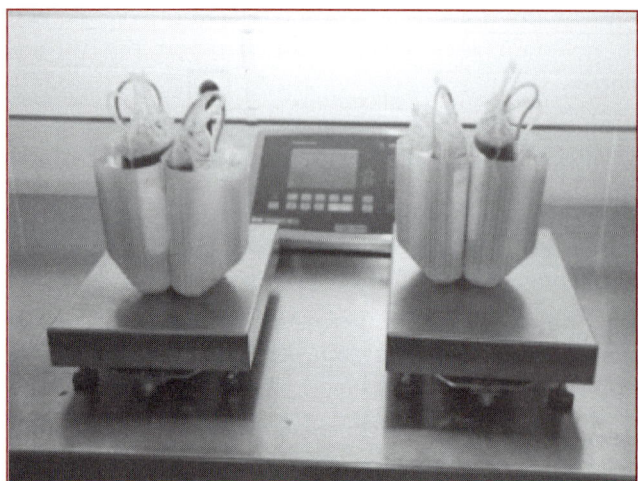

Figure 13. Balancing.
© EFS.

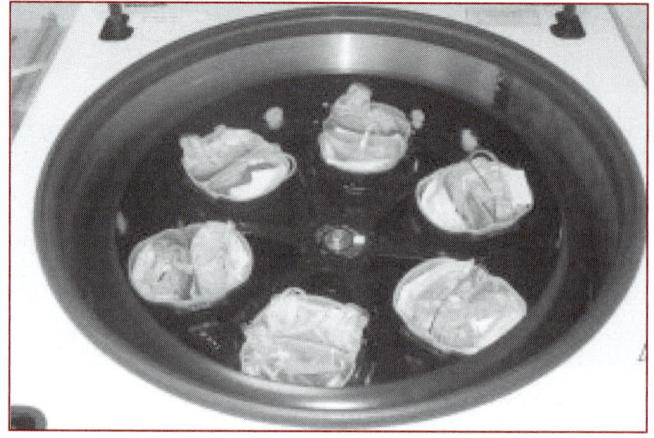

Figure 14. Centrifugation.
© EFS.

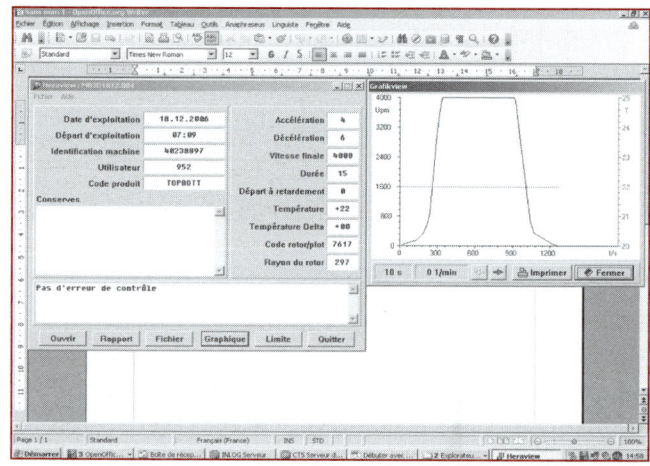

Figure 15. Centrifugation programme.

- **Mandatory information**

The label must show clear and legible information on the LBP: type of product, volume in mL, amount of active principle, ABO Rhesus Kell blood groups, expiry date and time, storage temperature, details of the establishment that prepared it, etc.

The blood groups, product code and donation number are shown alphanumerically and as barcodes. The format of the label was harmonized at national level on 31 December 2011.

- **Storing compliant products**

The storage containers are tailored to the requirements of each LBP. This vitally important equipment must be monitored at all times and fitted with high and low temperature alarms. A centralized temperature management system provides this round-the-clock monitoring and ensures that noncompliant temperatures are addressed quickly, thereby ensuring the safety and traceability of the storage conditions of stored products.

6. Preparation

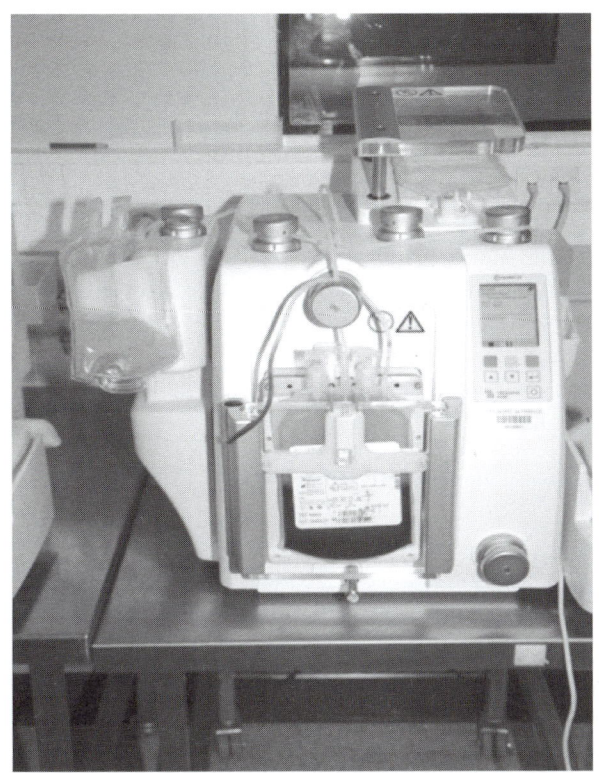
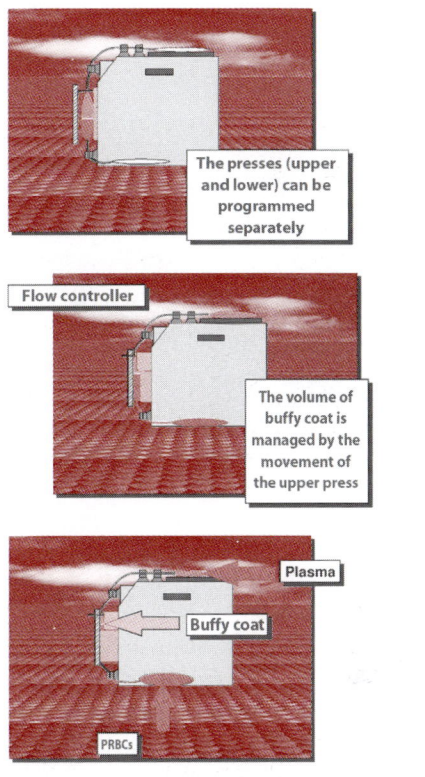

Figure 16. Separation machine.
PRBCs: packed red blood cells; BC: buffy coat.
© EFS.

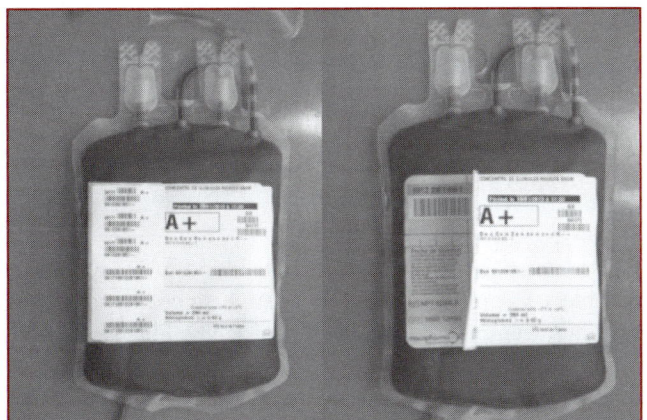

Figure 17. Labelling a compliant product.
© EFS.

• **Destroying noncompliant products**

Depending on the reason for noncompliance, noncompliant products are removed from the computer system and physically placed in containers for incineration. All the stages involved in product destruction are recorded, including confirmation of incineration.

Pathogen reduction

Pathogen reduction techniques are used to reduce the risk of transfusing any agents that may be found in the donation. Currently, this only applies to platelet concentrate and therapeutic plasma. The techniques for use with red blood cells are still in the experimental stage.

The preparation of packed red blood cells
Homologous PRBCs from whole blood

• **Product types**

There are 2 types of products:
– adult unit of leucocyte-depleted PRBCs;
– infant's unit of leucocyte-depleted PRBCs (depending on the haemoglobin content).

• **Preparation constraints**

Leucodepleting whole blood is difficult and requires control over various parameters, such as:
– the time between collection and filtration: filtration within 2 to 3 hours enables the phagocytosis of any microorganisms by macrophages. After this time, the earlier the filtration, the more effective it will be, ideally within 24 hours;
– the temperature of the whole blood: must be approved for the process at the time of leucodepletion;
– the filtration rate: the higher the filtration, the quicker the flow in the filter, reducing effectiveness (Figure 18).

Transfusion medicine: the French model

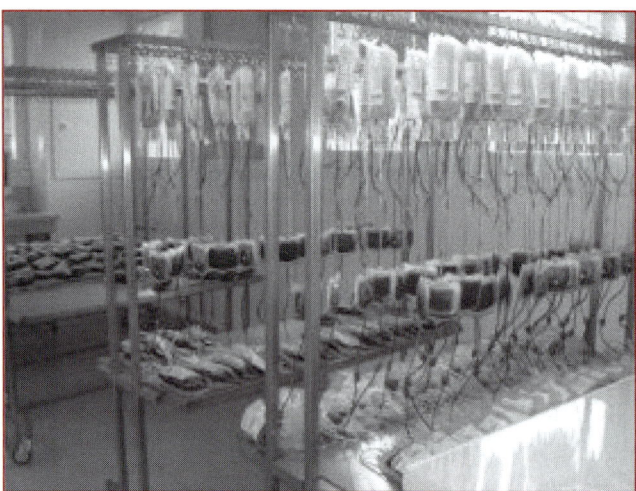

Figure 18. Leucodepletion of whole blood by gravity.
© EFS.

Leucocytes are removed from the PRBCs immediately after the separation stage.

All aspects of leucodepletion must first be defined and approved, addressing the critical points and limitations. This predetermined process makes it possible to obtain compliant and reproducible leucodepletion results.

- **Separation**

At the end of the separation stage, a preservative solution is added to the PRBCs, which extends the lifespan of red blood cells from 21 to 42 days (SAGM solution).

- **Regulatory characteristics of PRBCs**

Leucodepleted PRBCs have the following characteristics:

Appearance	Dark red liquid
Volume	A minimum volume is no longer specified
Haemoglobin	Adult unit: at least 40 g Infant's unit: at least 22 g
Haematocrit	Between 50% and 70%
Residual leucocytes	Less than 1×10^6 per unit
Storage conditions	Between +2 °C and +6 °C for 42 days

- **Post-labelling ABO check**

The ABO blood group shown on the product label is checked against the ABO blood group of the red blood cells in the bag for the final time. However, this safety measure is not regulatory required.

Homologous PRBCs from aphaeresis: erythrapheresis

Leucocytes are removed from the donated product in the preparation phase before it rejoins the same process as PRBCs from whole blood.

- **Regulatory characteristics**

These are the same as for PRBCs from whole blood.

Autologous PRBCs

- **Checking the information**

It is essential to check that information on the recipient, which is shown on the form accompanying the bag, is consistent with that on the product label (Figure 19).

The blood group is not shown on the product label alphanumerically but as a barcode, preventing its use by another patient.

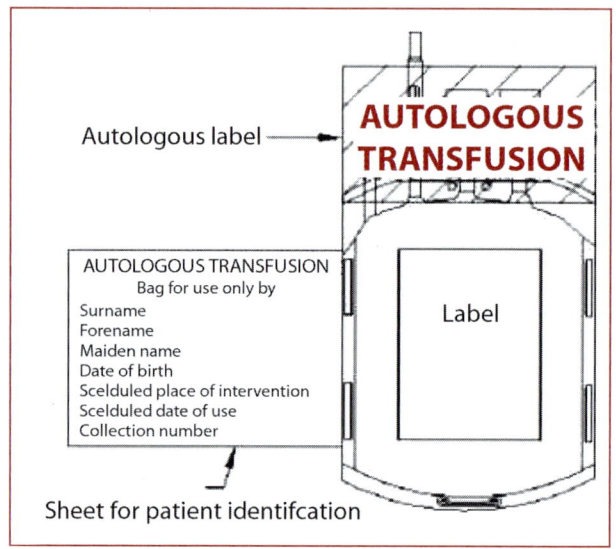

Figure 19. Checking the product label.

Pathogen reduction

This addition to preparation remains in the research-development phase for PRBCs.

The preparation of platelet concentrates

- **Mandatory leucodepletion**

PCs are prepared either from whole blood or by aphaeresis (simple or combined cytapheresis). Leucodepleting these LBP has been mandatory since April 1998. The use of combined aphaeresis in additive solution makes it possible to obtain a reasonable volume of plasma (300 to 550 mL) and PCs whose plasma protein content is reduced by two-thirds.

- **Mandatory rest phase**

Platelets are sensitive cells that react to impact and turbulence during the preparation phase. The preparation methods must prevent all unwanted changes and irreversible platelet activation. A rest phase without agitation after each stage can lessen this phenomenon.

PCs from whole blood

- **Product types**

There are 2 products:
- platelet concentrate, leucocyte depleted (PC-LD) for paediatric use;

6. Preparation

- pooled platelet concentrates, leucocyte depleted (P-PC-LD), which require several donors with the same ABO blood group, generally 5.

• **Preparation constraints**
- The donor must not have taken platelet antiaggregant or show signs of acute allergy.
- The bleed time must not exceed 12 minutes.
- The venipuncture must be clean to limit platelet and coagulation factor activation.
- The donations must be collected using a device suitable for platelet production, which rules out SUDs with integrated whole blood filters as these remove platelets.
- The volume collected must be sufficient to obtain a usable buffy coat.
- The whole blood must have been stored at room temperature and ideally left to rest for 10 to 15 hours.

• **Processing methods**

Two processing methods can be used, requiring 2 different collection devices:

- platelet-rich plasma method: seldom used;
- buffy coat method.

The latter technique requires two stages: centrifugation and separation. The first stage makes it possible to obtain 3 products: PRBCs, plasma and buffy coat.

Several compliant buffy coats from an identical ABO blood group are pooled, possibly with additive solution, using an appropriate device with a leucodepletion filter (method currently used by all preparation platforms).

• **The second centrifugation/separation stage**

This stage is particularly difficult. It makes it possible to extract P-PC-LD directly from the pool.

• **The semi-automated process for preparing P-PC-LD**

Using the pool of buffy coats, a machine combining the principles of a centrifuge and separator makes it possible to obtain blood platelets. The leucocytes are removed by in-line filtration during drainage into the final bag (Figure 20).

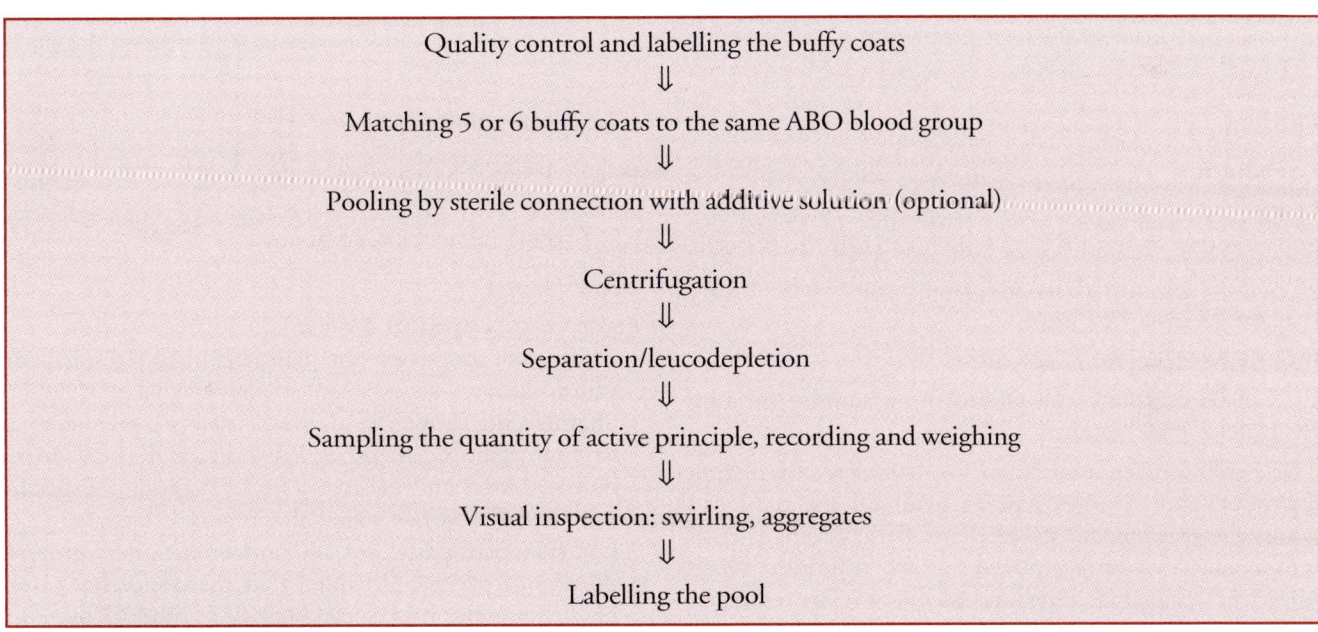

Quality control and labelling the buffy coats
⇓
Matching 5 or 6 buffy coats to the same ABO blood group
⇓
Pooling by sterile connection with additive solution (optional)
⇓
Centrifugation
⇓
Separation/leucodepletion
⇓
Sampling the quantity of active principle, recording and weighing
⇓
Visual inspection: swirling, aggregates
⇓
Labelling the pool

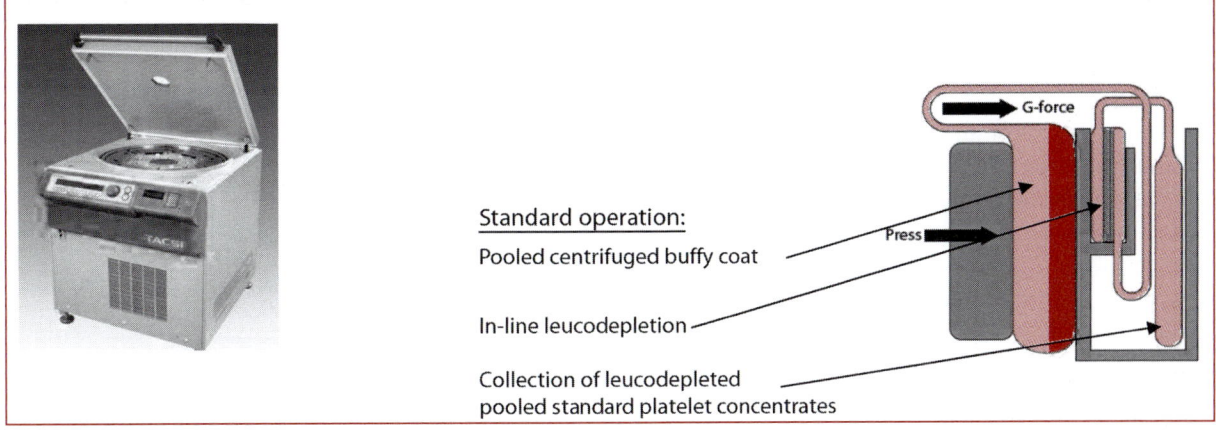

Standard operation:
Pooled centrifuged buffy coat
In-line leucodepletion
Collection of leucodepleted pooled standard platelet concentrates

Figure 20. P-SD-PC preparation machine.

PC from aphaeresis

The PC, which is from one donor, can generally be used to collect sufficient platelets for the recipient.

Regulatory characteristics

Depending on the type of aphaeresis separator, leucocytes are removed from the platelets either at the time of collection or by filtration on the preparation platform.

	SD-PC	P-SD-PC	APC	AI-PC
Appearance	Moiré pattern liquid with no signs of haemolysis			
Volume	≥ 40 mL	80 to 600 mL	< 600 mL*	P-SD-PC: 160 to 600 mL APC: < 600 mL
Minimum platelet count	0.375×10^{11}	1×10^{11}	2×10^{11}	P-SD-PC: 2.2 to 6×10^{11} APC: 2.2 to 6×10^{11}
Residual leucocytes	$< 1 \times 10^{6}$/unit	$< 1 \times 10^{6}$/unit		
Storage conditions	+20 °C to +24 °C in temperature-controlled containers 5 days, with slow and continuous agitation			
pH (at +22 °C)	≥ 6.4			
Residual amotosalen	-	-	-	≤ 2 µM

* No minimum volume, if content $< 2 \times 10^{11}$, the quantity/volume ratio must be approximately 1.2×10^{9} platelets/cm^3.
SD-PC: standard platelet concentrate; P-SD-PC: pooled standard platelet concentrates; APC: aphaeresis platelet concentrate; AI-PC: amotosalen-virus attenuation platelet concentrate.

Swirling

If we cause the platelets to move in a bag, we can see the shimmering swirls caused by the discoid shape. A qualitative and visual score makes it possible to record this phenomenon. A high score indicates usable PC with a good transfusion yield. In contrast, a negative score means that the PC will be destroyed.

Additive solution for preservation

PC can be prepared with plasma or an additive solution for platelet preservation.

These solutions contain citrate to neutralize coagulation activation and a buffer base to maintain the right pH whilst the platelets are stored. Part of the plasma is then removed (65%) and replaced by the solution, which improves recipients' tolerance to the PC by reducing chills/hyperthermia-type reactions.

Pathogen reduction

• **Technique**

Platelets from whole blood or aphaeresis, in preservative solution, are mixed with an amotosalen solution derived from psoralens, which will separate and bind to the nucleic acids of pathogens that may be found in the bag. The mix is exposed to UV light.

The treated products are then agitated with an adsorption device to reduce the amount of amotosalen (free and photoproducts).

• **Benefit**

This process is effective against viruses (enveloped and naked), bacteria and parasites.

The preparation of plasma

Plasma is prepared from whole blood or single/combined aphaeresis. This LBP has been leucocyte-depleted since April 1998.

Use of plasma

Plasma can be used in 3 ways:
– therapeutic use, where the plasma is intended solely for transfusion;
– pharmaceutical use: the plasma is used as a raw material to manufacture medicinal products derived from human blood and plasma. The LFB produces specifications defining raw material acceptance criteria;
– non-therapeutic use: not all "nonconformities" prevent the use of plasma. Provided that the donor has given his/her consent, plasma can be used to produce reagents that are extremely useful in transfusion and science.

Freezing technique

Irrespective of its use, prepared plasma must be deep-frozen as quickly as possible to preserve the labile coagulation factors.

There are 2 categories of plasma, depending on the time between collection and freezing:
– category 1: freezing within 24 hours after collection;
– category 2: freezing between 24 hours and 72 hours after collection.

Because of the way in which category 1 plasma is obtained, the activity of labile proteins is better maintained, which is why only this category of plasma is eligible for the purification of coagulation factors.

Category 2 plasma is primarily used in the production of immunoglobulin and albumin.

However, plasma can be downgraded to category 2 for reasons other than time of freezing:
– the time taken to collect the whole blood exceeds 15 minutes;
– the volume of plasma from whole blood is between 150 mL and 200 mL;
– the presence of clots in the whole blood or PRBCs.

To ensure that the plasma is frozen uniformly and its quality is not impaired, the temperature must be reduced quickly, to at least -30 °C. For category 1, at least 0.7 IU/mL of factor VIII is required.

Plasma for fractionation

• **Definition**

Leucodepleted fresh frozen plasma from whole blood or aphaeresis.

• **Technique**

The production stages are shown in Figure 21.

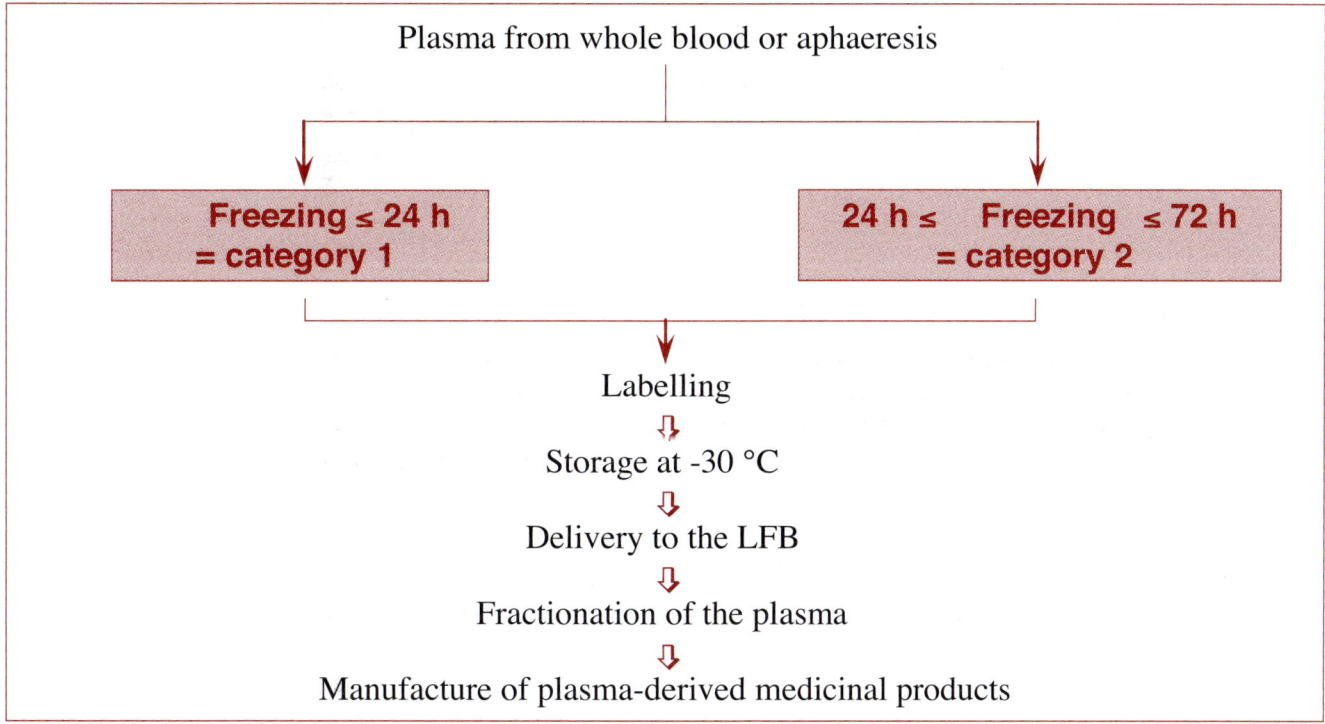

Figure 21. The stages in preparing plasma for fractionations.
LFB: French Fractionation Laboratory.

• **Benefit**

This plasma is used as a raw material to obtain the stable blood products that are medicinal products derived from human blood and plasma: albumin, immunoglobulins and coagulation factors. It is fractionated on an industrial scale by the LFB, which separates the various constitutive proteins using highly effective purification and safety assurance techniques (fractionated precipitation, chromatography, nanofiltration, inactivation, etc.). The presence of antitetanic antibodies and high-titre anti-HBs makes it possible to select hyperimmune plasma for the production of specific immunoglobulins by the LFB.

Therapeutic plasma

The safety of manufactured plasma is increased before it is made available for therapeutic use:
– quarantine plasma: quarantined prior to release;
– solvent/detergent-treated plasma: physicochemical treatment;
– amotosalen-treated plasma: treatment by a photo-reactive agent;
– "linked" plasma: transfusion of plasma with red cells from the same donor.

- **Quarantine plasma**

- *Definition*

Aphaeresis plasma is quarantined for at least 60 days. It is released from quarantine if a further donation by the same donor is found to be compliant.

- *Technique*

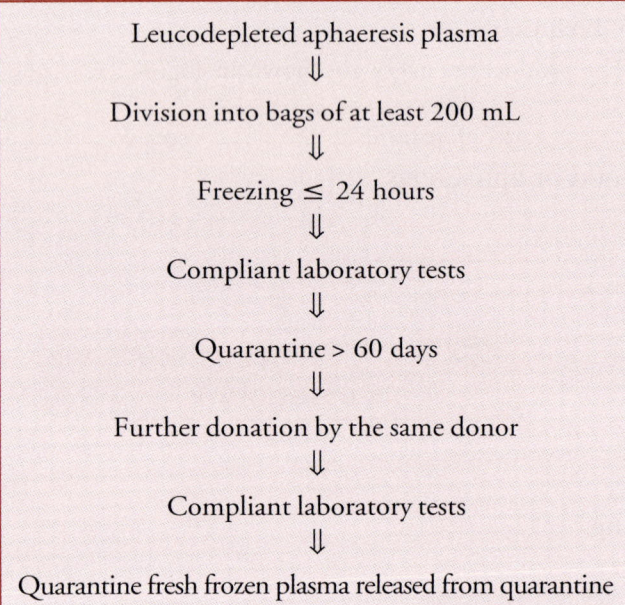

- *Benefit*

Quarantine covers the window period preceding the seroconversion of certain infectious diseases (HIV and hepatises B or C in particular). The safety assurance provided by quarantining only applies to the pathogens sought in donation testing.

NB: the widespread availability of nucleic acid testing (NAT) for HIV, HBV and HCV has made it possible to reduce the quarantine period from 120 to 60 days.

- **Solvent/detergent-treated plasma**

- *Definition*

Plasma prepared from a pool of 100 aphaeresis plasma donations, which undergoes a chemical pathogen reduction process.

The raw plasma material is provided by the EFS in accordance with the specifications defined by the pathogen reduction unity of EFS Aquitaine-Limousin (Bordeaux site).

- *Technique*

Use of solvent and detergent combined with heat.

- *Benefit*

The process destroys enveloped viruses that may be present.

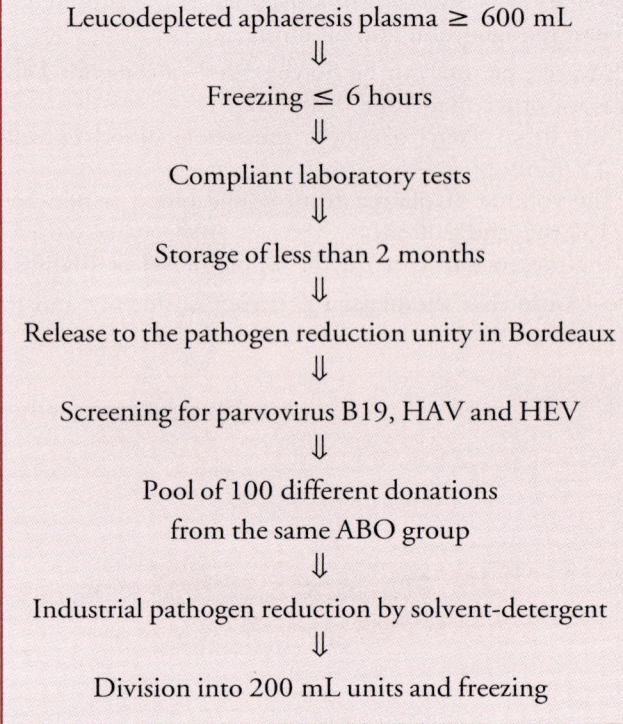

HAV: hepatitis A virus; HEV: hepatitis E virus.

- **Amotosalen-treated plasma**

- *Definition*

Aphaeresis plasma is pathogen reduced by the addition of amotosalen (when used with UV light, this photoreactive compound blocks the replication of pathogens found in the LBP).

- *Technique*

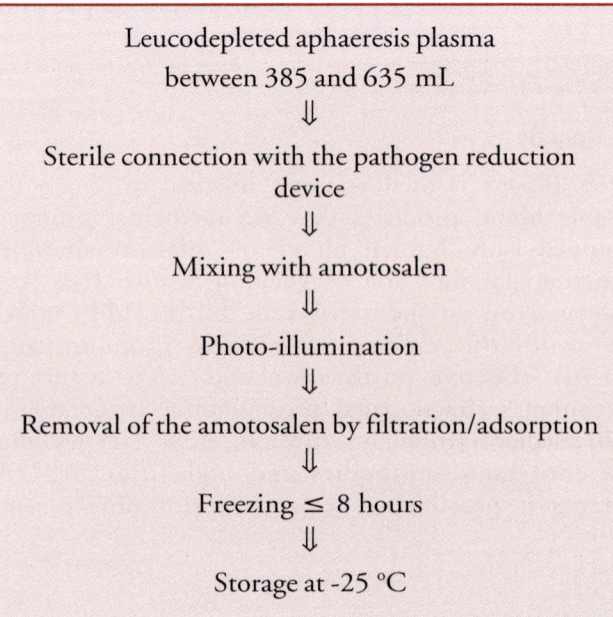

6. Preparation

- *Benefits*
- This process is effective against viruses (enveloped and naked), bacteria and parasites.
- The preparation technique makes it a "single-donor" product.

- **"Linked" plasma**
- *Definition*

Plasma obtained from a unit of whole blood and intended for the recipient of the PRBCs from the same donation.

- *Technique*

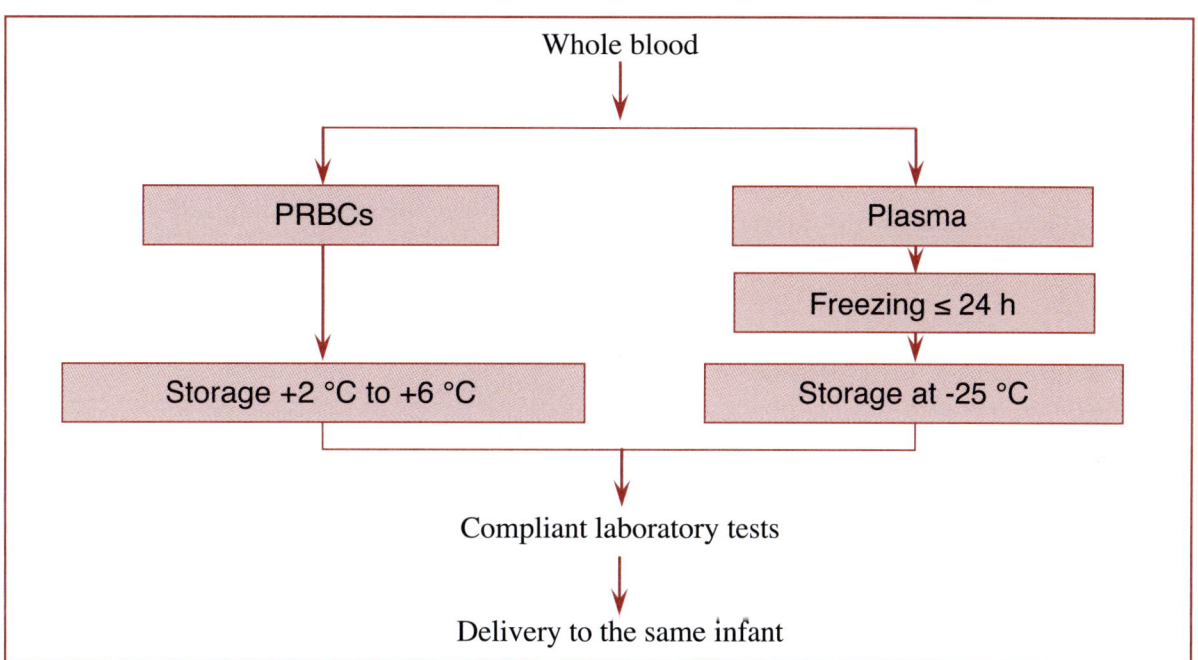

PRBCs: packed red blood cells.

- *Benefit*

Reduces the donor transfusion risk by providing plasma and PRBCs from the same donation to the same infant.

- *Regulatory characteristics*

	Plasma for fractionation	Therapeutic plasma		
		SD-FFP	AI-FFP	Q-FFP
Appearance	Clear to slightly cloudy liquid with no visible signs of haemolysis			
Volume	150 to 875 mL	Over 200 mL		
Factor VIII levels	0.7 IU/mL	0.5 IU/mL	0.5 IU/mL	0.7 IU/mL
Fibrinogen g/L	-	≥ 2 g/L	≥ 2 g/L	-
Proteins	50 g/L	-	-	-
Residual red blood cells	-	≤ 6 × 10^9/L		
Residual platelets	-	≤ 25 × 10^9/L		
Residual leucocytes	≤ 1 × 10^6/L	≤ 1 × 10^4/L		
Storage conditions	≤ -30 °C for one year	≤ -25 °C for one year from the preparation date	≤ -25 °C for one year	
Residual amotosalen	-	-	≤ 2 µM	-

SD-FFP: fresh frozen plasma pathogen reduced by solvent/detergent; AI-FFP: fresh frozen plasma pathogen reduced with amotosalen; Q-FFP: quarantine fresh frozen plasma
NB: there is a lyophilized presentation in the "therapeutic plasma" category. The pooling of plasma formed by groups A, B and AB and free from anti-A and anti-B immune antibodies confers universal status. The plasma is first quarantined or pathogen reduced with amotosalen. It is prepared by the French Armed Forces Blood Transfusion Centre (CTSA) and specifically authorized.

The preparation of granulocyte concentrates by aphaeresis

This LBP is seldom prepared, except in emergencies. It requires corticosteroid premedication of the donor, which increases the concentration of cells of the granulocytic series in the blood (mobilization of the marginal pool).

Manufacturing constraints

- The medical questionnaire must confirm that there are no contraindications to corticosteroid therapy (infections, ulcers, etc.) and obtain the donor's informed consent to the injection of corticosteroids.
- The laboratory tests must allow the donation: coagulation workup (prothrombine time, activated cephalin time) and complete blood count.

Technique

- There is little involvement by the preparation service.

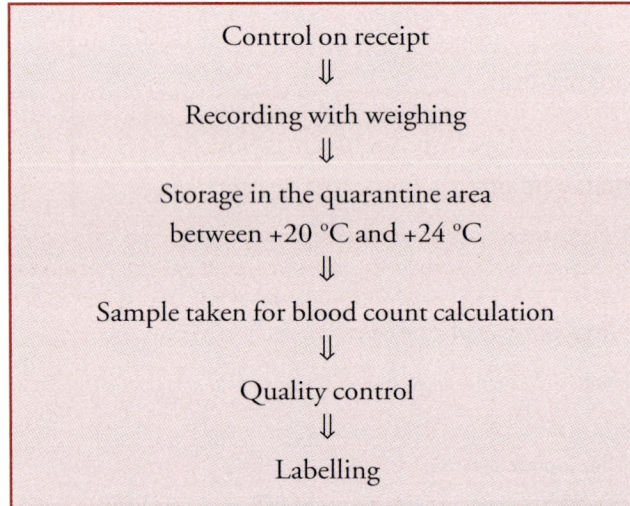

Regulatory characteristics

Appearance	Suspension with no signs of haemolysis
Volume	≤ 650 mL
Granulocytes count	> 2×10^{10}
Storage conditions	+20 °C to +24 °C for 12 hours. If the closed system is intentionally opened: +20 °C to +24 °C for 6 hours

Additional processing of labile blood products

Paediatric preparation

- *Definition:* involves dividing LBP for therapeutic use into several units aseptically by sterile connection.
- *Scope:* PRBCs, APC, quarantine plasma, granulocyte concentrates by aphaeresis (GCA).
- *Technique:* the LBP is divided, in a closed system, by sterile connection.
- *Regulatory characteristics*

Volume	More than or equal to 50 mL
Shelf life	Identical to the initial product

- *Benefit:* provides several units from the same donation to reduce the number of donors involved in repeated transfusions in children.

Plasma removal

- *Definition:* involves removing aseptically most of the plasma from a homologous cellular LBP for therapeutic use.
- *Scope:* PRBCs, PC and GCA.
- *Technique:* comprises one or more washing stages, either manual by centrifugation or automatic with a cell washer, with resuspension of the cell elements in an injectable solution (*e.g.* sodium chloride).
- *Regulatory characteristics*

Product	Haematocrit	Quantity of active principle	Shelf life	Total residual plasma proteins
PRBCs (in a closed system with additive solution)	40 to 70%	≥ 35 g	10 days	≤ 0.5 g
PRBCs (without additive solution)	50 to 80%	≥ 35 g	24 hours	≤ 0.5 g
GCA	-	≥ 80% initial quantity	6 hours	≤ 0.5 g
APC	-	≥ 1.5×10^{11} per unit	6 hours	≤ 0.5 g
SD-PC	-	≥ 0.375×10^{11} per unit	6 hours	≤ 0.5 g
P-SD-PC	-	≥ 1.25×10^{11}/mL	6 hours	≤ 0.5 g

PRBCs: packed red blood cells; GCA: granulocyte concentrates by aphaeresis; APC: aphaeresis platelet concentrate; SD-PC: standard platelet concentrate; P-SD-PC: pooled standard platelet concentrates.

6. Preparation

- *Benefit:* removes the maximum amount of plasma proteins (found in plasma) in the event of intolerance or history of post-transfusion purpura.

Volume reduction

- *Definition:* involves removing aseptically part of the suspension medium of a cellular LBP for therapeutic use.
- *Scope:* PRBCs, PC and GCA.
- *Technique:* after centrifugation, resuspension in a limited quantity of plasma, depending on the recipient.
- *Regulatory characteristics*

Quantity of active principle	PRBCs	Haematocrit ≥ 70%
	PC and GCA	Platelet and granulocyte count ≥ 80% of the initial product
Shelf life	PRBCs	24 hours
	PC and GCA	6 hours

PRBCs: packed red blood cells; PC: platelet concentrate; GCA: granulocyte concentrates by aphaeresis.

- *Benefit:* reduces the LBP's volume in the event of restricted volume intake for resuscitation reasons.

Cryopreservation

- *Definition:* involves freezing, storing and thawing aseptically a cellular LBP for direct therapeutic use with a cryoprotectant.
- *Scope:* phenotyped APC, phenotyped PRBCs
- *Technique:* the cryoprotectant added before freezing (glycerol or dimethylsulfoxide) is removed by washing after thawing.
- *Regulatory characteristics*

Quantity of active principle	PRBCs	Haematocrit: 50–80% without the addition of preservative solution 40–70% with the addition of preservative solution Haemoglobin ≥ 35 g Haemolysis level ≤ 1.2% of the cell volumes
	APC	Minimum platelets count after thawing ≥ 2×10^{11}
Residual cryoprotectant	PRBCs	Residual glycerol ≤ 1 g
Shelf life (frozen)	PRBCs	Below -60 °C: over 10 years Between -30 °C and -60 °C: 4 months
	APC	Below -130 °C: 3 years Between -60 °C and -85 °C: 2 years
Shelf life (thawed)	PRBCs	24 hours, 7 days if automated machine + preservative solution
	APC	6 hours

NB: the APC must be frozen within 24 hours of the collection.

- *Benefit:* makes it possible to build stocks of rare LBP.

Irradiation

- *Definition:* involves exposing a cellular LBP for therapeutic use to a source of ionizing radiation. The dose received by the LBP, which can be measured at every point in the irradiation area, must be between 25 and 45 gray.
- *Scope:* PRBCs, PC and GCA.
- *Technique:* using an irradiator, attaching an irradiation indicator to the bag and maintaining an irradiation register.
- *Regulatory characteristics*

Shelf life	PRBCs of less than 15 days	Adult unit: unchanged Infant's unit: 28 days
	PRBCs of more than 15 days	24 hours
	PC or GCA	Unchanged

- *Benefit:* inactivates the T lymphocytes transfused and associated with the graft-versus-host (GVH) reaction.

Reconstituted blood for paediatric use

- *Definition:* involves mixing aseptically PRBCs with thawed fresh single-donor plasma, thawed pathogen reduced or quarantined plasma, or physiological albumin solution, depending on the clinical indication.
- *Scope:* PRBCs.
- *Technique:* in an authorized, closed, sterile and apyrogenic recipient.
- *Regulatory characteristics*

Haematocrit	Between 35% and 50%
Shelf life	6 hours
Irregular antibodies	None

- *Benefit:* exchange transfusion or extracorporeal life support in newborns.

Additional qualifications of labile blood products

These tests supplement donation testing.

Phenotyping

- *Definition:* applies to cellular LBP for which one or more antigens of blood group systems have been determined in addition to the ABO-RH1 KEL1 groups.

PRBCs	Systematic determination of the RH-KEL1 phenotype. Phenotype extended: if other red cell antigens (Duffy, Kidd, MNS, etc.)
PC	Class I HLA antigens or HPA-specific platelets
GCA	Class I HLA antigens or specific granular systems

- *Regulatory characteristics:* details of each antigen determined followed by the result are stated on the LBP's label.
- *Benefit:* greater understanding of the LBP's blood group systems, enabling appropriate transfusion to recipients and preventing immunization.

Cross-matching

- *Definition:* applies to homologous cellular LBP for direct therapeutic use and their processed products for which the recipient's serum has been cross-matched against the donor's blood. The LBP can only be referred to as cross-matched if the product is fully compatible.
- *Regulatory characteristics:* "cross-matched on [date]", identity of the recipient, identity of the laboratory and test validity period, if shorter than the product life-span, are stated on the LBP's label.
- *Benefit:* compatibility between the LBP to be transfused and the recipient.

CMV negative

- *Definition:* applies to cellular LBP for direct therapeutic use and their processed products whose donor tested negative for anti-cytomegalovirus antibodies (CMV) at the time of the donation.
- *Regulatory characteristics:* "CMV negative" to be stated on the LBP's label.
- *Benefit:* avoids introducing CMV to a weakened, CMV-negative recipient (bone marrow allograft, pre-term birth, lung transplant, etc.).

Conclusion and development prospects

Current activity volumes in mainland France vary, according to the ETS, between 140,000 and over 350,000 annual collections.

"Preparation" was initially a manual phase. Tools were limited to the traditional centrifuge and manual extraction press, which led to the use of many different processes.

In the last 20 years, countless innovations have been made within preparation services: separation machines were followed by sterile connection systems and later by closed-circuit cell washers. Automated machines preparing leucocyte-depleted pooled platelet concentrates were recently introduced and are now widely used.

Very soon, machines that are able to produce LBP directly from whole blood will arrive on the market.

Alongside this, several developments are in the pipeline:

- the design, development and use of systems with increased ergonomics, user-friendliness, safety, efficiency and standardization;
- the use of new communication and traceability tools such as radio-frequency identification (RFID): this technique, which makes it possible to memorize and recover data remotely, is currently used to manage plasma for the LFB and is being introduced on all preparation sites. Its use is set to be extended to other LBP.

In the context of increased safety, new pathogen detection or reduction techniques are being assessed. The most effective will be selected and brought into mainstream use alongside or in replacement of less effective techniques.

Individual information systems are being overhauled and replaced by an identical system for all, which everyone can use, under the responsibility of the EFS.

The implementation of specifications from national contracts is also reducing the number of parties involved and streamlining preparation practices.

The rollout of these initiatives is enabling the EFS, the sole provider of blood transfusion services in France, to standardize its preparation platforms whilst harmonizing its techniques, equipment and methods in a context of maximum quality and safety.

6. Preparation

Key points

1. Flowchart of preparation operations

```
                    Receive the bags and verify
                            consistency
                                │
                                ▼
              no          Bag in-line filtered        yes
         ┌──────────────   whole blood   ──────────────┐
         ▼                                             ▼
    Leave to rest                              Filter the whole blood
         │                                             │
         ▼                                             ▼
  Put the bags into buckets                   Put the bags into buckets
   and centrifuge the bags                     and centrifuge the bags
         │                                             │
         ▼                                             ▼
  Separate the components                     Separate the components
  and add SAGM solution                       and add SAGM solution
     to the PRBCs                                to the PRBCs
         │         └──────────┐                        │
         ▼                    ▼                        │
                   Filter the packed red blood         │
                      cells and plasma                 │
         │                    │                        │
         ▼                    ▼                        ▼
     Buffy coat      Leucocyte-depleted        Leucocyte-depleted
                          plasma              packed red blood cells
                            │
                            ▼
                   Identify and affix
                  the RFID tag (optional)
                            │
                            ▼
                     Freeze the plasma
         │                    │                        │
         ▼                    ▼                        ▼
  Store at room temperature   Store in the cold room   Store in the cold room
       (quarantine)           -30°C (quarantine)       +2°C to +6°C (quarantine)
         │                    │                        │
         ▼         no         ▼         no             ▼
    Compatibility ────── Compatibility ──────    Compatibility
       testing              testing                  testing
         │ yes                │ yes                    │ yes
         ▼                    ▼                        ▼
  Mix the buffy coat with  Label and affix the        Label
  additive solution,       RFID tag (if not already    │
  centrifugation-separation done so)                   ▼
         │                    │                   Check the labeling
         ▼                    ▼                        │
  Obtain standard leucocyte- Encode the RIFD tag       │
  depleted pooled plasma          │                    │
      concetrates                 ▼                    │
         │                 Package the plasma bags     │
         ▼                        │                    ▼
    Samples / test                ▼              Store with a view to
         │                 Store at -30 °C       distribution (+2°C to +6°C)
         ▼                 with a view to distribution
    Label / check                 │
         │                        │
         ▼                        │
    Inspect visually              │
   (swirling index)               │
         │                        ▼                    ▼
         ▼                     Destroy              Destroy
  Store with a view to
  distribution (+20 °C to
  +24 °C whilst being agitated)
```

PRBCs: packed red blood cells; SAGM: saline-adenine-glucose-mannitol; RFID: radiofrequency identification; BC: buffy coat; P-PC-LD: pooled platelet concentrates, leucocyte depleted

2. The transport conditions of raw material products

Raw material product	Transport temperature
Whole blood from within 24 hours	+18 °C to +24 °C
Whole blood from between 24 and 72 hours	+2 °C to +10 °C
Packed red blood cells	+2 °C to +10 °C for a maximum of 24 hours
Packed red blood cells cryopreserved at: < -130 °C < -60 °C to -85 °C < -30 °C	< -130 °C < -40 °C for a maximum of 24 hours < -30 °C
Platelet concentrate	+20 °C to +24 °C for a maximum of 24 hours
APC cryopreserved at: < -130 °C < -60 °C to -85 °C	< -130 °C < -40 °C for a maximum of 24 hours
Granulocyte concentrate	+20 °C to +24 °C
Fresh frozen plasma	< -25 °C for a maximum of 24 hours
Fresh thawed plasma	+18 °C to +24 °C for a maximum of 6 hours

7. Donation testing

Azzedine Assal, Cécile Corbi, Pierre Gallian

Introduction

Donation testing has progressed considerably over the last 2 decades. It has benefitted from technological advances in microbiology testing, the increasing automation of technical processes and the computerization of laboratory data. Combined with concerted efforts to improve quality, these aspects have made a significant contribution to improving safety levels in donation testing services.

In accordance with good practice, donation testing has several aims, which are to:
- lessen the risk of immuno haematologic incompatibility and blood-borne diseases in recipients;
- inform donors when anomalies or peculiarities are identified by the tests;
- contribute to the protection of public health.

For that reason, the testing of donated blood and blood components includes:
- all mandatory microbiology tests, systematic or otherwise, conducted on the samples provided by the collection phase;
- the processing of available information on the donation or donor which is relevant to the testing, particularly the donor's administrative and laboratory data, data from the pre-donation interview, post-donation information, safety data and the results of the quality follow-up;
- other non-mandatory tests providing additional qualifications of labile blood products (LBP) for specific therapeutic uses.

All the data provided by donation testing laboratories (LQBD) are used to establish the status of the donation.

Azzedine Assal, azzedine.assal@efs.sante.fr
Cécile Corbi, cecile.corbi@efs.sante.fr
Pierre Gallian, pierre.gallian@efs.sante.fr

Mandatory tests

Table VII presents the list of immunohaematology and infection screening tests that are mandatory in the context of blood donation, with their date of introduction.

Since 2008, a hemogram has been conducted on every donation to determine haemoglobin levels and prevent anaemia. In a departure from the European directive, the reference values are 12 g/dL in women and 13 g/dL in men.

In 2010, the introduction of multiplex nucleic acid testing (NAT; Ultrio Novartis) in mainland France made it possible to screen the DNA of the hepatitis B virus (HBV). The automated NAT systems in LQBD are also able to screen for West Nile virus RNA, if necessary.

Finally, it is worth mentioning that nucleic acid testing for parvovirus B19 and hepatitis A and E viruses in plasma for fractionation and solvent/detergent-treated therapeutic plasma is conducted on pools of raw material.

General organisation of donation testing laboratories

The LQBD are managed by a clinical biologist, either a doctor of medicine or a pharmacist, whose education and training meet strict criteria defined by regulations. He/she leads a team of laboratory technicians and clerical staff, and reports to the director of the blood establishment (ETS) to which the LQBD belongs.

Almost 350 full-time equivalent staff are employed in EFS donation testing laboratories.

Donation testing services are currently being restructured in France, with plans to reduce the number of LQBD in mainland France from 14 (one per ETS) to 4.

The 4 future specialized platforms to be located in Montpellier (QBD Grand-Sud), which opened in 2011, Lille (QBD Grand-Nord), opening in 2013, and Angers (QBD Grand-Ouest) and Metz-Tessy (QBD Grand-Est), both scheduled to open in 2014, have been allocated equal resources. They are to have the most effective automated equipment and sufficient staff numbers to cover the most common causes of system downtime (failure, maintenance, etc.). If one of the 4 laboratories were to cease functioning altogether, it would also be possible to redistribute the services amongst the other 2. These new laboratories are designed to test an average of 2,500 to 2,700 donations each day, up to a possible 3,200–3,500 donations. The services are organized to provide results before 2.30 pm the following day for urgent platelet donations and by 6.30 pm for other donations.

Table VII. Mandatory tests.			
Date of introduction	Tests		
	Immunohaematology	Serology	NAT
1947		Syphilis	
1956	Haematocrit or haemoglobin		
1959	Anti-A and anti-B immune		
1971		HBs Ag	
1985	RCAS	Anti-HIV I/II AB	
1986		Anti-malaria AB*	
1988		ALAT** Anti-HBc AB	
1989		Anti-HTLV I/II AB French Antilles/Guiana	
1990		Anti-HCV AB	
1991		Anti-HTLV I/II AB other *départements*	
2001			NAT HIV-1 NAT HCV
2007		Anti-*Trypanosoma cruzi* AB*	

* If risk of the parasitic infection.
** ALAT screening was abolished in January 2004.
RCAS: red cell antibody screening; ALAT: alanine transaminase; NAT: nucleic acid test; HTLV: Human T Leukemia Virus; AB: antibody.

7. Donation testing

Donation testing in the mapping of the transfusion process

"Donation testing" services are the link in the transfusion chain which, along with the "preparation" phase, starts with the receipt of samples.

Upstream: the "collection" link

Donation collection services, the first link in the chain, collect the blood and preselect donors *via* the pre-donation interview. They order tests on the donations and provide the LQBD with the sample tubes needed for that purpose. If they are mandatory, these tests are conducted automatically. Others are requested by the physician in the blood establishment to ascertain donor suitability: testing for malaria, Chagas disease (for donors who may carry these parasitic infections) or anti-HLA antibodies (in multiparous women).

Downstream: the "distribution" link

This link receives, stores and shares out the end products pending issue to transfusion sites, other ETS or the hospital blood banks.

Medico-technical description of "donation testing" services

We will describe the various stages in donation testing, from receiving the blood samples to providing the results to the "preparation" phase, when they will be used to label the products, or to the physician in the blood establishment, who will then inform the donor (Figure 22).

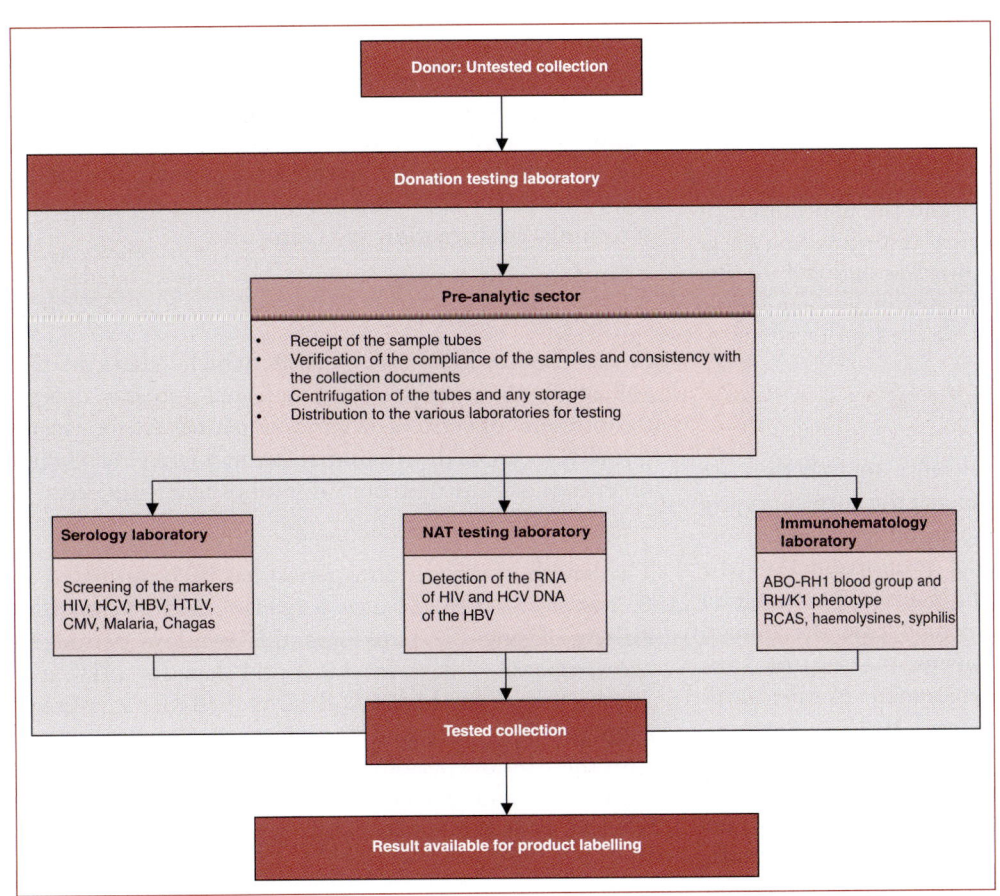

Figure 22. Diagram showing the organisation of the donation testing laboratories.

NAT: nucleic acid test; RCAS: red cell antibody screening.

Pre-analysis

Several types of sample tubes are sent to the LQBD by the donation collection services: 2 dried tubes for serological testing; one EDTA tube for immunohaematology testing, one EDTA tube for nucleic acid testing and one EDTA tube for determining the blood count.

Receiving and centrifuging the sample tubes

The sample tubes are provided with collection transmittal forms, which are used to check the number and type of tubes collected against those actually received by the laboratory. Any inconsistencies in the number, type or quality of tubes is notified to the collection services in an anomaly report. The samples are sorted manually depending on the type of donation: priority is given to platelets (identified by coloured labels).

Centrifuging and sorting the samples

The tubes are centrifuged; the speed and length of centrifugation depends on the tests to be conducted. After centrifugation, automated analyzers uncap and sort the samples by type, placing them into racks. They also check the number of tubes per donation prior to analysis.

Tests conducted in the donation testing laboratory
Screening for transfusion-transmissible infections

- **Main principles underpinning blood-borne infection screening methods**

The direct method involves detecting a pathogen or one of its components (antigen or nucleic acid).

The indirect method involves detecting the immune response specifically directed against the pathogen or one of its components. In essence, serological techniques are used to identify antibodies.

The time between first infection and the appearance of antibodies detectable by serological testing is known as the "window period". This limitation has led to the introduction of NAT testing, which reduces the window period.

- **Serological techniques**

- *Basic criteria*

The antibodies produced in response to infection are able to bind *in vitro* to the antigens of the corresponding pathogenic agent. This binding can be revealed by various processes, creating a signal proportional to the amount of antibodies present. This makes it possible to detect either the antibody, in which case the known value is the antigen, or the antigens, making the antibody the known value. The development of fully automated enzyme immunoassays, and ELISA (enzyme-linked immunosorbent assay) in particular, was a huge step forward. It can be used to screen for all the infectious agents sought in blood transfusion. In the new laboratories, screening for parasitic infections and antibody to cytomegalovirus (anti-CMV) uses ELISA test kits. Antibody testing for major viruses is conducted on automated Prism machines, which use similar enzyme chimioLuminescent immunoassay (chLIA) technology to ELISA but with microparticles and chemiluminescence as signal detection.

- *Interpreting the results of a serological test*

The intensity of the reactions observed is expressed as a signal-to-cutoff (s/co) ratio, using the values recommended by the supplier. An area of uncertainty, known as the "grey zone", is defined below the cutoff (Figure 23), reflecting the intrinsic variability of the technique. The diagram in Figure 23 shows the interpretation of ELISA test results depending on the grey zone defined (*e.g.* 20%).

- *Confirmation test*

The detection of antibodies by serological testing requires a further test to confirm or infirm the specificity of the antibodies directed against an infectious agent and so rule out the possibility of a false-positive result. We will mention 2 types of tests:
– Western Blot (WB) and immunoblot (IB) testing for human immunodeficiency virus (HIV) 1+2, human T-lymphotropic virus (HTLV) I–II, hepatitis C virus (HCV) and treponema;
– neutralization test for hepatitis B surface antigen (HBsAg).

- *Serology algorithms*

Algorithms (*e.g.* screening of anti-HIV antibodies, Figure 24) can be used to establish the outcome of testing by considering the results of screening and additional tests (different test kit to the one used for the screening, confirmation tests, etc.).

- **Nucleic acid testing**

- *Source of residual risk*

A very low residual risk persists, which relates to the collection of donations from infected subjects during the pre-seroconversion or window period. More exceptionally, it can be due to human error, a rare viral variant or immunocompetent but "immunosilent" subjects.

- *Reduction of the window period*

The length of the window period has been estimated at 66 days fors HCV, 22 days fors HIV, and 38 days fors HBsAg. Using NAT reduces this window period to approximately 7 days for HCV, 11 days for HIV and 20 to 30 days for hepatitis B virus (HBV), *i.e.* average gains of 89%, 50% and 45% respectively. By analogy with the window period, the time between the first contamination and detection of nucleic acid by NAT is referred to as the "serologically silent window".

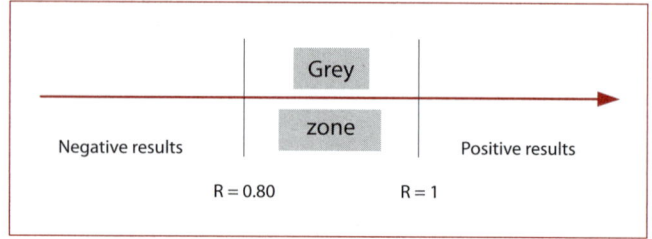

Figure 23. Interpretation of the results and grey zone.
s/co: signal-to-cutoff ratio.

7. Donation testing

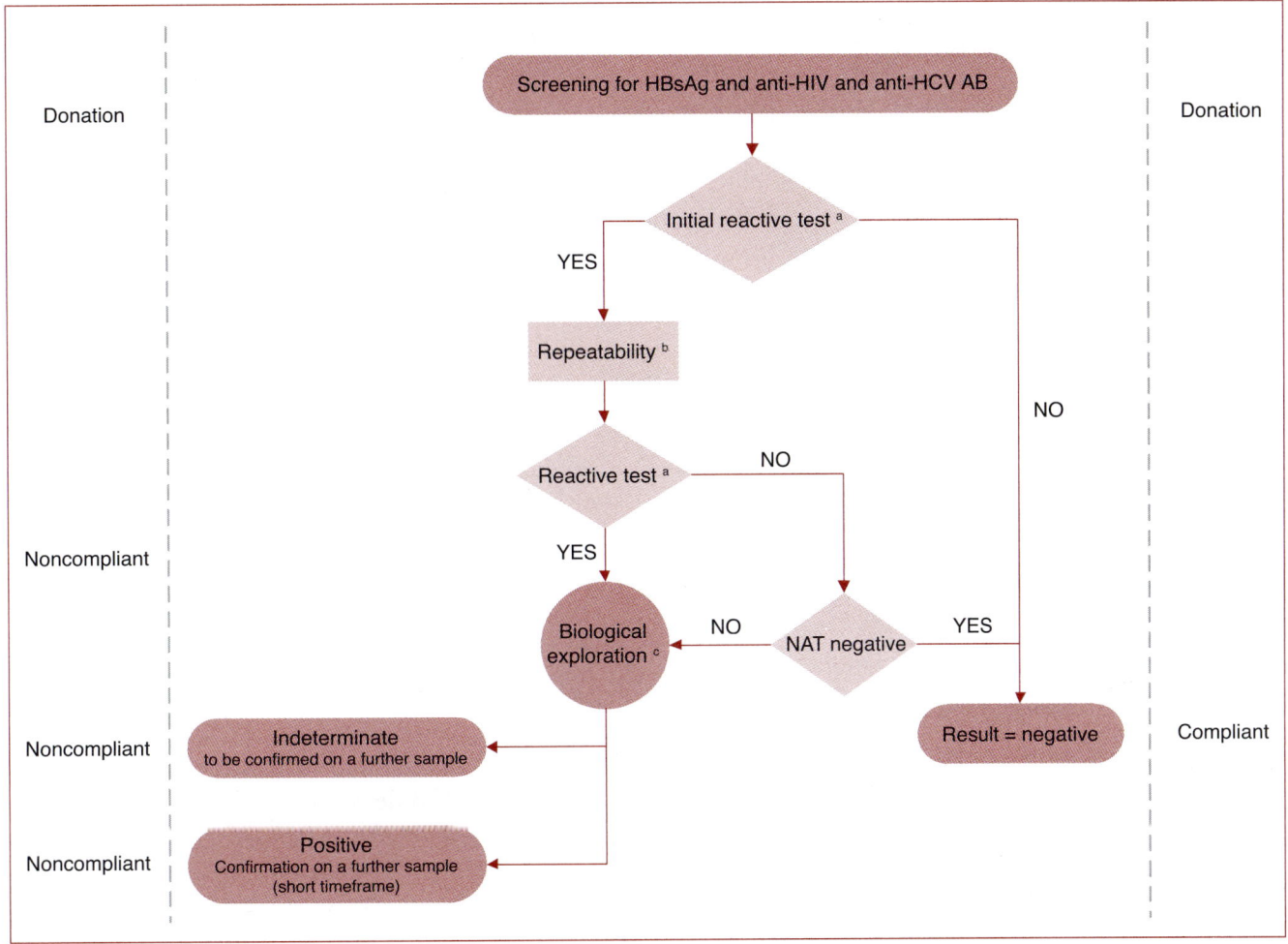

Figure 24. Homologous donation: algorithm for individual nucleic acid testing.
Ag: antigen; AB: antibody; HCV: hepatitis C virus; NAT: nucleic acid test.
– a: reaction signal > laboratory cutoff.
– b: retested in duplicate by the same assay.
– c: complementary testing procedure.

Various NAT techniques can be used. They make it possible to detect the viral genome following *in vitro* amplification of a "target" area chosen for its specificity and lack of variability. In the case of HIV, 2 target regions can be sought simultaneously. The automated testing systems suitable for blood transfusion use either the PCR (Polymerase Chain Reaction), *i.e.* Cobas S201, or TMA (Transcription-Mediated Amplification) technique. This technology (Procleix Ultrio) is currently being used on pools of 8 samples (eSAS) in 4 laboratories in mainland France, which are earmarked for closure, and on individual donations in other EFS laboratories (Tigris system Novartis). The techniques relevant to donation testing can detect the genomes of the 3 viruses simultaneously. These tests are said to be multiplex and, in the event of positive screening, require the conduct of 3 discriminatory tests to identify the virus in question.

Between 1 July 2001 (the date when HIV-1 and HCV NAT was introduced in France) and 1 January 2012, 16 and 13 donations infected by HIV and HCV respectively were identified using NAT.

- **Mandatory systemic markers**
- *Syphilis*

Syphilis screening, the first test introduced to blood transfusion in 1947, involves detecting the antibodies directed against *Treponema pallidum*, the bacterium responsible for syphilis, which is transmitted by sexual and parenteral route. The routine screening test in blood transfusion is TPHA (Treponema Pallidum Haemagglutination Assay). It involves exposing sensitized red blood cells (covered with *Treponema pallidum* antigens) to the subject's plasma (or serum). In the presence of specific antibodies, the cells aggregate on the surface of a test dish. A negative test result shows a tight button

Transfusion medicine: the French model

Table VIII. Interpretation of hepatitis B markers.							
	HBsAg	Anti-HBc AB		HBeAg	Anti-HBe AB	Anti-HBs AB	DNA
		IgM	IgG				
Acute hepatitis	+	+	+/-	+	-	-	+
Cleared hepatitis	-	-	+	-	+/-	+	-
Chronic replicative hepatitis	+	-	+	+	-	-	+
Chronic non-replicative hepatitis HBe seroconversion	+	-	+	-	+	-	-
Pre-core chronic hepatitis	+	-	+	-	-	-	+

Ag: antigen; AB: antibody.

of red blood cells on the same surface. Although a serological test for bacteria, syphilis screening is performed in immunohaematology laboratories due to the nature of the reagent (sensitized red blood cells) and technique (haemagglutination) used. The test is conducted using the blood grouping analyser PK 7300.

In 2011, 358 donors (1.14/10,000 donors) tested positive for this infection.

• *Hepatitis B virus*

Three HBV markers are sought in blood donors: HBsAg, the anti-HBc antibody and HBV DNA. The virus is transmitted by parenteral, sexual and interfamilial route.

HBsAg is the first detectable viral marker to appear in the blood. HBsAg screening in blood donors became mandatory in 1971. The disappearance of the HBsAg is a promising sign and the presence of anti-HBs protective antibodies indicates that the infection has been cleared. When the HBsAg remains in the body for over 6 months, reference is made to chronic hepatitis B.

Anti-HBc is the antibody directed against the capsid, a protein coat enclosing the viral DNA. This antibody appears a few weeks after HBsAg and remains for life. It can, therefore, be found in both acute and chronic hepatitis B. In some chronic hepatitis B cases, concentrations of HBsAg are low and cannot be detected by the serological techniques available to us (occult hepatitis B). In this case, the presence of the anti-HBc antibody, often associated with low HBV DNA viral loads, blocks the use of the infected product. Screening for other hepatitis B markers (HBeAg and anti-HBe antibodies) is not routine but can help to clarify the stage of the infection and the donor's HBV immune status (Table VIII).

NAT for HBV was introduced in ETS in overseas *départements* (French Antilles and Reunion Island) in 2005 due to the much greater prevalence of HBV in these areas and because NAT testing is performed on individual donations.

Screening for HBV DNA has been carried out in mainland France since December 2010.

In 2011, 264 donors (0.84/10,000 donors) tested positive for this infection (257 new donors and 7 known donors).

• *Human immunodeficiency virus*

HIV is an enveloped RNA virus in the retrovirus family. It is the causative agent of acquired immunodeficiency syndrome (AIDS) and is transmitted by sexual and parenteral route. Knowledge of its structure (Figure 25) is useful for understanding its physiology and the diagnostic tests used to detect it.

HIV screening in blood donations relies on the detection of anti-HIV 1+2 antibodies by serological techniques and the viral genome by NAT. Figure 26 summarizes the kinetics of HIV infection markers.

Viral RNA can be detected by NAT around the 10th day after contamination. The p24 antigen appears, meanwhile, around the 16th day. It is only around the 22nd day on average that anti-HIV antibodies can be detected by serological tests. Currently, so-called "combined" screening tests are able to detect the p24 antibody and antigen simultaneously. Therefore, the use of these tests shortens the "serologically silent window" during the primo-infection.

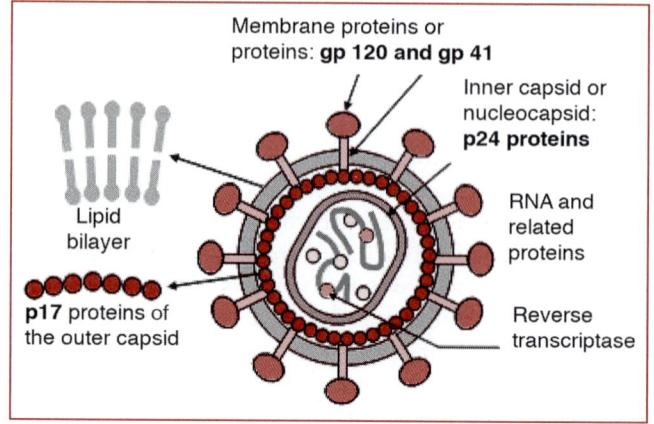

Figure 25. Simplified diagram of HIV.

7. Donation testing

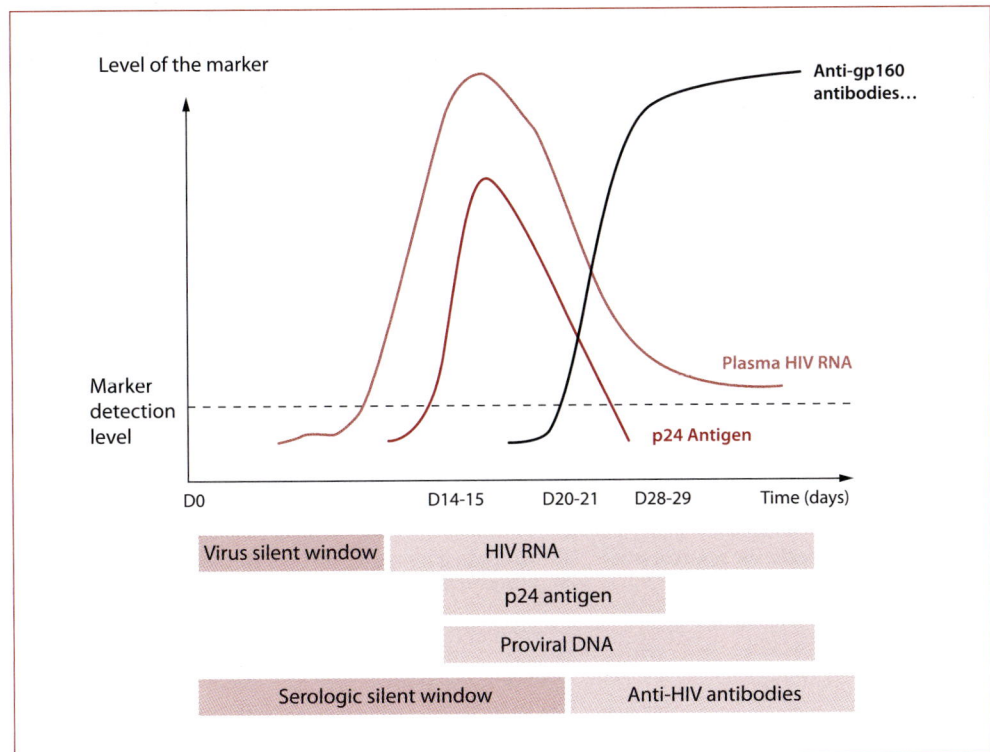

Figure 26. Schematic development of the markers of HIV infection.

In the event of positive screening, a WB or IB test is systematically conducted to confirm the results, clarify the specificity of the anti-HIV antibody and determine the virus type, HIV-1 or HIV-2.

In 2011, 36 donors (0.11/10,000 donors) tested positive for this infection (16 new donors and 20 known donors).

• *Hepatitis C virus*

HCV, an enveloped RNA virus in the *flaviviridae* family, was discovered in 1988. In 60 to 80% of cases, HCV is responsible for chronic hepatitis, leading to cirrhosis after 10 to 20 years and possibly liver cancer. Although HCV is transmitted primarily by parenteral route, nosocomial contaminations have been reported. As for HIV, HCV screening in blood donors uses both serological tests and NAT.

In the event of positive screening by the ELISA test, the confirmation test is an immunoblot.

In 2011, 140 donors (0.44/10,000 donors) tested positive for this infection (124 new donors and 16 known donors).

• *Human T-lymphotropic virus (HTLV-I and II)*

HTLV-I, the first known retrovirus, is responsible for various conditions, of which the best known are a neurological disorder, tropical spastic paraparesis and a type of cancer referred to as T-cell leukaemia or lymphoma. The virus is endemic in the Caribbean, Southeast Japan, Sub-Saharan Africa and South America. It is also found in the overseas *départements* of the French Antilles and French Guiana. It is transmitted by parenteral route, sexual route and breastfeeding.

HTLV-II is an orphan virus (not specifically associated with a known disease). HTLV serological tests have been mandatory in the French Antilles and French Guiana since 1989 and in mainland France since 1991. The confirmation test is a WB or IB. The window period is estimated at 51 days.

In 2011, 21 donors (0.07/10,000 donors) tested positive for this infection (19 new donors and 2 known donors).

• **Mandatory markers in certain situations**

• *Malaria*

Of the 4 plasmodium species, *plasmodium falciparum* is the most feared during post-transfusion accidents, as this species is responsible for serious forms of the disease in LBP recipients, leading to a significant proportion of deaths. The 3 other species are rarely fatal. Preventing transfusion-transmitted malaria requires temporary and definitive contraindications, as well as detecting malarial antibodies by serological testing in the subjects judged to be at risk in the Order on donor selection (Table IX). Indirect immunofluorescence (IFI) was replaced as the screening technique by the ELISA test in 2005, which is easier to use, fully automated and more objective. The additional techniques used are IFI and/or antigen testing and/or PCR.

Transfusion medicine: the French model

Table IX. Malaria-related contraindications (Decree of 18 January 2009).

Questions to ask the donor/measures/tests		Steps to take depending on the responses
History of malaria, malaria attack		Contraindicated for 3 years after the end of treatment. After 3 years, can donate if no symptom evident and first donation serological test negative
Returned from an endemic area in the last 4 months		Contraindicated for 4 months after returning
Returned from an endemic area between 4 months and 3 years ago	Born or lived in an endemic area in the first 5 years of life	Can donate if no symptom evident and serological tests negative for all donations in this period
	Stayed in an endemic area for over 6 consecutive months	Can donate if no symptom evident and serological tests negative for all donations in this period
	Other	Can donate if no symptom evident and first donation serological test negative
Returned from an endemic area over three years ago	Born or lived in an endemic area in the first 5 years of life	Can donate if no symptom evident and first donation serological test negative
	Stayed in an endemic area for over 6 consecutive months	Can donate if no symptom evident and first donation serological test negative
	Other	Can donate if no symptom evident

• *Chagas disease*

Chagas disease, or American trypanosomiasis, is caused by the flagellate protozoan *Trypanosoma cruzi*. The disease is endemic in Central and South America, and found in French Guiana. It can be transmitted during pregnancy, by blood transfusion or following organ donation. In France, screening for the disease in at-risk subjects, meaning donors who originate from endemic areas, or have lived or travelled in South America, as well as donors whose mother was born or lived in that region, was introduced into donation testing in May 2007. Screening is based on the use of an ELISA test. In the event of a positive or indeterminate result, further tests employ IFI and/or PCR.

• **Non-mandatory markers**

• *Anti-CMV antibodies*

Only the donations needed to meet demand for CMV-negative products are screened for anti-CMV antibodies. These products are indicated in pregnant women, premature babies whose mother's CMV status is seronegative or unknown, subjects receiving, or about to receive, a bone marrow transplant and lung transplantees. CMV screening uses an ELISA technique that is able to detect antibodies in the IgG and IgM classes.

• *Additional qualification of plasma*

The LQBD conduct non-mandatory tests on plasma intended for the LFB ahead of the production of specific immunoglobulin. The tests in question involve tetanus and anti-HBs antibodies.

Immunohaematology tests

• **Prevention of immunological risk**

The second role of the LQBD, alongside screening for blood-borne infections, involves determining the main immunohaematological characteristics of donors and blood products from their donation. The genetic polymorphism and immunogenicity of blood group antigens can be an obstacle to transfusion. The fixation of an antibody onto the corresponding blood group antigen very often leads to the destruction of red blood cells, which can in turn lead to serious pathological complications and even the death of the patient.

The donor immunohaematology laboratory determines the ABO-RH1 blood groups in all donations and the RH-KEL1 phenotypes in the first 2 donations. In some donors, other antigens may be determined: this is the extended phenotype.

As well as determining red cell antigens, the donor immunohaematology laboratory screens plasma for any dangerous irregular antibodies and anti-A/anti-B immune antibodies (haemolysins) that may cause haemolytic complications in the event of ABO-compatible transfusions from different blood groups.

• **Tests conducted and principles underpinning the diagnostic methods**

• *ABO blood grouping*

The ABO system is characterized by the presence or lack of A and/or B antigens on the surface of red blood cells, and the presence or lack of so-called natural anti-A and/or anti-B antibodies in plasma. In the ABO system, we regularly find the natural antibody corresponding to the antigen that we do not have (Table X).

ABO blood grouping includes two further tests:

– a cells test (forward grouping), which involves screening for antigens A (ABO1) and B (ABO2) with the following monoclonal reagents: anti-A (anti-ABO1), anti-B (anti-ABO2) and anti-AB (anti-ABO3). The anti-A and anti-AB reagents must recognize Ax subgroups;

– a plasma or serum test (reverse grouping), which involves screening for anti-A and anti-B antibodies with A1 and B test cells.

Table X. The four main ABO blood groups.			
Blood group	Antigen present on the red blood cells	Antibodies present in the plasma	Percentage in France
A	A	Anti-B	45%
B	B	Anti-A	9%
O	Not A or B	Anti-A and anti-B	43%
AB	A and B	Not anti-A or anti-B	3%

Concordance between the 2 tests, cells and serum, is essential to confirm a blood group.

• *RH1 (or RhD) phenotype*

The RH (Rhesus) blood group system brings together almost 50 different antigens. Among them, the RH1 (D) antigen is by far the most immunogenic. Eighty-five percent of Europeans have it: they are said to be RH1 or RhD positive. Due to its strong immunogenicity, its determination cannot be separated from ABO blood grouping. RH1 blood grouping includes the use of anti-RH1 monoclonal reagent. A small percentage of individuals express the RH1 antigen more weakly than others, which is then referred to as weak RH1 or formerly weak D or D^u. The RH1 antigen is more difficult to detect in these cases but it is essential to do so as many of them are immunogenic and cells carrying a weak RH1 antigen can be hemolyzed by an anti-RH1 antibody in the recipient. Additional techniques aiming to identify a weakened expression of the RH1 antigen are therefore used in donors who were initially found to be RH1 negative. The anti-RH1 monoclonal reagent must be able to detect most RH1 variants, particularly the partial RH1 antigens in category VI and weak, RH1 type 2.

• *RH-KEL1 phenotypes*

The determination of RH-KEL1 phenotypes involves using specific monoclonal serum tests to identify the RH2 (C), RH3 (E), RH4 (c), RH5 (e) antigens of the RH system and the KEL1 (K) antigen of the KEL system. Outside RH1, these antigens are the target of most dangerous irregular antibodies. For the first donation, determining the RH-KEL1 phenotype is based on two tests, with the technician using two lots of reagents. Two reagents of the same specificity should originate from separate clones. For a second donation, determination is based on at least one test. For subsequent donations, further determinations are optional.

• *Extended phenotypes*

They correspond to determining the presence of blood group antigens other than those referred to above. The FY1, FY2 (Duffy system), JK1, JK2 (Kidd system), MNS3 and MNS4 (MNS system) antigens are frequently involved. This determination makes compatible packed red blood cells (PRBCs) available to the issuing services for transfusion in a patient who has one of these irregular antibodies, which may be responsible for severe post-transfusion haemolytic complications. Determining extended phenotypes follows the same principles as for RH-KEL1 phenotypes: 2 determinations on 2 different donations, after which testing is optional.

• *Red cell antibody screening*

Every donation is systematically tested, which involves identifying the antibodies directed against red cell antigens other than A and B in the plasma or serum of donors. In practical terms, it involves bringing the sample into contact with group O test cells. The range of test cells used is defined by regulations and must include the following antigens: RH1, RH2, RH3, RH4, RH5, KEL1, KEL2, FY1, FY2, JK1, JK2, MNS1, MNS2, MNS3, MNS4, LE1, LE2 and LU2.

If the test is positive, the relevant red cell antibodies must be identified. Any antibodies thus identified which may impact on the donor's medical, transfusion or obstetrical future must be notified to the physician in the blood establishment so that he/she can inform the donor.

• *Anti-A and anti-B immune antibodies (haemolysins)*

These antibodies may result from alloimmunization by pregnancy or, more rarely, an incompatible transfusion. In most cases, however, they originate from heteroimmunization after the body comes into contact with substances of animal or bacterial origin. It involves IgG, which can cause haemolytic complications. The test, which detects the anti-A and anti-B antibodies likely to reduce the lifespan of the red blood cells in recipients carrying the corresponding antigens, is conducted on every blood donation.

All donor immunohaematology testing uses haemagglutination techniques. The tests on each donation are conducted with automated analyzers and in microplate format (PK 7300 for the ABO-RH1 groups, RH-KEL1 phenotypes, immune anti-A/B antibodies and syphilis serology, Figure 27, and Galileo for red cell antibody screening).

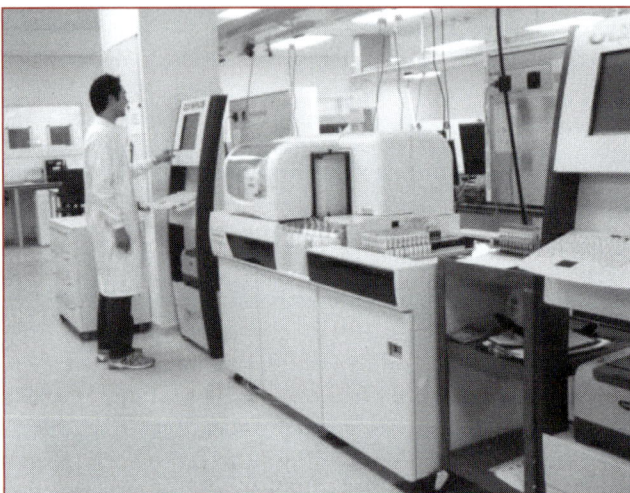

Figure 27. Olympus PK 7300.
© EFS.

The organisation of the laboratory and data management

The primary aim of donation testing laboratories is to provide test results (markers of infection and immunohaematology) in timeframes enabling the rapid labelling of LBP, particularly platelet concentrates.

Data management

The LQBD have their own central computer system into which all data is entered, including the data generated by the laboratory (primarily test results) and that provided by the information system or blood management software (LMT) of the ETS.

- **Data transfer**

Each collection has a unique 11-digit barcode, which is first matched against the donor number and then identified and checked by the automated analyzers. Figure 28 illustrates the first stage in transferring information between the 2 systems. It involves transferring a file containing information on the donations to be processed, which were collected the previous day and recorded in the LMT by the collection staff, from the LMT to the laboratory information management system (IL). As well as the number and type of donation, this file includes information on the donor, number of previous donations, any past results and the tests to be conducted. Entering the file into the IL launches specific algorithms dependent on the information from the LMT, particularly past results. This might lead to the conduct of further tests, for example, or block the use of a donation.

- **Approval and transfer of the results**

Once the tests are complete, the lab technicians approve the analysis of the results in accordance with the criteria defined by the laboratory manager. The results are then transferred from the automated analyzers to the IL for biological validation under the responsibility of the laboratory director, who is a clinical biologist. This follows the steps laid down in the results interpretation algorithms. Once the biological validation is complete, the biologist authorizes the transfer of the results from the IL to the LMT, where they can be consulted and used by other departments in the establishment, particularly the preparation services and blood collection physicians (Figure 29).

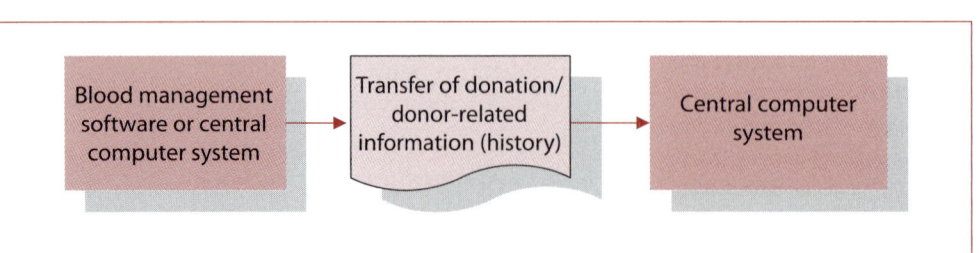

Figure 28. Transfer of information on the donation and donor between the central computer system and laboratory information management system.

7. Donation testing

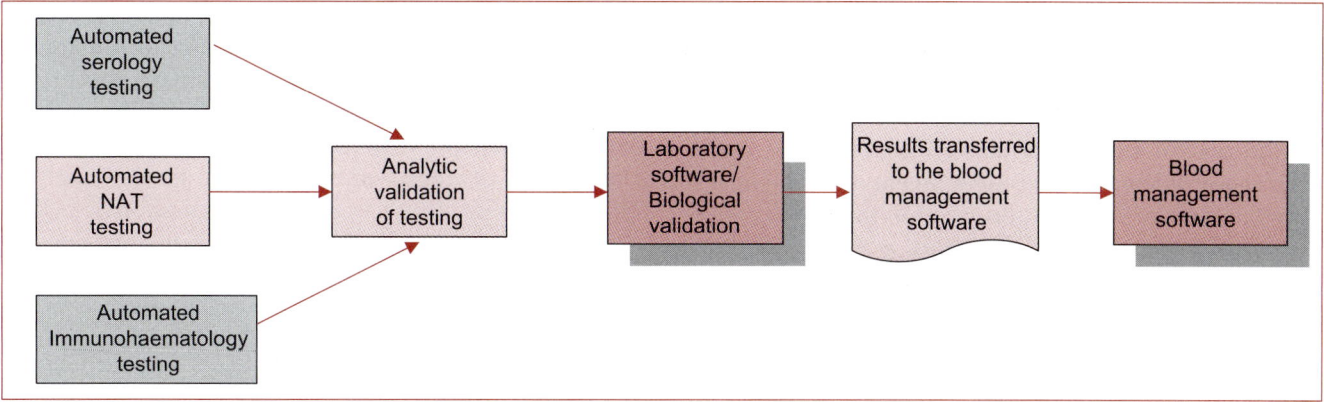

Figure 29. Validation and transfer of the results to the central computer system.
NAT: nucleic acid test; DIH: donor immunohaematology; LMT: blood management software.

Within the central computer system, decision-making trees authorize or block the labelling and distribution of LBP, depending on the results of donations testing, as well as donor eligibility and information.

Different types of results and action on abnormal results

• **Immunohaematology results**

The results of blood grouping, phenotyping and irregular antibody testing must be coherent and consistent with the donor's previous results, if any. If not, the central computer system blocks the abnormal results and prevents product labelling. Internal procedures indicate the steps to be taken to clarify any incoherencies and inconsistencies, determine the ultimate results, and decide how blood products from the donation will be used.

• **Results of markers for infection**

There are 3 possible conclusions for each marker in the central computer system:
- *Negative results:* when the marker screening results are negative, the LMT authorizes the labelling of the product (if the immunohaematology results are also compliant);
- *Positive results:* any positive marker screening result will block the blood products and lead to their destruction, with the following exceptions:
  – positive CMV serology does not prevent product labelling. A CMV-negative product is selected at a later stage, depending on the prescription,
  – the LFB accepts plasma that has tested positive for anti-HBc antibodies as a raw material, provided that levels of anti-HBs are more than 0.5 IU/mL,
  – in planned autologous transfusion, positive serology for the following markers: syphilis, malaria antibodies, and positive anti-HBc antibodies if anti-HBs positive. The decision to take blood from and transfuse patients is taken jointly by the prescribing physician and ETS physician in charge of blood collection based on the patient's medical history and additional diagnostic data from clinical and biological testing;
- *Indeterminate results:* when an initially positive test is not confirmed by further or confirmation testing, it is deemed to be "indeterminate". The corresponding products are destroyed and the donor is recalled for follow-up.

Informing donors

A national procedure outlines the steps taken when an abnormal result is found in a blood donor. The laboratory manager forwards the abnormal results to the blood collection physician, who informs the donor. The blood collection physician is responsible for choosing the most appropriate means of contacting and managing the donor in line with the type of anomaly found. Donor follow-up must provide the quickest and most suitable medical response to the anomaly, reflecting the need to safeguard the health of the donor or his/her friends and family.

Alongside this, the information system of the ETS is updated with all relevant safety data generated by investigation of the anomaly.

The steps taken when a positive marker for infection is found depend on whether it involves a new or regular donor. A new donor is asked to undergo further testing, epidemiological investigation and assessment to determine the appropriate medical care. A positive result in a regular donor also requires tests in the recipient(s) of LBP from the last negative donation and an LFB alert if the donor's plasma has been provided for fractionation.

Conclusion

The "donation testing" phase is the most automated in the transfusion process, thanks to advances in the

Transfusion medicine: the French model

techniques. In the future, it aims to standardize its facilities and homogenize the practices and techniques used, whilst continuing to provide results that enable the rapid availability of LBP.

At the present time, controlling the emergence or re-emergence of infectious agents remains a public health issue. For example, significant and increasingly frequent epidemics of West Nile virus, which causes neurological conditions in recipients, are affecting several countries in the Mediterranean region and North America. For many years, the US, Italian and Greek transfusion systems have performed NAT screening for its viral RNA. Donation testing must remain open to the possibility of screening for other viruses that may be relevant in blood transfusion, such as Dengue, Chikungunya and hepatitis E.

In the midterm, the challenges facing donation testing services necessitate regular scientific and technological surveillance. The prospect of using new techniques (nucleic acid tags enabling the simultaneous detection of several pathogens, nanotechnologies, etc.) will address the issue of pathogen emergence, but are also likely to change laboratory services and the organisation of LQBD considerably. In immunohaematology, the introduction of automated genotyping should make it possible to select the most appropriate LBP for the phenotypes of recipients by indentifying antigens for which there are no serological tests (Dombrock, Colton, etc.) and genotyping the rare blood donors characterized by the lack of common antigens (Jsb, MNS5, RH18, RH34, RH46, RH31, RH59, etc.), which is particularly important in managing transfusions in drepanocytic patients of African origin.

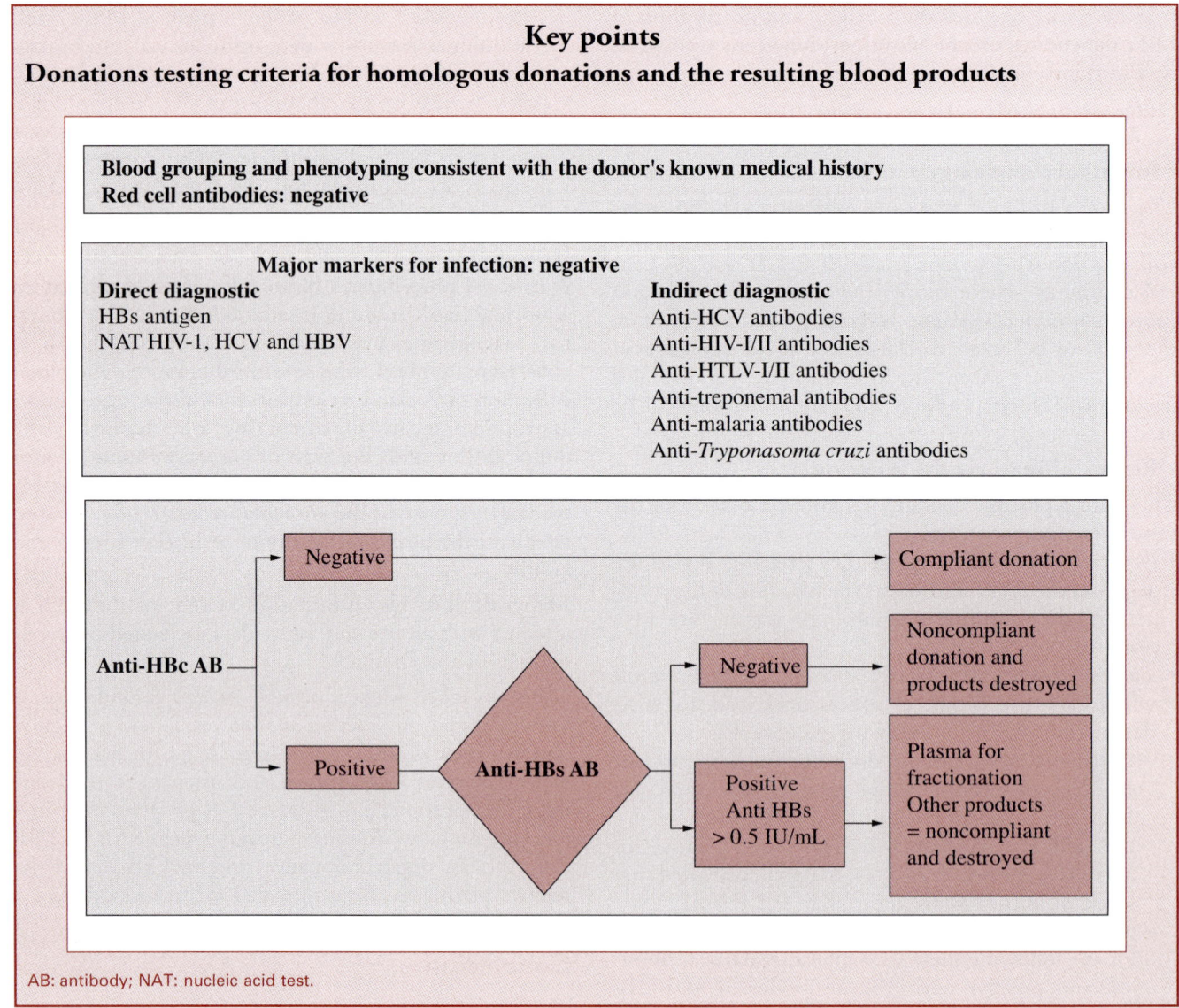

AB: antibody; NAT: nucleic acid test.

8. Patient testing

Françoise Hau, Claire Krause, Francis Roubinet

Outside donation testing, and exceptional circumstances, the laboratory services of the French Blood Establishment (EFS) are limited to the two highly specialized areas that are immunohaematology and histocompatibility.

The sole objective of immunohaematology testing is to ensure the safety of blood transfusion for patients (selecting the right product for the right patient) and the immunological safety of pregnant women and their unborn infant. In the particular case of pregnancy, immunohaematology tests aim, firstly, to detect any alloimmunization against a blood group antigen which may have serious consequences, even death, and require transfusions in the foetus *(in utero)* or newborn, and secondly, to prevent alloimmunization against the D (RH1) antigen of the Rhesus system, which could compromise future pregnancies, through anti-D injection in Rh-negative women. Immunohaematology tests have no direct "clinical" impact but are needed to determine the appropriate treatment for a given patient. They are inseparable from the provision of medical care and have no "utility" outside this sphere. It is an increasingly common form of "personalized" medicine, in which ascertaining the right product for the right patient demands a specific investigation. Testing is often provided at the same time as the product, in a jointly financed treatment package. In July 2012, the French National Authority for Health (HAS) described this notion for medicinal products as "companion testing". Immunohaematology clearly meets this description. We can question the historical reasons that have led to the development of current processes in which pre-transfusion immunohaematology tests are "valued" in exactly the same way as standard diagnostic tests, leading to confusion over their clinical justification and leaving the EFS to defend the importance of the "companion testing" link between immunohaematology and the delivery of labile blood

Françoise Hau, francoise.hau@efs.sante.fr
Claire Krause, claire.krause@efs.sante.fr
Francis Roubinet, francis.roubinet@efs.sante.fr

products (LBP). This link is a major part of blood transfusion safety, as was reaffirmed by the Directorate-General for Care Provision (DGOS) in a recommendation to the Regional Health Agencies (ARS) in 2010. The primary purpose of blood transfusion testing is therefore the delivery of products, of which 86% are provided by the EFS's delivery sites and 14% by the hospital blood banks that are not located near the EFS's transfusion sites. Immunohaematology testing is an indispensable and mandatory prerequisite for patient safety, ensuring immunological compatibility between LBP and patient. It is a local service provided round the clock by the EFS. It should also be noted that, in a large majority of cases, immunohaematology tests are conducted in emergency situations due to urgent needs for LBP. The link between immunohaematology, transfusion support and the delivery of LBP is essential to health safety and is the foundation of the French blood transfusion model. The importance of the link between immunohaematology and the delivery of LBP is, however, recognized by almost all industrialized countries, as was emphasized by a report submitted to the National Union of Health Insurance Funds (UNCAM) by the French National Blood Transfusion Institute in 2009. This consensus recognizes the importance of a consolidated structure providing blood transfusion testing and delivering LBP. Given the 1998 Blood Act, which reasserted that LBP should be delivered by the EFS's sites and, where necessary, the hospital blood banks to better manage the strategic resource that are LBP, these same sites should be conducting the immunohaematology tests required.

Histocompatibility (HLA) is another highly specialized form of testing, which makes it possible to characterize the antigens and antibodies of HLA systems and, to a lesser extent, platelet systems for the purpose of analyzing the compatibility between donor and recipient prior to grafts or transplants. These tests are also conducted in studies of associations between certain phenotypes, genotypes and diseases, as well as in the prevention and exploration of TRALI (transfusion-related acute lung injury). The tests ordered for allografts of haematopoietic stem cells (HSCs) essentially use molecular biology typing techniques, HLA A*, B*, C*, DRB1*, and DQB1*, to identify a compatible donor. For organ transplants, the workup includes HLA class I and II typing, supplemented by regular screening for anti-HLA antibodies. The HLA laboratories enter these data into the records of patients on the transplant waiting list maintained by the French Biomedicine Agency (ABM), which organizes the distribution of organs throughout the country. Updating these records ensures the best possible immunological response to transplanted organs, reducing the risk of humoral rejection, and equal access to transplantation.

Medico-technical description of "patient testing" services

General organisation of EFS laboratories

The EFS's immunohaematology services are provided within 137 sites belonging to multisite laboratories, which are being created in line with the reform of clinical biology. Reflecting the immunohaematology-delivery link referred to above, all these immunohaematology sites are "associated" with one of the EFS's LBP delivery sites. The number of immunohaematology tests conducted per annum has been growing steadily over the last 6 years, rising from 331 million B in 2005 to 376 million B in 2011. (Any act of biomedical analysis is identified by a code number which is a factor identified by the key letter B: *e.g.* ABO-RH1 blood group = B 35).

Histocompatibility and immunogenetics testing is conducted within 32 laboratories, which provide public services. The geographical distribution of HLA laboratories reflects the locations of transplantation centres: seventeen sites within the EFS and fifteen in hospitals. Following Prof. Jean Dausset's efforts to establish links and cooperation between immunology laboratories and transfusion centres, HLA knowledge and practices within the EFS have been advanced by the teams' expertise in collecting and storing biological materials, managing donors' records and increasing blood, organ, tissue and cell donation. EFS sites conducted 106 million B in patients in 2011, a figure that has been rising significantly for several years. Transplant-related testing is increasing by approximately 3.5% annually. Combined with maintaining an HSC register [voluntary donors of bone marrow and placenta blood] and transfusion-related testing, the services provided by HLA laboratories increased by 30% between 2008 and 2012.

The general organisation of these laboratory services mirrors the EFS's own organisation into regional establishments, generally covering 1 or 2 administrative regions, under the umbrella of a national government agency. This gives each site of the EFS's multisite laboratories access to general, support and quality services in their area, which is essential if they are to obtain ISO 15189 certification, as well as a pyramid structure for complex immunohaematology tests, making it possible to resolve almost all issues in timeframes compatible with patient safety and optimal efficiency. Overall consistency is ensured by national meetings of the regional managers of these services.

As we have just seen, the EFS's laboratories are seeking to achieve ISO 15189 certification. All our laboratories will be certified or have submitted their application to the French Certification Committee (Cofrac) by

8. Patient testing

the end of 2013. The seventeen EFS sites providing histocompatibility testing are already accredited under the European Federation for Immunogenetics (EFI) system.

In 2012, the services employed near 1,400 full-time equivalent for immunohaematology testing and 260 for HLA testing.

Description of the principles underpinning the tests

In both areas, some tests determine a phenotype or genotype, meaning the presence or absence of an antigen (on red blood cells for immunohaematology and on white blood cells or platelets for histocompatibility) or the corresponding gene, whilst others detect antibodies in patients' serum or plasma which recognize the corresponding antigens that may lead to difficulties in a transfusion or graft.

It should also be noted that, irrespective of the techniques, the 2 areas of testing are becoming increasingly automated. In practical terms, the tests use serological or molecular methods.

Serological methods

These involve detecting any contact between an antigen and the corresponding specific antibody. If the presence of an antigen is sought, an antibody is used as the reagent (serum test) and if an antibody is sought, red blood cells or cells carrying the corresponding antigen are used.

The method of demonstrating the antigen-antibody reaction can vary with the technique.

In immunohaematology, the agglutination reaction of the red blood cells is demonstrated using either a microfiltration or microplate adherence technique (Figure 32).

In histocompatibility, antigen typing often uses the lymphocytotoxicity technique (LCT) after isolating the mononuclear cells by density gradient (Ficoll) or separating the lymphocytes. The reaction is demonstrated with special Terasaki plates and the antiserums of known specificities. In the presence of the target antigen and complement, the antibody causes cell lysis. The use of a vital stain and microscope reveals the percentage of lysed cells (Figure 30). This technique makes it possible to type HLA class I, A and B, quickly and easily. HLA typing of the HLA DR and DQ antigens by LCT, meanwhile, requires the separation of the B lymphocytes expressing HLA class II antigens. This practice is being replaced by molecular biology determinations of the corresponding HLA genes.

The same principles are used in antibody screening but the development of solid-phase techniques has improved the detection of anti-HLA antibodies compared with complement-dependant techniques, particularly in histocompatibility. LCT nevertheless remains the primary technique for pre-transplant or lymphocyte cross-matching. Even more recently, screening for anti-HLA antibodies, whether in transplantation or transfusion, has been based on multiplexing techniques with Luminex fluorescent microspheres or beads (Figure 31). The beads demonstrating the reaction are coated with purified HLA antigens. The combinations of fluorophores highlight the beads in the reading and identify the antigens on which the antibodies of the test serum are fixed. Because these techniques are highly sensitive, the positive thresholds must reflect the indications, whether the objective is immunological follow-up and rejection prevention in a patient awaiting transplant or the non-transmission of anti-HLA antibodies in the prevention of TRALI.

Molecular methods

Immunohaematology and histocompatibility are also benefitting from the considerable advances provided by molecular biology techniques, which are making it possible to examine human genetic polymorphism more closely.

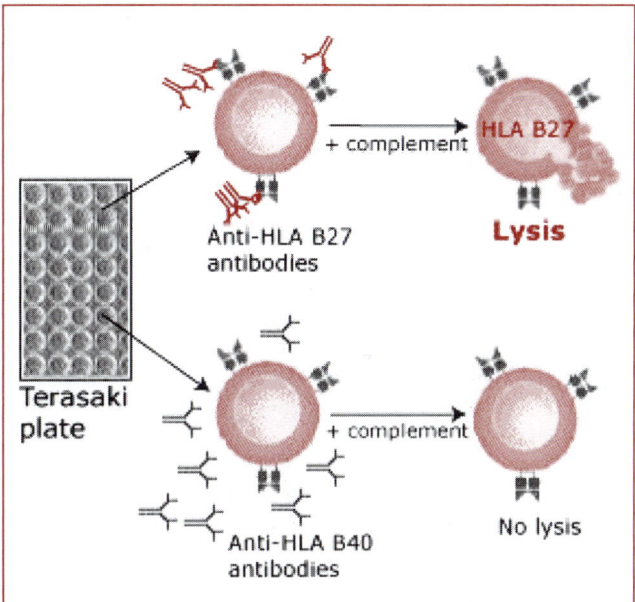

Figure 30. Principle of the lymphocytotoxicity technique.

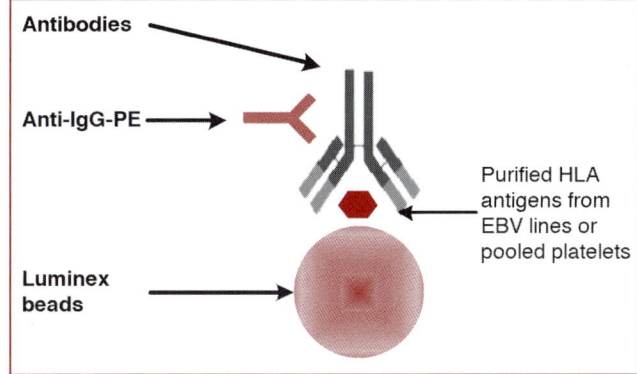

Figure 31. Principle of the Luminex technique.
PE: phycoerythrin.

Transfusion medicine: the French model

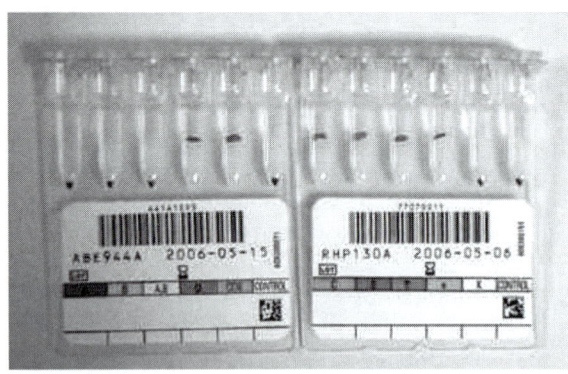

A. Microtube filtration techniques

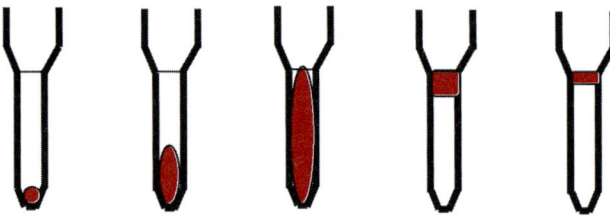

Negative reaction   Positive reactions of various intensities

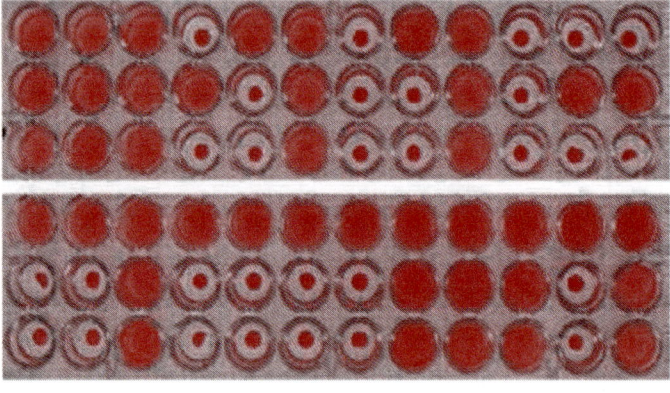

B. Solid-phase immune adherence techniques

Side view

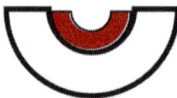 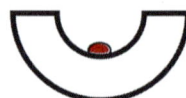

Birdside view

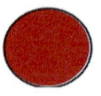 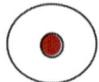

Positive reaction   Negative reaction

Figure 32. Serological methods in immunohaematology.

8. Patient testing

The main methods used are not specific to these fields and involve various techniques after DNA extraction and generally an amplification phase with Polymerase Chain Reaction (PCR), as for HLA:
- PCR-Sequence Specific Primer (SSP);
- PCR-Sequence Specific Oligoprobe reverse (SSOr), when the Luminex beads are coated in known-sequence oligonucleotides;
- PCR-Sequence Based Typing (SBT): sequencing the exons and typing the variants of HLA class 1 and 2 chains.

Type, volume and circumstances to prescribe tests
Immunohaematology tests

Immunohaematology tests can be subdivided into two major categories:

- **So-called "standard" tests**, which are ABO/RH1 blood grouping, RH/KEL1 phenotyping, irregular antibody screening, cross-matching and the direct antiglobulin test (DAT). In numbers, the EFS conducts the following standard tests each year:
  - ABO/RH1 blood grouping: approximately 2.4 million tests p.a.;
  - RH/KEL1 phenotyping (antigens that may cause alloimmunization): approximately 2.4 million tests p.a.;
  - irregular antibody screening: approximately 2.5 million tests p.a.;
  - DAT, a test that demonstrates *in vivo* antibody binding to the patient's red blood cells: approximately 300,000 tests p.a.;
  - cross-matching (testing directly associated with the delivery of LBP): approximately 270,000 tests p.a.

These tests ensure the safety of transfusion recipients and pregnant women:
- by regulations, ABO/RH1 blood groups and RH/KEL1 phenotypes must be determined twice before any transfusion and in pregnancy (except in life-threatening situations);
- for packed red blood cells (PRBCs), irregular antibody screening must take place within a validity period of less than 3 days or 3 weeks, depending on the patient's medical history. In pregnant women, irregular antibody screening must be repeated at intervals specified by regulations, which vary depending on the patient's medical history and RH1 phenotype. In the event of positive screening in pregnant women, the antibodies must be identified and possibly dosed or titred;
- cross-matching is mandatory in recipients presenting, or having presented, with anti-red cell alloantibodies and in newborns presenting with a positive DAT or born to an alloimmunized mother. By regulations, the period of validity of cross-matching is 3 days from collection.

Currently, EFS laboratories conduct just one-third of these standard tests, with approximately 15% conducted by hospital laboratories and 55% by private laboratories.

- **More complex immunohaematology tests**, which are essential to ensure the safety of blood transfusion for patients:
  - exact identification of the antibodies found in a patient's serum or plasma (mandatory when the screening is positive): approximately 220,000 tests are carried out by our laboratories each year;
  - determination of a red cell phenotype other than RH/KEL1 (approximately 270,000 tests p.a.) to confirm the identification of anti-red cell antibodies directed against 1 or more non-RH/KEL1 antigens. This test is mandatory in complex alloimmunization. It is also provided on a preventive basis in patients receiving repeated transfusions (sickle cell anaemia, thalassaemia, etc.). In these cases, it involves detecting the presence or absence of the FY1 and 2, JK1 and 2, MNS3 and 4 antigens;
  - exploration of haemolytic anaemia with characterization of the anti-red cell alloantibodies fixed to the surface of patients' red blood cells (elution) and free in the plasma, screening and titration of the serum cold agglutinins;
  - exploration of the adverse events occurring in recipients of an LBP transfusion;
  - follow-up of the pregnancy of immunized women, monitoring changes in the content (titration) and concentration (quantitation) of the antibody.

It is important to note that EFS laboratories conduct the vast majority of complex immunohaematology tests as most private laboratories conduct only simple tests and transfer the samples to the EFS laboratories in difficult cases. The laboratories of the EFS and those hospitals with delivery banks also conduct almost all the tests associated with an urgent request for LBP or immunohaematology tests ordered out of hours. Although the EFS only performs 25% of irregular antibody screening tests, its laboratories conduct nearly 60% of tests to identify irregular antibodies (which accurately characterize irregular antibodies that are dangerous in the context of transfusion or obstetrics). Only 35% of hospital laboratories and 11% of private laboratories conducted these tests in 2007. This situation is even more marked for the determination of extended red cell phenotypes. Of the 323,965 extended phenotypes performed in 2007, 267,278 were by the EFS (82.5%), 4,179 (1.3%) by hospital laboratories and 52,508 (16.2%) by private laboratories.

Histocompatibility tests

Table XI presents the main HLA tests and their indications in transfusions or transplantations, as well as the strategies adopted in France. These indications are provided as guidance only, with various typing techniques in particular often being used in combination, depending on the organisations of the laboratories.

In numbers, the main tests conducted by the EFS are:
- 139,000 HLA typing tests (excluding voluntary bone marrow donors), broken down into the following techniques:
  – 22,000 typing tests using LCT serological techniques,
  – 117,000 by molecular biology, of which 38% by allele resolution;
- 103,000 anti-HLA antibody screenings, including 25,000 identifications by sensitive techniques and 16,000 screenings in donors as part of TRALI prevention;
- the EFS conducts over 50% of tests linked to the transplant of organs and HSCs in France. In 2012, 77% of voluntary bone marrow donors on the "bone marrow transplant" register were registered and typed by the EFS, resulting in 11,818 new HSCs donors. The EFS's 6 placental blood banks have collated over 7,000 units, whose typing is managed by our HLA laboratories. Transplant-related services – organs, HSCs, registering voluntary bone marrow donors and managing placental blood banks – account for over 90% of the tests conducted in our histocompatibility laboratories;
- 10 laboratories within the EFS provide leucocyte-platelet immunology testing: HPA genotyping plus screening and identifying antiplatelet antibodies in the exploration of neonatal thrombocytopenia and ineffective transfusions linked to HPA immunization, accounting for over 5,000 genotyping tests and 10,500 antibody screening tests each year;
- one laboratory has expertise in HNA granulocyte immunology, whose indications are restricted and account for nearly 300 genotyping tests and 2,700 antibody screening tests.

Table XI. Main histocompatibility tests.

Choice of techniques		Main indications	
		Donors	Recipients
Immuno-serological methods	HLA A, B typing in LCT	Donor of phenotype-compatible APC Organ transplant donor	Transfusion of HLA-compatible APC Organ transplant recipient
	Anti-HLA antibody screening by LCT	Lymphocyte cross-matching in the exploration of TRALI	Exploration of inefficiencies in platelet transfusion Organ transplant recipient: IgM detection Pre-graft lymphocyte cross-matching
	Anti-HLA antibody screening by sensitive Luminex-type method	Female donors of APC, non-nulliparous: TRALI prevention	Exploration of inefficiencies in platelet transfusion Organ transplant recipient
Molecular methods	Genetic genotyping: HLA A*, B* HLA DRB1*, DQB1* (SSP, reverse SSO)	Organ transplant donor	Organ transplant recipient
	Allelic genotyping: HLA A*, B* C* HLA DRB1*, QB1* (SSP, reverse SSO HD, SBT)	Inclusion of VBMD in the FGM register Donor of HSCs	HSC transplant recipient
	Genetic genotyping: HLA A*, B* Allelic genotyping: HLA DRB1*	Placental blood transfusion	

LCT: lymphocytotoxicity; APC: aphaeresis platelet concentrates; TRALI: transfusion related acute lung injury; VBMD: voluntary bone marrow donor; FGM: French Bone Marrow Registry; HSCs: haematopoietic stem cells.

Importance of quality management in testing

Irrespective of the area, immunohaematology or HLA, tests are conducted in the framework of a certification programme demonstrating the quality of testing and reliability of the results.

According to the ongoing reform of clinical biology, which is yet to be finally approved by France's political bodies, medical testing has 3 stages: pre-analytical, analytical and post-analytical. The laboratory providing the testing is responsible for all these stages. It would be inappropriate to cover the analytical phase here, which

8. Patient testing

is a specialist area, but we would like to examine major points in the pre- or post-analytical stages which can affect patient safety.

Clarifying the collection phase, identifying samples and ordering tests

Collections must be taken and identified in conditions prescribed by regulations. Particular care should be taken when identifying collections, which must provide an accurate link between the sample tube(s), the patient and the tests ordered. This link is now secure in laboratories with the blind double data entry of the identification details noted on the test order and on the tube(s). Laboratories do not check the data entered, however, and numerous inconsistencies are encountered on a daily basis, causing delays and even cancellations in testing. The tubes should be identified by the collection staff immediately after the collection and in the presence of the patient. The information marked on the label should then be verified by asking the patient to confirm his/her identity (open question: "can you tell me your name?"). Failing this, several document types or identity details should be compared. This identification stage can be complicated in emergency or life-threatening situations. It is therefore essential that an internal procedure within the hospital, which is approved by the EFS delivery site or hospital blood bank, makes provision for a temporary method of identification in emergency or life-threatening situations, in which it is sometimes impossible to obtain all personal details immediately. This procedure must also make it possible to link this temporary identity to an LBP prescription and confirm the details as quickly as possible. Despite the training of state-registered nurses and awareness-raising on the subject, cross-checks against immunohaematology or HLA data reveal this type of error all too frequently, which can have very serious consequences in patients. This is why French legislation still requires two blood grouping tests to be conducted on two separate collections prior to transfusion.

As with all medical testing, immunohaematology or HLA tests are ordered by prescription which must bear the prescriber's name and signature. The data shown on the prescription must be precise, legible and accurate, which is often facilitated by the test order forms provided to wards, although it can be written on a blank prescription sheet. The data required by French regulations are:
– surname (surname at birth);
– any other surname (*e.g.* married name);
– date of birth;
– forename(s);
– sex (essential for gender-neutral, unusual or foreign forenames);
– the exact type of tests required;
– essential clinical data: indication of pregnancy with date of the last period, injection of anti-RH immunoglobulin; exact contact details of the mother if it involves a newborn, context of the transplant, etc.;
– the prescriber's name and signature;
– the identification of the hospital and ward;
– the level of emergency, which is not trivialized;
– the date and time of the collection as well as the number of samples provided;
– the name, job title and signature of the collector.

The quality of the samples is also a major point affecting the quality of the results generated.

Finally, before being sent by the collection services and when received by the laboratory, it is essential to compare the details on the test order against the sample tubes. An investigation must be launched in the event of inconsistencies.

Tables XII and XIII present the main nonconformities found in this area and the steps taken by the EFS in response.

Table XII. Nonconformities involving tests.		
Type of noncompliance	**Request refused?**	**Rapid correction possible?**
No tests ordered	No	Yes
Surname and/or forename and/or date of birth not provided (or illegible)	Yes	No
Name of the prescriber not provided (or illegible)	No	Yes
Name of the sampler not provided (or illegible)	No	Yes
Collection date not provided	Yes (except if date shown on the tube)	No
Type of tests not specified	No	Yes
Collection time or name of the sampler not provided / Different samplers for 2 tests ordered at the same time	Yes / One test is conducted / The second is refused	No

Transfusion medicine: the French model

Table XIII. Nonconformities involving samples.		
Type of noncompliance	Request refused?	Rapid correction possible?
No tube	Yes	Not applicable
Surname and/or forename and/or date of birth not provided (or illegible)	Yes	No
Duplicated labelling	Yes	Not applicable
Major discrepancy between the identity details on the prescription and tube	Yes	No
Major discrepancy between the identity details on the prescription, tube and in the records (s and ss, I and II, name ending with and without an s, etc.)	No	Yes
Collection date and time not provided	YES (except if date and time shown on the prescription)	No
Unsuitable tubes	Yes	No
Hemolyzed sample	YES (except transfusion incident or clinical context)	Not applicable
Coagulated sample	YES (if red blood cells required for testing)	Not applicable
Settled serum or plasma	NO (reported on the result)	Not applicable
Insufficient quantity	Yes	Not applicable
Soiled prescription and/or tubes	Yes	No

Transport of samples and timeframe for delivery to the laboratory

Once collected, the samples must be sent to the laboratories in conditions that maintain the quality of the goods and safety of the handlers. Tubes containing biological samples must be placed in an airtight container, covered in an absorbent material and wrapped in protective outer packaging showing the names and addresses of the recipient laboratory and sender. In the event of road transport, the labelling and packaging must comply with current regulations on transporting hazardous materials.

The transfer of samples, conduct of tests and provision of results to the prescriber are essential parameters to ensure patient safety, particularly in the context of urgent transfusions or grafts. The EFS conducts immunohaematology and HLA tests on behalf of many hospital. In standard practice, which has proven effective, the hospital practitioner prescribes the immunohaematology test that may be associated with a LBP request, takes the collection from the patient and sends the sample directly to the EFS laboratory. It performs the final part of the pre-analytical phase, the analytical phase ordered by the prescription and the post-analytical phase, and then sends the result to the prescriber with any opinions, interpretations and recommendations. It is essential that future changes to the regulations do not compromise this chain of events, as it is best suited to managing tests and results in timeframes compatible with safe blood transfusion in patients.

The notion of emergency in laboratory services in general, but especially in the context of urgent transfusions in immunohaematology, and urgent transplants or grafts in HLA, must not be trivialized. The level of emergency must be specified on the test order. It requires the laboratory to conduct the tests as a matter of priority, often within complex and onerous organisational processes, and sometimes to the detriment of other tests. Unfortunately, we can see that the notion of emergency is not always clear, either though misuse or omission.

Availability of the results for the prescriber and cost management

Test results must include a series of informations, which is now fully inscribed in law and provided at the same time especially accompanied as any opinions, interpretations or recommendations. The regulations also allow LBP to be delivered on the basis of a document summarizing the patient's immunohaematology results, which is called the "blood group card".

This blood group card serves to report results and summarize the patient's haematological data, ensuring the immunological safety of transfusion. Pursuant to current French regulations, it must show on one side all the information stipulated in the Order of 26 April 2002, namely (Figure 33):

8. Patient testing

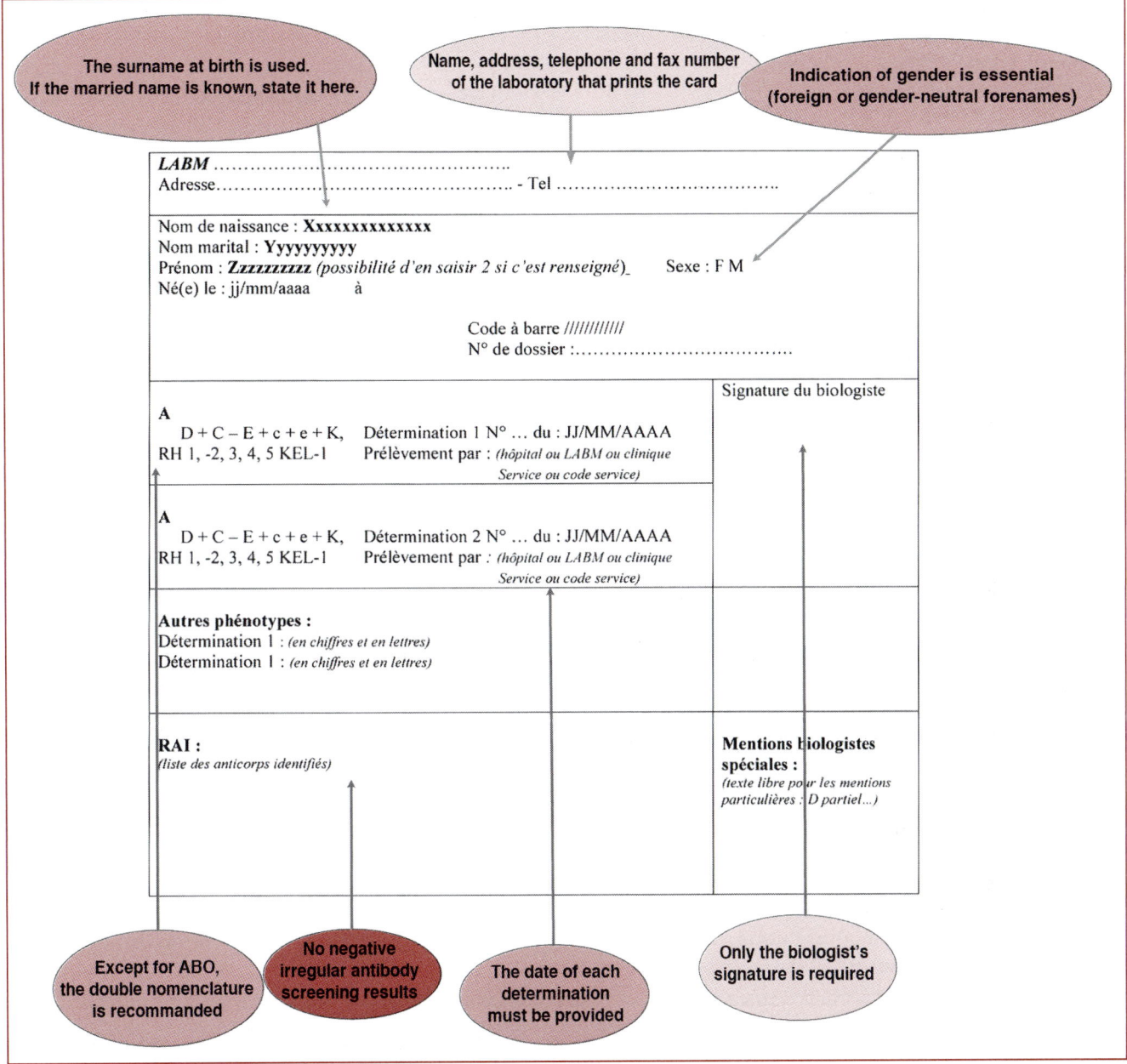

Figure 33. Blood group card.

- details of the laboratory that printed the card (name, address and telephone number);
- details of the patient (surname at birth, followed by any married name, forename(s), sex and date of birth). If the married name changes but all other details remain the same, the card is still valid;
- the result and date of each ABO/RH1 blood grouping and RH/KEL1 phenotyping;
- the presence of one or more irregular antibodies;
- the biologist's signature.

It should be reiterated, however, that blood group cards are not mandatory for the delivery of LBP: delivery can be based on test results. The card must not, in addition, show any handwritten annotations or self-adhesive labels presenting only some of the information. This last point is an important one. When all the information is printed on a single self-adhesive label affixed to a blank index card, the document then complies with the Order of 26 April 2002. A negative irregular antibody screening result should not be shown on a blood group card as this is a *permanent* summary, whilst a negative irregular antibody screening result is potentially transitory. In contrast, if an antibody is identified at any time, it must be stated on the blood group card, even if it becomes undetectable (negative irregular antibody screening), as this may affect a future transfusion.

For the secure transfer of test results to the prescriber or from the prescriber to LBP delivery sites, and data storage in an accessible and permanent computer system, electronic data exchanges are developing rapidly. For technical, strategic and policy-related reasons, however, these exchanges only involve patients within the same hospital. Yet it would make sense to give prescribers across the country access to permanent data such as red cell phenotypes or HLA, which would boost efficiency. The rollout of such a tool would require the prior implementation of a unique national identification number and reliable patient authentication system, as well as a cap on the number of laboratories that can enter data into the system, which could be managed by the EFS. In this area, the savings in immunohaematology and possibly HLA tests should be significant.

Conclusion

The EFS's laboratories are highly specialized, only conducting immunohaematology tests relating to the delivery of LBP and histocompatibility tests that are often prompted directly by a potential graft or transplant. These testing services are provided round the clock across France.

Although the tests are laboratory services, they remain very specific and are not conducted by private laboratories in most cases, particularly complex or out-of-hours tests.

The EFS's laboratories have been involved in a continuous improvement and quality management initiative for some time, enabling them to exceed regulatory requirements in the certification process.

In the French transfusion model, given the organisation of LBP delivery which was laid down by lawmakers in the 1998 Act, the operation of the EFS's laboratories is indispensable to the immunological safety of transfused and grafted patients, and it is essential to remain aware of any regulatory changes that could compromise the current structure and patient safety. Any organisation aiming to establish or strengthen the immunohaematology/delivery link should, however, be promoted.

Key points of the services

The EFS's laboratory services are unique insofar as they are limited to areas linked, for immunohaematology, to the immunological safety of blood transfusion and the monitoring and prevention of prenatal alloimmunization and, for histocompatibility, to providing grafts or transplants. Therefore, all cases involve specialist tests.

Although the EFS currently conducts just under 30% (370 million B) of all immunohaematology testing in France, its 137 sites manage the vast majority of complex, urgent or out-of-hours tests. This internationally recognized management ensures the safety of the immunohaematology/delivery link in LBP, which is essential for transfusion safety.

In histocompatibility, the EFS conducts approximately 50% of tests relating to transplantation, with the remainder managed by hospital laboratories. All these laboratories provide 24-hour services, conducting the tests needed after organ donation and contributing, with the French Biomedicine Agency, to meeting the needs of patients who are awaiting transplant.

The EFS sites conducting immunohaematology or histocompatibility tests are organized within multisite laboratories mirroring the regional organisation of blood establishments and national organisation of the EFS. All support, technical, IT and quality services are also regional, optimizing efficiency. The regional structure of immunohaematology services makes it possible to conduct all the tests needed to ensure the safety of transfused patients in quality assured conditions.

The EFS is ISO 9001 certified and its laboratories have been involved in the 17025 and later the 15189 certification process for many years. By 2013, all the EFS's laboratories will be certified or have submitted their application to Cofrac.

9. Distribution, delivery and transfusion support

Suzanne Assari, Anne François, Francis Roubinet

The primary role of the French Blood Establishment (EFS) is to provide the labile blood products (LBP) needed by patients throughout the country. Product availability can be measured in both quantity and quality terms, *i.e.* a sufficient number and variety of LBP to meet requirements.

To achieve these objectives, pursuant to Act 98-535 of 1 July 1998 on increased health monitoring and greater control over medicinal products for human use, and in line with the plans organizing blood transfusion services (SOTS), the EFS distributes processed blood products from its preparation platforms to patients across France via its 156 delivery sites, representing nearly 850 full-time equivalent staff in the EFS, in addition to the 185 delivery banks, or 443 emergency banks of health facilities. This **"distribution"** must supply the necessary LBP in timeframes compatible with transfusion safety, as well as manage these precious products to reduce wastage and prevent shortages wherever possible. Distribution services also include providing raw plasma material to the French Fractionation Laboratory (LFB), which has a monopoly over the fractionation of voluntary plasma donations in France under the Order of 28 July 2005, so that it can manufacture medicinal products derived from human blood and plasma. The preparation platforms also supply raw plasma material for the manufacture of pathogen reduced fresh frozen plasma by solvent/detergent (SD-FFP).

Staff at the EFS's delivery sites, or who are responsible for providing LBP via delivery or emergency banks, select blood products for a patient on the basis of medical prescription, taking into account the results of essential immunohaematology tests and known patient data (transfusion protocols or instructions) to ensure immunological safety. The selection of LBP for a given patient is called **delivery**. The products transferred to the

Suzanne Assari, suzanne.assari@efs.sante.fr
Anne François, anne.francois@efs.sante.fr
Francis Roubinet, francis.roubinet@efs.sante.fr

prescribing ward must be transfused as quickly as possible, within 6 hours of receipt.

To tailor the prescription to the patient, or if special circumstances arise, the prescribing practitioner can utilize the **transfusion support services** provided by the EFS's transfusion professionals, as required by law.

In the transfusion chain, the **"distribution, delivery and transfusion support"** link is therefore located immediately downstream of the "collection", "preparation" and "testing" phases. Patients' needs dictate the quantity and quality of products to be collected, and coordination with the collection services is indispensable in anticipating needs and possible difficulties. Close relationships are also required with the EFS's specialized preparation and testing platforms to organize the availability of LBP, particularly those with a short lifespan, such as platelet or specific products, and those which undergo secondary processing (*e.g.* plasma removal).

Distribution/delivery also works in synergy with the "patient testing" phase to have, as and when required, the test results needed to select LBP. Their complementarity is one of the key elements of blood transfusion safety.

Optimal use of prepared products and their availability throughout the country was finally achieved using a "stock management" process regulating LBP stock levels primarily in the regions but also nationwide, and a "logistics" process organizing the transport of LBP and maintaining the cold chain whenever they are taken to the sites that need them most.

Distribution/delivery services provide the final link in the donor to recipient chain, taking LBP to patients, recording confirmation of the transfusion in hospital and enabling the downstream "haemovigilance" process to manage follow-up and analyze any adverse reactions.

Medico-technical description of "distribution, delivery and transfusion support" services

Pursuant to European directive 2002/98/EC, "distributing LBP" is defined in the transposing decree of 1 February 2006 as "the supply of labile blood products by a blood establishment to other blood establishments, health facilities managing blood banks, and manufacturers of health products derived from human blood or blood components".

According to this transposing decree, "the delivery of labile blood products is understood to mean making labile blood products available on medical prescription ahead of administration to a given patient". Deliveries must therefore be made on the basis of prescriptions, whilst ensuring the immunological compatibility of the patient and compliance with existing transfusion protocols. By regulations, delivery services can only be provided by an EFS delivery site or the authorized delivery and emergency bank of a hospital blood bank.

The EFS is required to provide transfusion support services to hospitals. The decision of 6 November 2006 defining the principles of good practice outlined in Article L. 1223-3 of the French Public Health Code defines transfusion support as "assistance with choosing treatment by transfusion, prescribing labile blood products, performing transfusions, monitoring recipients and providing the appropriate storage and transport conditions for blood products".

Distribution of labile blood products

Distribution services are provided by two areas of activity:
- preparation platforms, which distribute raw plasma material to the LFB or EFS Aquitaine-Limousin (SD-FFP) and LBP to the various delivery sites of blood establishments (ETS);
- delivery/distribution sites, which generally distribute LBP to the hospital blood banks.

The intraregional distribution of therapeutic LBP, or amongst the various regional ETS, mirrors the organisation of one of these areas of activity.

Distributing raw plasma material to the LFB

A multiannual contract is agreed between the EFS and the LFB to meet the needs of French patients. This contract covers the quantity, quality and specificities of the plasma delivered to the LFB. It also ensures compliance with the "LFB leucocyte-depleted plasma for fractionation" specifications.

Table XIV shows changes in the overall supply of raw plasma material to the LFB since 2006.

Table XIV. Volumes of plasma delivered to the LFB (actual figures).		
	Plasma supplied to the LFB	Change (%)
2006	649,164 L	
2007	694,052 L	6.9%
2008	769,931 L	10.9%
2009	827,740 L	7.5%
2010	854,676 L	3.3%
2011	914,750 L	7.0%
2012	862,074 L	-5.8%

9. Distribution, delivery and transfusion support

The EFS's preparation platforms also distribute raw plasma material to the SD-FFP production unit of EFS Aquitaine-Limousin in Bordeaux. The volume of raw plasma material provided increased by 40% between 2006 and 2012 (Table XV).

Table XV. Number of litres of plasma distributed to the blood establishment of Aquitaine-Limousin to manufacture solvent/detergent-treated plasma (actual figures).		
	Plasma supplied to Bordeaux	Change (%)
2006	26,741 L	
2007	31,417 L	17.5%
2008	34,821 L	10.8%
2009	41,042 L	17.9%
2010	30,418 L	-25.9%
2011	34,765 L	14.3%
2012	37,477 L	7.8%

Distributing labile blood products between blood establishments

- Some ETS (EFS Île-de-France and EFS Alpes-Méditerranée) are unable to collect sufficient LBP to cover the varying needs of their hospitals, which are instead met by ETS with surplus stocks in an annual programme managed at national level.
- In addition, unforeseeable events, bad weather, periods of very high demand and viral outbreaks can destabilize a region, which will then be assisted by another.
- Finally, a fall in demand combined with a rise in donations may lead to LBP being moved from one region to another to avoid wasting these vital products.

To ensure self-sufficiency in every part of the country, national regulation of LBP stocks has been introduced. The distribution of LBP between ETS is therefore organized around the principle of *solidarité*. A national regulation unit based at the EFS's head office monitors the stock levels available across the country. Every day, each ETS provides the regulation unit with details of its stocks of packed red blood cells (PRBCs) per ABO-RH1 group, generating real-time information on the levels in France. ETS are also required to provide the following figures per ABO-RH1 group for the week W-1 and forecasts for the following 8 weeks:
– the number of PRBCs labelled per group;
– the number of PRBCs received or distributed to other regions;
– the number of PRBCs delivered/distributed to hospitals;
– the number of outdated PRBCs.

Figure 34 shows changes in national stock levels over a year as a graph, with forecasts for the following 8 weeks in dotted lines and a long-term simulation based on figures from previous years. Columns represent the stock levels converted into a number of days of distribution/delivery.

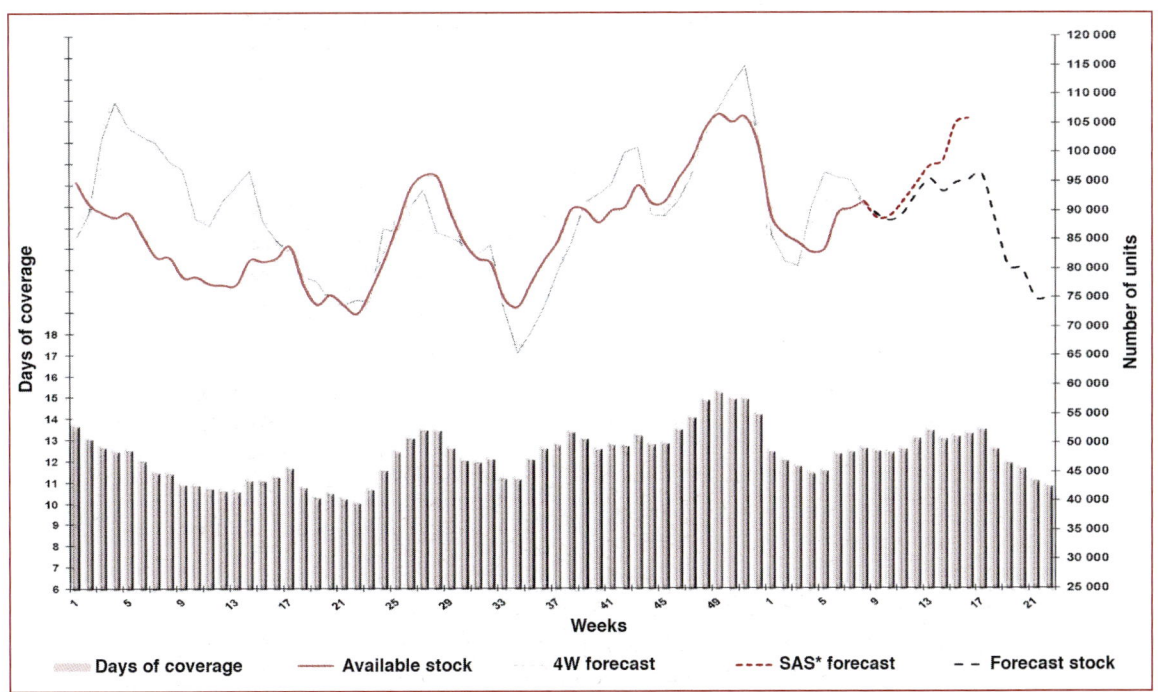

Figure 34. Changes in the national stock levels of packed red blood cells (week 1 in 2012 to week 22 in 2013).
* Stock Supply Software.

Transfusion medicine: the French model

The eight-week forecasts of national stock levels are broken down by region and analyzed. In the event of an extended shortfall in requirements (whether quantitative or qualitative, and in each group), appropriate steps are taken: possible changes to the supply chain, transfer of LBP from one ETS to another, regional or national appeals for blood donors, etc.

In 2012, inter-ETS exchanges of PRBCs represented a volume of just over 250,000 PRBCs.

Distributing LBP within a same ETS

An ETS has between 4 and 25 delivery sites. The supply of LBP from preparation platforms to transfusion sites is organized very differently in each region but always aims to ensure both the quantitative and qualitative availability of LBP to all sites in accordance with established guidelines. Minimum and maximum stock levels are determined for each LBP type and delivery site, which are closely monitored by the distribution services and resupplied as and when required, in line with the availability and frequency of intersite transport.

Transport logistics are of major importance. Managing transportation between the various sites within each regional ETS is a daily challenge. Transport is provided either by ETS drivers or external service providers, which are chosen on the basis of strict criteria. Depending on the distances between the sites and the size of their output, intersite shuttles may run once or several times daily, 5 or 7 days a week. In exceptional circumstances, the use of alternative methods of transport such as taxis may be arranged by the distribution services.

Distributing labile blood products to the blood banks of health facilities

The law allows hospitals to store and deliver LBP with the authorization of the director of the Regional Health Agency (ARS), which is based on the opinion of the French National Agency for Medicines and Health Products Safety (ANSM) and the EFS on the storage and delivery conditions and compliance with SOTS.

A blood bank stores ready-to-use therapeutic LBP under the responsibility of a physician or pharmacist. Authorization to operate a blood bank, which is granted by the director of the ARS, is subject to:
– a signed agreement between the EFS and hospitals;
– written standard operating procedures and the use of suitable equipment;
– a satisfactory inspection at least every 5 years by decentralized government services (ARS), which is often conducted jointly by the Public Health Inspector and Regional Haemovigilance Coordinator.

There are 3 types of blood banks:
- delivery banks, which store the LBP distributed by their referent ETS and deliver them for a patient hospitalized. In 2011, there were 185 delivery banks. They are found in hospitals that provide significant transfusion services (> 500 PRBCs per annum) and are located at some distance from an EFS delivery site (or in areas that are difficult to reach quickly due to heavy traffic);
- emergency banks, which store group O PRBCs and, if necessary, the group AB plasma distributed by their referent ETS, and deliver them for a patient hospitalized in life-threatening situations only. They are found in hospitals that provide complex obstetrical or surgical services and cannot obtain LBP in timeframes compatible with the transfusion-related emergencies they treat. France had 443 emergency banks in 2011;
- holding banks, which store the LBP delivered by their referent ETS for a patient hospitalized and transfer them to the wards at their request.

Only the first 2 types of banks are affected by the distribution process.

For a delivery bank, the composition of stocks is specified in an annex to the agreement and is dependent on the transfusion services provided. Target and minimum stock levels are determined. Similarly, the breakdown of stocks by group and by phenotype is designed to reflect that of the population being served, i.e. transfused patients.

For an emergency bank, the stock of PRBCs is formed by group O PRBCs (RH: -1, -2, -3, 4, 5 KEL: -1; and RH: 1, 2, -3, -4, 5 KEL: -1) to ensure access to products that are compatible for most patients in emergency situations, pending those that will be selected by the delivery site. If the bank stores therapeutic plasma, it is group AB. The quantity of LBP depends on the medicine, surgery, obstetrics and transfusion services provided, as well as the timeframes for supply by the referent ETS.

These LBP banks, which are subject to regulatory monitoring, must work closely with their referent EFS site:
– LBP stocks: the aim is to reduce wastage and destructions insofar as possible;
– premises: access must be limited to authorized personnel and subject to strict hygiene procedures;
– storage equipment: must be maintained, cleaned and its temperature regulation checked on a regular basis. Alarms must be centralized (centralized management technique);
– staff training: employees must be regularly trained and assessed. They must be authorized to perform their duties;
– standard operating procedures, which must be written and recorded.

The referral site inspects the bank annually to check that it is being operated correctly.

9. Distribution, delivery and transfusion support

To optimize availability and protect the resource, it is possible but not recommended to return unused PRBCs. To do this, the PRBCs are placed in temperature-controlled containers providing the appropriate storage conditions. Distributed or delivered LBP can only be returned to stock if there is evidence that they have been stored in regulatory conditions (unbroken cold chain in particular). For blood banks, the agreement outlines the management of returned products. The partners are liable for returning the products to stock, which is detailed in a procedure.

Outside these situations, the LBP can be returned to the ETS in 2 circumstances:
- the LBP are no longer compliant. This involves outdated, spoiled, damaged or soiled LBP, or LBP that have not been used in the regulatory timeframes. These products should be returned to the referent ETS by which they were distributed for destruction. Failing this, the hospital provides the referent ETS with details of the number and type of products, the reason for noncompliance and the date of destruction;
- the LBP are withdrawn by the referent ETS (batch recall of single-use devices, post-donation information, etc.). Depending on the reason for withdrawal, the products are returned to stock, quarantined or destroyed.

LBP stocks within blood banks represent a significant product volume that cannot be mobilized by the EFS (group O RH: -1 in particular). To maintain the resource and safeguard the health of donors, stocks should therefore be kept at strictly essential levels.

Delivery of labile blood products

This aims to "provide *the right product, at the right time* for *the right patient*". To ensure blood transfusion safety, LBP are selected based on the characteristics of the available products, known patient data (immunohaematology and transfusion protocols or instructions) and prescription requirements. The LBP chosen are then cross-matched in the computer system against the patient's immunohaematological status, packaged, provided to the courier and delivered to the hospital ward.

Immunohaematology test results are required for LBP delivery; the collection of samples and ordering of tests must now meet the guidelines outlined in ISO 15189 certification. These tests must also comply with the Order of 26 April 2002 on good laboratory practice in immunohaematology.

At this stage it is worth reiterating the importance of the link between immunohaematology and LBP delivery in safety assurance. The conduct of immunohaematology tests by the same structure that provides delivery makes it possible to have data on recipients in real time and meet the legal requirement that immunohaematology data are transferred electronically to the delivery services. The tests will be conducted on the basis of consistent and confirmed identification data, avoiding any potential delay caused by failure to provide the right documents for the patient in question. The discovery of a rare antibody or phenotype in a patient can considerably extend the delivery timescales due to the unavailability of suitable products. Anticipating and assessing these requirements with the transfusion services and ascertaining the number of compatible LBP available as soon as the discovery is made will make the transfusion easier to organize. If crossmatching is necessary, the possibility of accessing the sample onsite shortens the testing timeframes and removes the need for further patient samples. Similarly, if an adverse reaction occurs during or after the transfusion, the availability of pre- and post-transfusion samples as well as the LBP transfused in a same structure makes it possible to conduct all necessary tests.

Transfusion emergencies

To improve the management of transfusions in postpartum haemorrhage, 3 levels of emergency, which were recommended by multidisciplinary experts in 2002, are now established in law and must be shown on the LBP prescription.

These levels define the availability timeframes of LBP and how they should be selected if immunohaematology tests are unavailable:
- **immediate life-threatening emergency:** situations in which LBP must be provided ***without delay***. If immunohaematology tests are not available, the LBP are delivered before the results are known. The PRBCs given are group O, either RH: -1, KEL: -1 or RH: 1, KEL: -1;
- **life-threatening emergency:** situations in which LBP must be provided in **less than 30 minutes**. If immunohaematology tests are not available, the LBP are delivered insofar as possible with the confirmed ABO-RH1 groups and RH-KEL1 phenotypes. The results of irregular antibody screening will be known at a later stage (allocation of PRBCs). The PRBCs given will be ABO, possibly RH-KEL1 phenotype, identical or compatible;
- **relative emergency:** situations in which LBP are often provided within *2 to 3 hours*. This timeframe makes it possible to conduct all immunohaematology tests:
  – confirmed ABO-RH1 groups;
  – confirmed RH-KEL1 phenotypes;
  – irregular antibody screening.

The LBP provided will be ABO identical or compatible, and perhaps cross-matched in the event of positive irregular antibody screening.

The level of emergency, particularly life-threatening and immediate life-threatening emergencies, must be specified on the prescription. Whenever possible, the prescribing ward will telephone the delivery service or blood bank to check that the prescription has been received and the level of emergency understood. Finally, the number of transfusion emergencies must, insofar as possible, be limited to confirmed cases.

It is therefore important to implement a system for organizing product delivery in emergency situations, particularly life-threatening emergencies. The hospital must produce a written procedure, which is approved by the ETS delivery site or hospital blood bank, detailing the means of obtaining LBP (telephone number, fax number, materials and means of transport, particularly if there is no transfusion site in the vicinity of the hospital or delivery bank onsite). Some establishments, particularly maternity hospitals, may encounter these emergency situations very rarely – just 1% of women experience postpartum haemorrhage and not all require transfusions – and only the availability of an updated procedure can guarantee effective transfusion management.

One essential point is to make provision for a temporary means of identification in immediate life-threatening emergencies or disaster situations in which personal details cannot always be accessed immediately. This procedure must also make it possible to link this temporary identity to an LBP prescription and update it as soon as the details are known.

Receiving the prescription of labile blood products and immunohaematology results

On receiving the prescription, the delivery service staff timestamp the paperwork and check very attentively:
– the consistency between the prescription and immunohaematology documents;
– the compliance of the prescription;
– the validity of the immunohaematology documents;
– the consistency between the personal details shown on the LBP prescription and on the immunohaematology documents provided.

Incorrect merging of records and incomplete verifications, which cause delays in transfusions, are frequent errors in wards.

Medical testing laboratories are often asked to provide replacement blood group cards. This is unfortunate as there is still no reliable patient identification and authentication system, meaning that there is a real risk of mistakenly printing the results of patients with the same name, which could ultimately lead to a haemolytic accident.

Particular attention is required if prescriptions and immunohaematology documents are sent by fax.

Compliance of the prescription

An LBP prescription is a medical document for which the prescriber is liable. It is often written on a pre-printed document but nothing prevents the use of a blank prescription sheet. It is essential to identify the patient on the prescription: surname at birth; any other surname (*e.g.* married name); forename(s); date of birth; and sex. The prescription also states:
- the number, type and any preparation or processing of the LBP requested;
- for the prescription of platelets: the date and result of the last platelet count, the patient's weight and the required posology;
- for the prescription of plasma, the indication for which the prescription is written;
- the name of the ward and requesting establishment (and telephone number);
- the prescriber's name;
- the level of emergency, if any;
- the date of prescription;
- in non-emergencies, the required date and time of delivery.

The request is provided, where appropriate, with useful clinical and biological information, in line with patient confidentiality, and any transfusion protocols. Pending the widespread use of software making it possible to receive only fully completed and wholly legible prescriptions, many of these requests are noncompliant and require the delivery staff to contact the ward to obtain essential information.

The sooner the prescription is sent after being written, the longer the delivery services will have to correct non-conformities and, if necessary, arrange the supply of suitable products.

Validity of the immunohaematology documents and transfer

Immunohaematology documents must meet the legal requirements and be transferred to the delivery unit electronically. To compare the patient's immunohaematology data and the LBP automatically on the computer system, it is essential that these data are available in the software of the delivery services (ETS transfusion site or hospital blood bank). The simplest scenario is when the same structure conducts the immunohaematology tests and delivers the LBP. The data are then automatically available through blood transfusion software. The situation is much more complicated when the tests are conducted by a separate laboratory and must then be transferred by the ERA system, which imports the results into the patient database. This system provides vital services but requires a specific connection between each laboratory and delivery site. This connection may only be used after several validation tests conforming that

9. Distribution, delivery and transfusion support

data are transferred correctly. Some regions have managed to implement this system to a large extent, but many laboratories in France seldom or never use it. Analysis of the risk that the supplier reconfigures or updates the software, leaving the laboratory with a new and unfamiliar version, has shown that errors could be generated in the messages sent. The ANSM has only authorized use of the system if the data import by ERA is based on the laboratory's paper results and once these have been checked against the imported results.

On "Reservation" prescriptions: the decision of 6 November 2006 states that "if LBP are reserved prior to delivery, a clear procedure outlines the reservation process and the checks to be made before the products are provided to staff in the health facility or service provider responsible for transportation". To ensure the availability of LBP, many hospitals wards write "reservation" prescriptions for LBP, particularly platelet concentrates. This reservation also makes it possible to check that the records are complete and that the delivery could be made immediately when triggered. The practice should be interpreted as cooperation between the hospitals and EFS to optimize the management of LBP and best meet patients' needs.

Any noncompliance at this stage should be managed with the help of the prescribing ward. Some nonconformities are major and block delivery (*e.g.* number or type of LBP not specified), whilst others only require additional information and must not delay delivery in life-threatening situations.

Selecting or creating the patient in the delivery site's blood management software

Locating and selecting the patient's records in the computer system are complex tasks and no method is entirely secure. In databases with several million files, many patients have the same surname and date of birth, or the same surname, forename and very similar date of birth. Therefore, some files are duplicates with different ABO-RH1 groups or RH-KEL1 phenotypes. Incorrectly recording name changes, *i.e.* after marriage, adds to the complexity of the problem, as do spelling mistakes. One solution would be the use of a unique, permanent, national and accessible patient ID number. The French Agency for Shared Health Information Systems (ASIP) is currently developing a health system ID number. The implementation of such a system will be an important factor in blood transfusion safety in coming years.

There are 2 possible scenarios:
- either the patient is not recognized in the computer system, in which case the delivery staff create a record and enter the results of immunohaematology tests by ERA import or manual double data entry;
- or the patient is recognized in the computer system, in which case the immunohaematology results are matched against those that have already been entered in the blood management software (LMT), and the products prescribed are compared with any transfusion protocols or instructions. Any discrepancy between the prescription and protocol will prompt contact with the prescribing ward to check the validity of the request, supplement the protocol if the indication is justified or amend the prescription if a mistake has been made.

Selecting labile blood products

Staff then select the LBP in accordance with the quantitative and qualitative criteria specified in the prescription. Limiting matched RH-KEL1 phenotypes to young people, particularly women, and subjects who may receive repeated transfusions is very common in France (over 70% of deliveries) but not systematic as the median age of recipients is sixty-nine. Outside protocols that require the use of specific LBP, the LBP with the shortest expiry date will be chosen. LBP storage areas should be organized to reflect this practice, optimize stock management and reduce wastage, which is unacceptable financially and moreover ethically.

Some protocols require LBP that have undergone secondary processing, such as irradiation or plasma removal. The organisation must create process flows for these products as stocks may be formed. These transformations on the processing site or on a specific site that is also a distribution/delivery unit or preparation platform.

The barcodes of selected products are scanned and entered into the patient's records, and the immunohaematology data on the LBP are automatically compared to the patient's test results. If incompatibilities are detected, the delivery is blocked in the system and an investigation is launched.

If, however, the system validates the delivery, delivery form(s) are automatically printed. The delivery form is a legally required document presenting data on both the patient and delivery in the same format, which is used to create a paper trail of the use of LBP. It shows the patient's personal and administrative details as well as summarizing essential information on his/her immunohaematological status and any transfusion protocols or instructions. Every LBP that is delivered is identified alphanumerically with its number, description, ABO/RH1 groups and RH-KEL1 phenotypes, in addition to the date and time of release by the computer system. A delivery form is printed for each product type as it must remain with the products and different LBP have different storage requirements. This delivery form includes a space for recording receipt by the ward and reiterates that two further controls are required by regulations to be made in the presence of the patient prior to the transfusion (document consistency check and final compatibility check for PRBCs). The ward can use several designated areas to confirm the transfusion, record the date and time, and show that the final control was made at the patient's bedside. Several copies of the delivery form are printed, on carbon paper or otherwise, with the exact number dependent on how many are needed by the hospitals to manage the transfusion records and haemovigilance data. At least one copy is returned or faxed to the EFS to enter the complete product traceability details into the computer system and another is filed in the patient's transfusion records. Electronic tools transferring the traceability data contained in the delivery form are being developed and introduced.

A final check of the coherency and consistency of all the information and documents is made when the "package" is delivered, matching the medical prescription data, delivery form and immunohaematology test results against the LBP delivered for the last time. This final check is recorded and initialled by the person who makes it. Once delivered, the form must be stamped to show the actual time of delivery if the order has been prepared in advance.

In practice, 2 situations are then possible:
- the LBP are quickly provided to the courier sent to collect them and packaged for transport (in suitable containers, eutectic if necessary, depending on the method of transport and journey time);
- the LBP are put on standby and stored at the appropriate temperature, often with the aforementioned documents.

Providing labile blood products to the courier

Providing LBP to the courier for transportation to the prescribing ward is an important stage. Good delivery practice states that the person authorized by the prescribing ward presents a document specifying which LBP are to be collected and identifying the recipient (prescription, copy of the prescription, blood group card, waybill, etc.). The phased introduction of patient data transfer systems has considerably increased the likelihood of having such a document. Yet records of the mistakes made at this point, which remains one of the most critical, show that, although available, the document is poorly verified, if at all. Analysis of incidents in the transfusion chain shows that mistakenly providing the courier with products prepared for another patient is the initial error that, through carelessness and failure to follow the checking procedures, leads to inappropriate transfusion.

Volumes of labile blood products delivered in France

Figures 35, 36 and 37 show changes in the delivery of PRBCs, plasmas and platelets over the last 6 years.

We can note a constant rise in PRBC deliveries in the last 6 years, giving a total increase of +20.5% over that period.

In 2011, 86.2% of PRBCs were delivered by the EFS's delivery sites and 13.8% by hospital blood banks.

The delivery of therapeutic plasma and platelet products (in number of bags) also increased significantly by +32% and +28.9% between 2006 and 2012.

Furthermore, the proportion of pools of standard platelet concentrates (P-SD-PC) in total platelet deliveries rose dramatically from +18.4% in 2006 to +51.3% in 2012.

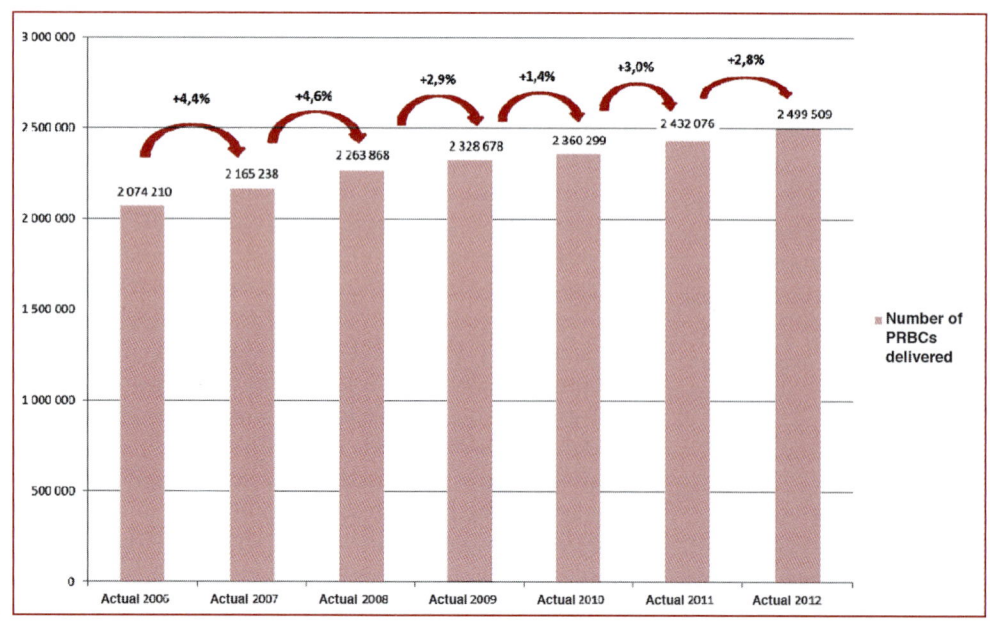

Figure 35. Changes in the number of packed red blood cells delivered.

9. Distribution, delivery and transfusion support

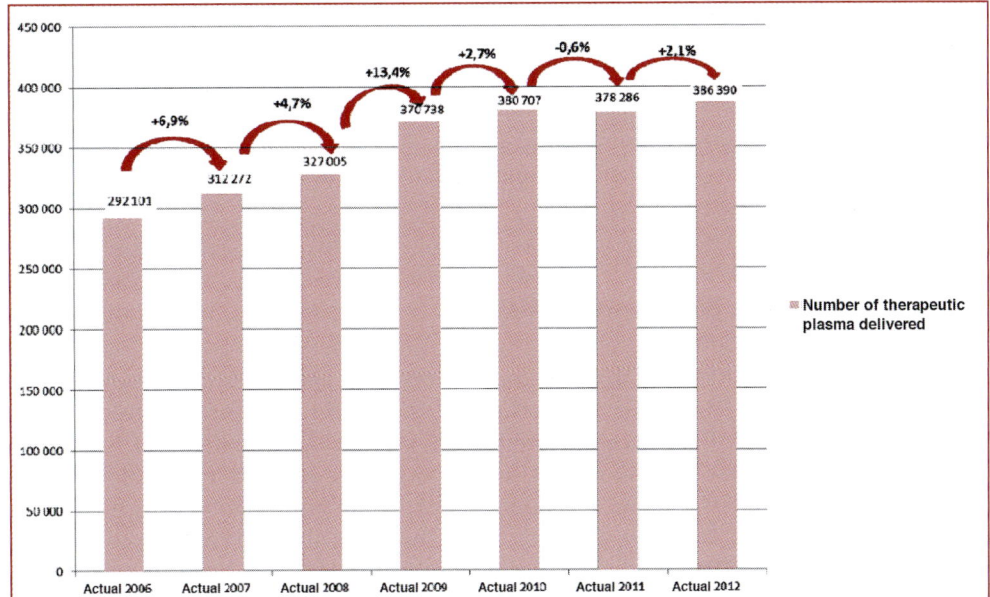

Figure 36. Changes in the amount of therapeutic plasma delivered.

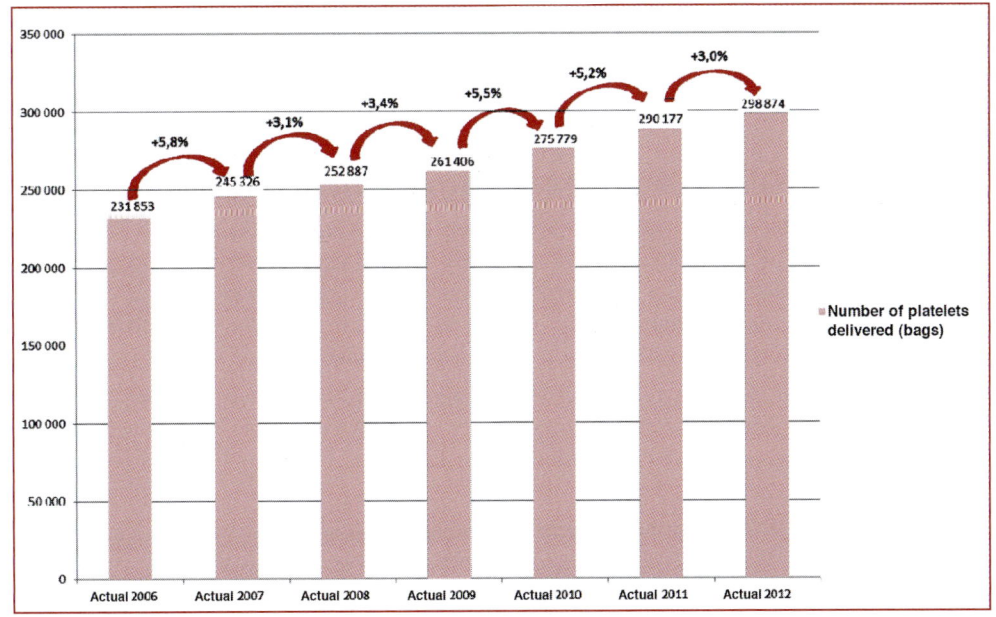

Figure 37. Changes in the platelets delivered (in number of bags).

Transfusion support

Transfusion support provides personalized assistance within the transfusion sector, i.e. the right product at the right time, which is suitable for the patient and/or the condition. It also fulfils a public health role, with consistent support across the country limiting the quality and quantity of products delivered to the strict minimum in order to guarantee the availability and optimal use of this rare and precious resource.

Good practice makes provision for the constant availability of transfusion support provided by physicians who specialize in blood transfusion (postgraduate qualification in haematology, transfusion medicine or proficiency in transfusion technology).

This transfusion support is made available to prescribers and health professionals to bring them everything they need to ensure blood transfusion safety (guidance on prescriptions, information on the various LBP, managing transfusion incidents, etc.), as well as delivery sites, to suggest changing a prescription to better meet patients' needs, or even to recommend withholding transfusions. By law, transfusion support is a very broad field. All the staff in the EFS's delivery services help the healthcare professionals in hospitals provide transfusion services on a daily basis, often sharing data with prescribers and proposing, with the approval of a physician, different LBP to those prescribed. Finally, in the framework of Transfusion Safety and Haemovigilance Committees (CSTH), working with the EFS to develop transfusion protocols on emergency situations and manage conditions for which recommended clinical practices are not formally recorded should be encouraged.

In its public health role, transfusion support must be consistent across the country, with the same education provided to the different stakeholders. This education must make them aware of their contribution to the correct use of LBP and only in indications that require them. Our aim is to meet approved indications and embrace therapeutic innovations but also to safeguard the ethical donation model based on anonymous, voluntary and unpaid blood donors, which can only exist and continue in a context of permanent national self-sufficiency. If the growing demand for LBP is warranted, significant steps should be taken with blood donors to maintain this self-sufficiency. Transfusion support providers must realize that they too are links in the ethical donation chain and contribute to maintaining self-sufficiency through the appropriate prescription and delivery of LBP.

Conclusion

LBP distribution, delivery and transfusion support are the last actions of the ETS's transfusion site or blood bank before the transfusion. They are subject to specific regulation, which must be adhered to at all times to ensure patient safety. Strict compliance with guidelines by delivery staff should reduce immunological risk, which is the biggest risk in blood transfusion, considerably.

Key points of the services

Act 98-535 of 1 July 1998 on increased health monitoring and greater control over medicinal products for human use gave the EFS authority over the management and delivery of LBP across France, with the primary aim that any patient can receive the right blood products at the right time anywhere in the country.

The EFS's services are structured pursuit to the decree on plans organizing blood transfusion services (SOTS). In line with the SOTS, the EFS delivers 86% of PRBCs from 156 sites throughout the country. The remaining 14% are provided by 185 delivery hospital blood banks that provide significant transfusion services but are located at some distance from an EFS site. The management of LBP within these delivery banks is shared between the EFS and the hospitals, which regularly exchange unused products to limit wastage.

Finally, the needs of patients who require LBP as a matter of extreme urgency are also met by 443 emergency banks, whose role is limited to immediately life-threatening emergencies and covering the time needed for immunohaematology tests to be conducted and other LBP provided by an EFS site. In terms of quantity, these services are very small.

The EFS is also responsible for providing transfusion support via its specialist physicians and so contributing to managing the use of LBP (already among the lowest levels in Europe) and tailoring the transfused product to the specific needs of patients.

Impact of the ageing of the population on the use of packed red blood cells in France

Since 2002, the EFS's annual reports have revealed an increase in the issue of PRBCs following more than fifteen years of decline. This increase appears to be permanent and is accelerating year on year, bringing the patterns of blood collection and LBP issue closer together. In this context, there is a risk of shortage if collections are unable to meet additional needs in PRBCs.

The EFS conducted a national, retrospective, observational study to examine the impact of population growth, particularly the ageing of the population, on changes to the use of PRBCs and the number of transfusion recipients (2002-2010). It also aimed to provide forecasts of these indicators for coming years (2011-2020).

For the study period and all transfusion regions, the number of recipients who received at least one PRBC per annum (by age and sex) was obtained from the EFS database. The breakdown of the French population by age, sex and *département* for the years in question and population forecasts for 2010 to 2020 were provided by the French National Institute for Statistics and Economic Studies (INSEE). Changes in the use of PRBCs, number of recipients and average number of PRBCs transfused per patient were analyzed by age group, thousand inhabitants and region.

The results of the study show that the number of PRBCs transfused rose from 1,830,540 in 2002 to 2,324,001 in 2010 and the number of recipients from 366,162 to 491,406, giving increases of 27% and 34.2% respectively. These figures can be explained, in part, by population growth with 14.5% of the increase in the number of PRBCs transfused and 16% of the increase in the number of recipients linked thereto.

If all the factors determining the use of PRBCs were to remain stable between 2010 and 2020, population growth would lead to a 14.8% rise in the number of PRBCs transfused and a 16% rise in the number of recipients. These increases would be generated primarily by the 60–74 age group, as well as people aged 85 and over.

Many factors affect the use of PRBCs and population growth only explains part of the increase. To better gauge future needs, we must consider the rise in morbidity and changing transfusion and treatment practices, particularly those based on professional guidelines and consensus. The reorganisation of the health system and the impact of certain conditions, with a specific geographic split, should also be taken into account.

In conclusion, this study provides an accurate snapshot of the demography of transfused patients in France. It should be followed by more specialist studies on the role of transfusion support in the therapeutic strategies of various diseases.

10. Transfusion

Jacques Chiaroni, Rémi Courbil, Suzanne Mathieu-Nafissi, Jean-François Quaranta

The development of medicine and surgery has always been dependent on blood transfusion. In France, the users of labile blood products (LBP) are the wards of public, private, semi-private and even military health facilities (ES). A small number of LBP transfusions are also carried out in the health centres of the French Blood Establishment (EFS).

Over 550,000 patients are transfused in France each year, using over 3,000,000 LBP. Most LBP are supplied by the EFS's delivery sites.

> **Key figures on transfusion services in France**
>
> The main figures on transfusion services in 2011 show:
> - 568,513 patients transfused in nearly 1,900 ES;
> - 3,122,330 LBP delivered with 99.45% traceability (records of how the LBP is used);
> - LBP are delivered:
>   – in 86.2% of cases by one of the EFS's 156 delivery sites;
>   – in 13.8% of cases by one of the 185 hospital delivery blood banks (amongst the 628 blood banks);
> - the ratio of transfused LBP is 49.37 per 1,000 inhabitants;
> - the rate of transfused patients is 8.7 per 1,000 inhabitants;
> - on average, each transfused patient receives 5.5 LBP.

In the transfusion mapping, the "transfusion" process is the finale link in the chain. However, this process cannot be safely provided without constant exchanges and shared knowledge with the "distribution, delivery and transfusion support" process. Relations between these two links should be particularly close.

Jacques Chiaroni, jacques.chiaroni@efs.sante.fr
Rémi Courbil, remi.courbil@efs.sante.fr
Suzanne Mathieu-Nafissi, suzanne.mathieu-nafissi@efs.sante.fr
Jean-François Quaranta, quaranta.jf@chu-nice.fr

EFS health centres

The physicians in blood establishments (ETS) have always performed procedures such as bloodletting, which is similar to blood donation in practical terms, as well as transfusing LBP.

Since 2009, patients who are treated by bloodletting have been able to give blood as donors if there is no contraindication to doing so. The bloodletting-cum-blood donation scheme contributes to national self-sufficiency in LBP.

Aphaeresis, a technique that was initially used to take plasma and platelets from blood donors via automated cell separators, has been developed in patients to treat or collect various blood components.

The creation of the EFS made it possible to form a network of health centres (CDS). Authority over the CDS changed hands with the publication of new laws on their operating licences in 2010, which are now granted by the Regional Health Agencies (ARS).

The CDS of the EFS are fully involved in the quality process: each one has ISO 9001 certification and most have JACIE accreditation [Joint Accreditation Committee-ISCT (Europe) & EBMT] for the collection of cells for cell therapy.

The EFS's medical care network is organized into 91 CDS across France. The services provided by the CDS include so-called minor procedures like bloodletting, transfusions or perfusions, and more complex procedures including therapeutic aphaeresis, plasma exchanges, low density lipoprotein (LDL) aphaeresis, red cell exchanges, erythrapheresis (hemodilution), leukapheresis and thrombapheresis, as well as taking haematopoietic stem cells (HSCs) and mononuclear cells (MNC) from patients and donors.

62 CDS solely provide bloodletting. Activities in the others are more varied. 23 CDS are multipurpose and located alongside hospitals, treating their patients either on the ETS site or on their own wards.

The total CDS workforce includes approximately 30 reception staff, 60 nurses and 40 physicians.

In 2012, the CDS of the EFS carried out **54,684 bloodlettings** and managed 16,439 others in the framework of blood donation, **6,367 transfusions of packed red blood cells and 889 of platelet concentrates**, 1,381 perfusions, 3,413 plasma exchanges, 3,275 collections of blood HSCs, including 430 collections of allogenic cells in related and unrelated donors, 160 autologous MNC and 88 allogenic MNC, 2,602 extracorporeal photochemotherapy procedures, of which 1,382 using the "closed" technique and 1,220 using the "open" technique, 1,243 red cell exchanges, 323 LDL aphaeresis, 298 erythrapheresis, 59 leukapheresis and 14 thrombapheresis, giving a total of **11,152 therapeutic aphaeresis procedures**. They also contributed to 542 donations for planned autologous transfusion and 16,293 samples for laboratory workups.

Bloodletting is aimed at iron overload patients – genetic haemochromatosis and metabolic syndromes – and more rarely other conditions such as polycythaemia or porphyria cutanea tarda.

Transfusions are performed in anaemia or thrombocytopenia of various causes but primarily in patients with haematological diseases.

Plasma exchanges remove the patient's plasma and replace it with healthy plasma (from blood donors), alone or in combination with ionic, macromolecules or other solutions such as human albumin. They are performed in a wide range of conditions such as thrombotic microangiopathies and various autoimmune diseases.

Red cell exchanges remove the patient's red blood cells and replace them with healthy red cells from donors. The main condition here is sickle-cell anaemia, a severe blood disorder that causes chronic pain and strokes in young subjects. Treatment is provided in an emergency setting during a sickle-cell crisis, preventively over the long term or on an ad-hoc basis, *e.g.* before surgery.

Other forms of therapeutic aphaeresis are less common. **Leukapheresis** removes excess white blood cells from patients, *e.g.* in leukaemia. **Thrombapheresis** removes excess platelets during thrombocythemia.

Cell separators can also collect **peripheral stem cells for cell therapy** and enable the conduct of HSC transplants.

Extracorporeal photochemotherapy collects the patient's MNC, which are exposed to UV light in the presence of a photoactivatable drug. These cells are then reinjected into the patient, where they provoke changes in immune cells. This technique is used in T-cell mediated diseases such as cutaneous T-cell lymphoma or graft-versus-host disease in HSC allograft recipients.

Therefore the EFS's CDS contribute, albeit modestly, to the transfusion of LBP in the same way as ES wards. Many of their services involve bloodletting but they also provide a wide range of medical procedures that benefit patients.

Medico-technical description of "transfusion" services

In France, transfusion is a medical procedure that can be delegated to midwives or State-registered nurses, provided that a physician is able to intervene at any time.

The physician is responsible for the transfusion he/she prescribes and must ensure that the person to whom he/she delegates the procedure is able to carry it out.

Justification of the transfusion of labile blood products

Transfusion is a replacement therapy that helps patient to overcome some long or short hurdle. Evaluation of the benefit-to-risk ratio must be repeated on each occasion. The decision to provide transfusions must always be based on individual circumstances, discussion and valid reasoning (Table XVI).

Transfusion of packed red blood cells

The primary aim of transfusing packed red blood cells (PRBCs) is to improve tissue oxygenation in a context of haemoglobin deficiency (anaemia).

The symptoms of anaemia depend on its intensity, speed of onset, and the age and health of the subject.

The main clinical signs are pallor (skin, musocal membranes, linings), asthenia (chronic anaemia), intense thirst (acute anaemia), rapid heartbeat with shortness of breath on exertion and then at rest, signs of cerebral anoxia: headaches, dizziness, ringing in the ears, floaters and even coma [haemoglobin (Hb) < 3 g/dL in a healthy subject].

Poor clinical tolerance of anaemia justifies the transfusion decision.

The following laboratory values, analyzed against the backdrop of the speed of blood loss and clinical tolerance, are used to determine the justification for transfusion:

- Hb ≥ 10 g/dL = no justification for transfusion;
- 6 g/dL < Hb < 10 g/dL = signs of anaemia intolerance, as well as certain surgical and obstetrical circumstances, justify the transfusion;
- Hb ≤ 6 g/dL = transfusion necessary (Figure 38).

Note that when Hb is < 8 g/dL, there is an increased risk of bleeding.

The quantity of PRBCs to transfuse is the minimum amount needed to alleviate signs of poor tolerance and/or to bring the Hb concentration up to acceptable levels.

There are various formulas for calculating the number of PRBCs to transfuse. However, as a general rule, we estimate that 1 PRBC increases Hb by 1 g/dL in adults and 4 g/dL in children.

Table XVI. Indication of the main determinations or processing of labile blood products.

Packed red blood cells (PRBCs)			Aphaeresis platelet concentrate (APC) and PRBCs		
RH/KEL1 phenotyping	Cross-matching	Extended phenotyping	Irradiation	CMV negative	Plasma removal
As a general rule, any patient with a reasonable life expectancy Otherwise, on a mandatory basis: women of childbearing age, recipients of multiple transfusions, immunized patients (IAS positive or previously shown to be positive)	Immunized patients (positive IAS and/or history of irregular antibodies)	Complex alloimmunization	Immunosuppression In utero or exsanguinous transfusion Massive transfusion in premature neonates Transplant of haematopoietic, autologous or allogenic stem cells	Pregnant women Newborns or foetuses Lung transplant Allograft of haematopoietic stem cells	Intolerance to plasma protein History of post-transfusion purpura

IAS: irregular antibody screening; CMV: cytomegalovirus.

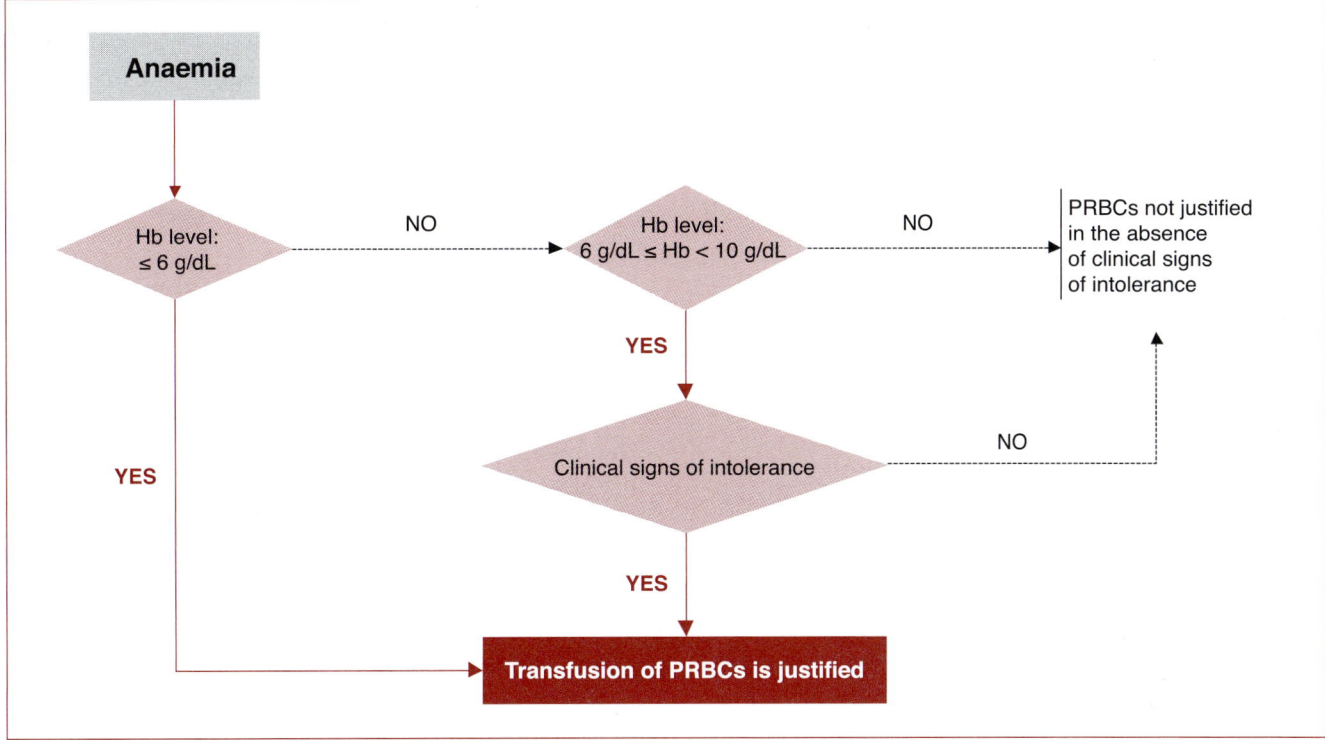

Figure 38. Criteria for transfusion of packed red blood cells.
Hb: haemoglobin; PRBCs: packed red blood cells.

Depending on the particular aim, the effectiveness of the transfusion can be measured in clinical and biological terms (alleviation of the signs of poor tolerance of anaemia and Hb levels after 24 hours).

Transfusion of platelet concentrates

The primary aim of transfusing platelet concentrates (from aphaeresis or whole blood) is to improve the haemostasis process in a context of decreased platelet production (central thrombocytopenia) or, more rarely, congenital platelet disorders.

The laboratory values for transfusion are different in a medical or surgical context.

In a surgical context:
- platelet count > 50 G/L = no justification for transfusion;
- 50 G/L ≤ platelet count ≤ 100 G/L = factors increasing the risk of haemorrhage and limiting the platelet yield (cf. text box 1) and certain surgical procedures (neurosurgery and ophthalmic or ENT surgery) justify the transfusion;
- platelet count < 50 G/L = transfusion necessary.

In a medical context (particularly in oncology):
- platelet count > 100 G/L = no justification for transfusion;
- 10 G/L ≤ platelet count ≤ 50 G/L = factors affecting the platelet yield and any invasive procedure (insertion of a central venous catheter, lumbar puncture, lymph node biopsy, etc.) justify the transfusion;
- platelet count < 10 G/L = transfusion necessary (Figure 39).

A preventive approach recommends systematic transfusions when the platelet level is < 10 G/L. A curative approach only considers transfusions when there are signs of haemorrhage, irrespective of the level (cf. text box 2).

Text box 1

Haemorrhage risk factors:
- Anticoagulant treatment (DIC, fibrinolysis): platelet transfusion for a cutoff ≤ 50 G/L;
- Invasive procedure (lumbar puncture, medullary biopsy, central catheter), digestive endoscopy with biopsy, bronchial endoscopy with bronchoalveolar lavage or brushing, liver biopsy, transbronchial biopsy, dental avulsion: platelet transfusion for a cutoff ≤ 50 G/L (the transfusion is given prior to the procedure and controlled with a platelet count);
- Fever ≥ 38.5 °C, infection, arterial hypertension, mucositis grade ≥ 2, potential bleeding lesions (brain tumour or invasion, endoluminal lesion or tumour), sudden drop in the platelet count in 72 hours: platelet transfusion for a cutoff ≤ 20 G/L.

The quantity of platelets to transfuse is 1 unit (0.5×10^{11} platelets) per 7 kg of weight in adults and 1 unit (0.5×10^{11} platelets) per 5 kg of weight in children.

There are various formulas for calculating the number of platelet units to transfuse. However, as a general rule, it is estimated that 1 unit per 7 kg of weight increases the platelet count by 30 G/L in adults (for the same result, the posology is doubled in children).

Depending on the particular aim, the effectiveness of the transfusion can be measured in clinical and biological terms (stoppage of bleeding and platelet count after 24 hours).

> **Text box 2**
> Clinical signs of bleeding justify transfusion:
> • External haemorrhage, irrespective of the source;
> • Petechiae purpura and extensive ecchymosis;
> • Extensive, painful and compressive haematoma;
> • Retinal haemorrhage visible at the back of the eye;
> • Haemorrhagic blisters in the mouth;
> • Disorders of consciousness, sudden vision problems, headache, other neurological signs of sudden onset (suspected cerebral haemorrhage).

Transfusion of therapeutic plasma

The primary aim of transfusing therapeutic plasma is to compensate for abnormal haemostasis in hemorrhagic shock.

Abnormal haemostasis is defined as fibrinogen < 1 g/L, a prothrombine ratio (PR) < 40% and an activated cephalin time (ACT) > 1.5 to 1.8 times the control value.

The benefit of therapeutic plasma has also been shown for plasma exchanges in thrombotic thrombocytopenic purpura and haemolytic-uremic syndrome in adults, as well as hemorrhagic disease of the newborn (Figure 40).

The quantity of plasma to transfuse is 10 to 15 mL/kg in adults and children (posology doubled or even tripled in the case of plasma exchanges).

The plasma is thawed to 37°C, requiring fifteen to twenty minutes for 200 mL of plasma.

The effectiveness of the transfusion can be measured in clinical and biological terms (stoppage of bleeding and normalization of the PR and ACT).

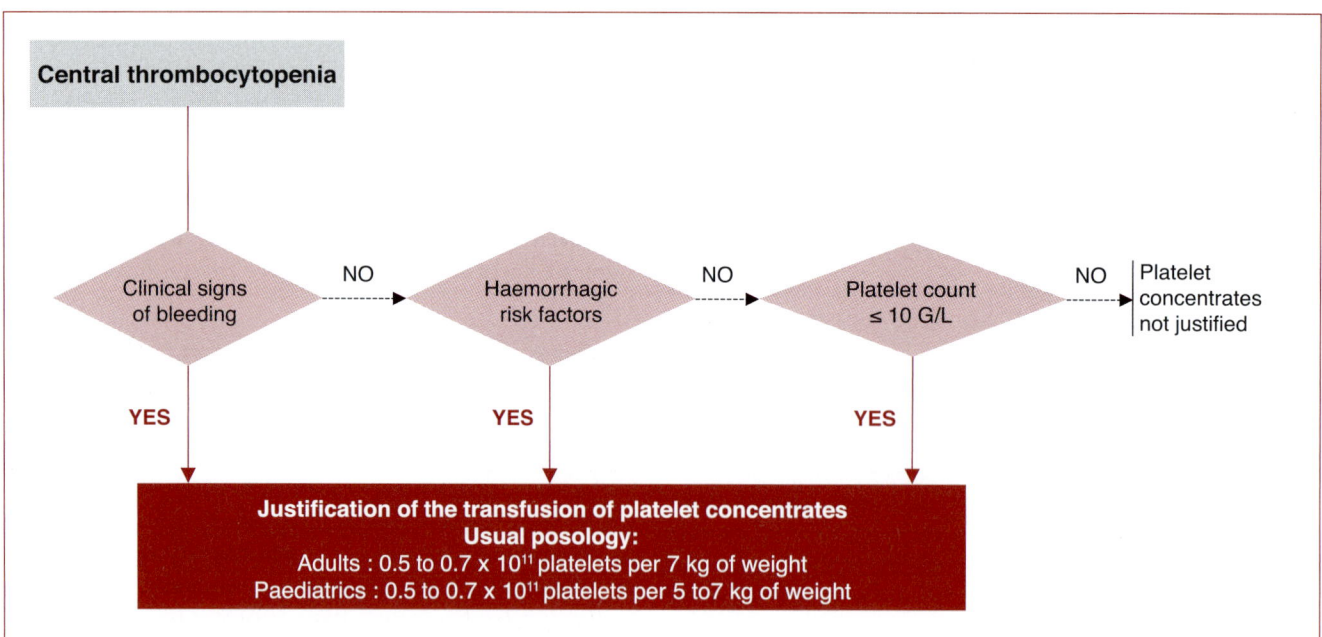

Figure 39. Criteria for transfusion of platelet concentrates.

10. Transfusion

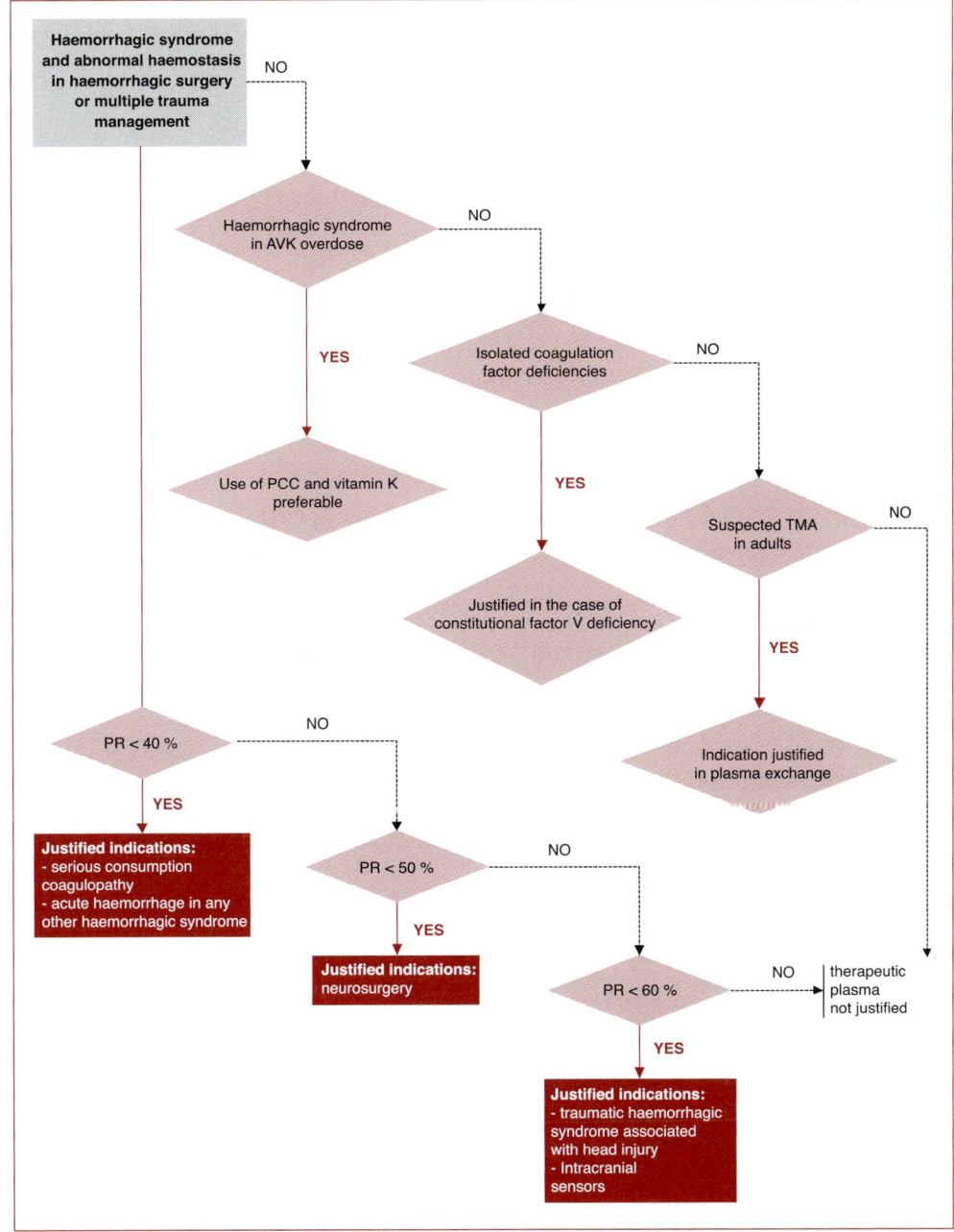

Figure 40. Criteria for transfusion of therapeutic plasmas. AVK: anti-vitamin K; PCC: phrothrombine complex concentrate; TMA: thrombotic microangiopathy; PR: prothrombine ratio.

Prescribing the main labile blood products

An LBP prescription is a medical document for which the prescriber is liable (*cf.* Chapter 9 page 87). The prescription of LBP is provided with confirmed immuno-haematology results (*cf.* Chapter 9 page 88).

Receiving and verifying labile blood products

The LBP must be checked when received by the ward irrespective of the method of delivery, *i.e.* by the ETS *via* a carrier or courier or by the hospital blood bank *via* a courier.

A staff member in the ward that receives the LBP will verify:
– that the patient for whom the LBP are intended is on the ward;
– the transport conditions;
– consistency between the prescription, LBP received and delivery form;
– the appearance of the LBP.

Rare blood groups

Providing compatible PRBCs for patients who carry a rare pheno (geno)type remains a challenge in transfusion medicine. There is no internationally agreed definition of rarity, which can vary hugely with the populations in question. Most countries have implemented a national system to meet these needs.

Blood group systems

In 2012, the International Society of Blood Transfusion (ISBT) identified over 330 red cell surface antigens, of which 292 are classified into 33 blood group systems. However, not all can be associated with a system due to the lack of genetic evidence. Low-incidence antigens (< 1%) are classified in the 700 series (By, Chr^a, Bi, etc.) whilst high-incidence antigens (> 90%) are listed in the 901 series (At^a, Emm, AnWj, Sid). If several antigens are classified together on the basis of genetic, serological and biochemical information, but cannot be associated with a new or existing system due to insufficient information, they form a collection (COST, I, ER, GLOB, VEL). All these antigens are recognized by specific, natural or alloimmune antibodies, which can be implicated to varying degrees in transfusion or foetomaternal conflicts. 38% of these antigens are found in over 99% of the general population [1].

The notion of a rare pheno (geno)type

There is no consensus over the incidence level at which a pheno (geno)type is said to be "rare" [2]. The American Association of Blood Banks (AABB) defines an incidence of 1/1,000 (0.1%) in the general population as "rare" and 1/10,000 (0.01%) as "very rare". In France, the figure is 4/1,000.

The notion of rarity varies with the populations

The breakdown of genetic diversity by area reveals that distribution varies with the geographical origin of the populations. Blood groups are no different and so it is logical that the same phenotype may be common or merely found in one population and rare, or even totally absent, in another. For example, the incidence of the "Rhesus" negative phenotype is 15% in Western European populations but falls as we move towards Asia and is almost nonexistent in the Far East. If there were insufficient reserves of this specific phenotype, a "Rhesus negative" individual in the Far East could therefore be considered untransfusable. We can see, then, that to ensure transfusion compatibility for certain blood groups, it is vital to seek donors in populations with the same geographical origin as the patients.

Migratory phenomena and sustainable supply

If an immigrant community presents with blood groups that are considered rare in the host population and significant cultural barriers to blood donation, a lack of compatible units may limit transfusions. Considering the evolutionary history of modern man, genetic variability appears more frequent and better established in Africa than elsewhere. In addition, as in other traditional societies, cultural barriers to voluntary and anonymous blood donation remain high in Africa due to the heavy symbolism of human material and the organisation of blood transfusion based primarily on replacement donation for a close relative. Communities of African descent (Sub-Saharan Africa, West Indies and Indian Ocean) face a particularly significant risk of transfusion issues due to this very high level of genetic variability, low participation in blood donation and prevalence of conditions that may require long-term LBP, such as sickle-cell anaemia. In France, the number of sickle-cell patients is estimated at 6,000 and the figure is set to double or triple over the next 10 years.

The characteristics of rare pheno (geno)types

The main rare blood groups can have various characteristics:
- the lack of an antigen that everyone has, which defines a phenotype as "antigen negative". Whilst their absence can be suspected in most cases (lack of 2 antithetical antigens), they remain difficult to detect as, given the unavailability of serological reagents on the market, molecular biology techniques must be used (Table XVII);
- the presence of incomplete or partial antigens for which patients can synthesize, following transfusion or pregnancy, an antibody recognizing the part they lack. This is the case for certain antigens of the RH system (RhD, RhC or Rhe) within African populations;
- the simultaneous lack of so-called "common" antigens, of which 2 combinations are worth reporting:
  – the first combination concerns the **simultaneous lack of antigens within the same system**. This is the case of the RH system, where a number of phenotypes are linked to the presence in double dose of rare or even

Table XVII. Rare blood groups.

Examples of commonly lacking antigens	Populations	Types of antibodies
H:-1 (Bombay) or H:W1	India, Reunion Island	Natural antibodies
P:-1 (formerly Pk, lack of the P antigen)		
GLOB:-1,-2 (Formerly Tja negative, lack of the P and Pk antigens)		
I:-1		
RH:-17 (D../D..)		Immune antibodies
RH:-29 (.../... (RH null)		
RH:-57 (ces340/ces340)	Sub-Saharan Africa	
RH:-31 and RH:-34 (with partial RhE) (ceAR/ceAR, ceEK/ceEK, ceBI/ceBI)	Sub-Saharan Africa	
RH:-31 and RH:-19 (with partial RhE) (ceMO/ceMO)	Sub-Saharan Africa	
RH:-31 and RH:-59 (with partial RhE) (ce254/ce254)	Sub-Saharan Africa	
RH:-46 (with partial RhC) (RN/RN)	Sub-Saharan Africa	
KEL:-2 (cellano negative)		
KEL:-4 (Kpb negative)		
KEL:-5 and KEL:-20 (Ko)	Reunion Island	
KEL:-7 (Jsb negative)	Sub-Saharan Africa (1%)	
XK:-1 (Mac Leod)		
JK:-3 (JK:-1, 2 (JK(a-b-))	Melanesia	
FY:-3 and FY:-5 (FY:-1,-2 / Fy(a-b-))	Sub-Saharan Africa (70%)	
MNS:-5 (U) (MNS:-3,-5 or Uvar)	Sub-Saharan Africa (1.5%)	
LU:-2 (Lub negative)		
YT:-1 (Yta negative)		
GE:-2,3,4 (Yus phenotype)	Mediterranean	
GE:-2,-3,4 (Gerbich phenotype)	Papua New Guinea	
GE:-2,-3,-4 (Leach phenotype)		
CO:-3 (CO:-1,-2 / Co(a-b-))		
Jr:-1 (Jra negative)	Travellers	
VEL:-1		

exceptional haplotypes (*RZRZ or DCE/DCE*, *r'r'* or *dCE/dCE*, *r'r'* or *dCe/dCe*, *r"r"* or *dcE/dcE*). A particular phenotype in the RH system called "R°", which has strong inter-population variation, is also worth reporting. It is characterized by the presence of the RhD antigen and simultaneous absence of the RhC and RhE antigens. This combination is found in approximately 60% of African populations but in only 1% to 2% outside Africa. Individuals carrying this phenotype can alternatively be transfused in RhD negative phenotype. Therefore, the lack of "R°" blood units increases the use of RhD negative units, contributing to the chronic lack of this group in national stock levels;

- the second combination is characterized by the **simultaneous lack of antigens in various systems**. This includes the Fya (FY1), Jkb (JK2) and S (MNS3) antigens, for example, which also have significant inter-population variability, with an incidence of 12% in Sub-Saharan Africa versus 1/5,000 to 1/10,000 individuals outside the continent. As for the "antigen negative" phenotype, transfusion issues may be caused here by the lack of compatible units, particularly in poly-immunized sickle-cell patients;

- the expression of certain antigens that are almost specific to African populations [RH10, RH20, KEL6 (Jsa)] but whose high incidence (10 to 20%) can cause problems in the event of intra-ethnic transfusions prompted by another rare blood group. Here too, given the unavailability of serological reagents on the market, detection involves genotyping.

Organisation in France

In France, donors and recipients presenting with a rare pheno (geno)type are listed in a national database. Bags from donors are frozen to -80°C in a National Rare Blood Bank (BNSR). The bank is supplied by regional ETS on the basis of the pheno (geno)type information provided by the laboratories of the EFS and the National Reference Centre for Blood Groups (CNRGS).

Supply strategy

Although compatible products can be provided in most cases, difficulties persist for certain phenotypes, including for the transfusion of sickle-cell patients. It is therefore essential to implement a rare blood supply strategy amongst the host population to maintain stock levels in the BNSR, especially of the pheno (geno)types characteristic of populations originating from Sub-Saharan Africa. This must include targeted awareness-raising of immigrant communities and detection of these variants in donors from Sub-Saharan Africa, particularly by genotyping.

Conclusion

Because of its history, France is a diverse, multicultural country in which equal access to healthcare is a fundamental principle. This also includes equal opportunities to find matches in treatments using products from the human body, with the necessary polymorphism enrichment strategy of "biological donations" of blood, bone marrow, placenta blood and even organs.

Références

1. Peyrard T, Pham BN, Le Pennec PY, Rouger P. The rare blood groups: a public health challenge. *Transfus Clin Biol* 2008; 15 (3): 109-19.

2. Reesink HW, Engelfriet CP, Schennach H, *et al.* Donors with a rare pheno (geno) type. *Vox Sang* 2008; 95 (3): 236-53.

He/she then stores the LBP on the ward.

The control procedure on receipt of the LBP in the ward is as follows:

1. Check
- that the product is intended for that ward;
- that the packaging used to transport the products is:
  - marked "labile blood products",
  - in good condition,
  - clean;
- that the packaging label shows the following information:
  - departure point,
  - delivery point and recipient,
  - type and number of products contained therein,
  - storage conditions;
- that a delivery form is attached to the packaging and shows:
  - the name of the recipient ward,
  - the name of the patient,
  - the date and time of delivery;
- that the storage conditions meet the requirements and timeframes outlined in health facilities procedures;
- that the LBP delivered match the order and the details on the delivery form.

2. Check the appearance of the product, integrity of the bag, expiry date and accuracy of particular claims (*e.g.* cross-matched PRBCs).

3. Validate the receipt. In the event of non-compliance, do not transfuse and alert the delivery services (EFS transfusion site or hospital blood bank).

4. Start the transfusion as soon as possible.

5. Store the products in optimal conditions pending transfusion.

All LBP must be used within 6 hours of receipt by the ward *if compatible with the processing.*

Only a written and co-signed agreement between the ETS and health facilities specifying storage conditions makes it possible to modify this rule for surgical procedures lasting longer than 6 hours.

As a safety measure, but also to limit the destruction of unused LBP, the prescribed LBP should be delivered by the ETS or hospital blood bank as and when required by the patient to prevent all storage on the hospital ward.

If the LBP are not used immediately on the ward, it is vital to maintain the correct storage temperatures.

Depending on the products, the minimum and maximum temperatures to maintain are the following:

- PRBCs: stored between + 2 °C and + 6 °C. All PRBCs must be transfused within 6 hours of receipt;
- platelet concentrates (P-SD-PC/aphaeresis platelet concentrates): stored between +20 °C and +24 °C on an agitator. To be transfused as soon as possible after receipt by the ward;
- therapeutic plasma: stored frozen to ≤ -25 °C, thawed to +37 °C in fifteen to twenty minutes and then transfused within 6 hours of thawing.

Preparing the transfusion of labile blood products

It is essential to have all the necessary documents and equipment beside the patient in order to follow the "one place" rule and not be forced to stop the transfusion preparation to locate missing items. Interruptions can lead to errors or omissions in a control stage.

In the treatment room, the professional who will perform the transfusion ascertains that he/she has all the necessary documents and equipment.

He/she prepares the equipment needed to insert a large-calibre peripheral venous line or, if the patient already has a venous line, he/she checks that it is intact and working correctly. In agreement with the physician, he/she always ensures that there is an isotonic solution on standby. If treatments are being administered by venous route, the possibility of discontinuing them during the transfusion should be discussed with the physician managing the patient.

The professional checks that there is a sufficient amount of tubing (one tube per bag transfused) with a 200 μm filter suitable for the administration of LBP (standard transfusers for PRBCs and therapeutic plasma, specific transfusers for P-SD-PC and aphaeresis platelet concentrates).

The validity (expiry date) of the test kits is checked. The professional must obtain a test kit for each PRBC to be transfused. As a safety measure, it is always wise to have several test kits so that the test can be repeated if there is any doubt over the result.

The documents required for the transfusion (transfusion records, delivery form, medical prescription of LBP, valid blood grouping and irregular antibody screening documents) are provided and removed at the same time as the equipment and the product to be transfused to the patient.

The equipment needed to monitor clinical parameters is provided and the availability of emergency equipment is systematically checked.

Before being transfused, the LBP is prepared. Simply leaving PRBCs at room temperature for 15 to 30 minutes is sufficient, or a specific heater can be used if time is of the essence; therapeutic plasma is thawed to +37 °C in a bain-marie by the EFS transfusion site or hospital blood bank. It must be transfused within 6 hours of thawing (thawing time marked on the label). For platelet concentrates, the transfusion must be immediate.

When the decision to transfuse the patient is made, the physician is required to give him/her clear, accurate and appropriate information.

This pre-transfusion information centres on the need to use transfusion therapy because of the patient's clinical and/or biological condition, the immunohaematology tests required by the transfusion, any unexpected adverse reactions associated with the treatment, how frequent they are and how they can be reduced.

The professional who performs the transfusion informs the patient of the transfusion regimen and the symptoms which may occur and should be reported.

The patient is given any necessary premedication prescribed in the transfusion records and is then placed in a comfortable position.

The vital signs (pulse, blood pressure and temperature) are taken and noted on the transfusion records. They will serve as guidance should an adverse reaction occur.

Performing and monitoring the transfusion of labile blood products

The transfusion must be prepared in the presence of the patient and performed:
- **in one place:** the patient's bedside;
- **at one time:** the LBP are checked against the recipient;
- **by one person:** just one person must prepare and perform the transfusion.

The final pre-transfusion control at the patient's bedside has 2 stages: a consistency check mandatory for all LBP and a final compatibility check mandatory for all allogenic or autologous PRBCs.

- Checking the recipient's identity:
  – asking the patient to confirm his/her full name and date of birth;
  – following an identification procedure defined by the health facilities if the patient cannot answer questions.
- Checking the recipient's identity against the details on:
  – the LBP prescription;
  – the blood grouping documents and, for the transfusion of PRBCs, the results of irregular antibody screening;
  – the delivery form.
- Checking that the blood group is consistent on:
  – the blood grouping document;
  – the delivery form (identical or compatible);
  – the label of the LBP (identical or compatible).

- Checking that information on the LBP (type of LBP, eleven-digit number, blood grouping, description) is consistent on:
  – the label of the LBP;
  – the delivery form.
- Checking the LBP expiry date and time.
- Checking compliance with the existing transfusion protocol for this patient.

> The final check of ABO compatibility, which is made at the patient's bedside before the administration of the PRBCs, is mandatory in France, even in emergencies, and must follow strict guidelines. The aim is to prevent an adverse reaction caused by incompatibility in the ABO system. Yet experience shows that it often detects an error in recipient identification.
>
> The final compatibility check, which involves both the units to be transfused and the patient, must be:
> - made immediately before each transfusion of allogenic and/or autologous PRBCs;
> - made in the presence of the patient, meaning in the patient's room on the ward or in the operating theatre;
> - made without any interruption by the professional performing the transfusion;
> - repeated for each bag of PRBCs in the presence of the patient, by the professional who connects the bag.

Once the final pre-transfusion control is complete, meaning the consistency check and compatibility check in the case of PRBCs, the LBP is transfused immediately, preferably using the primary route for transfusion (peripheral venous line, implantable port) or else by central venous route.

The flow rate must be slow (30 drops/minute for the first 50 mL in adults) for the first 10 minutes to assess the patient's clinical tolerance.

No medicinal product should be injected into the bag of LBP or tubing. Any other drips using the same line are, if possible, temporarily discontinued with the agreement of the medical team. The patient must be nil by mouth during the transfusion.

It is recommended that the professional remains with the patient during the transfusion of the first millilitres of the LBP, *i.e.* for at least 15 minutes, before constant monitoring reflecting the patient's clinical condition is provided. The professional reminds the patient that transfusions are generally well tolerated and that the slightest signs of intolerance must be reported immediately.

Measurements (pulse, blood pressure, temperature and if necessary respiration rate, diuresis, SaO_2, state of consciousness, skin colour, central venous pressure) are noted on the medical records or anaesthesia form. The permeability of the venous line, airtightness of the tubing links and transfusion flow rate are regularly controlled throughout the LBP transfusion.

The occurrence of dizziness, headache, shivering, hyperthermia, redness or paleness, difficulty breathing, cough, dyspnea, lower back pain, diarrhoea, nausea, vomiting, skin rash or any other abnormal symptom must systematically result in the immediate halt of the transfusion, leaving the venous line in place, and the physician is conducted to decide on what steps to take. The professional alerts the EFS transfusion site, notes the incident in the patient's records and reports it to the health facilities Haemovigilance Officer.

Clinical follow-up with monitoring of the vital signs (temperature, blood pressure, diuresis, etc.) must be continued for 2 hours after the end of the transfusion of the last LBP.

The transfusion yield must be assessed with a hemogram and/or haemostasis exploration, generally within 24 hours.

The empty bags, with the tubing clamped, and ABO compatibility test kits for PRBCs must be stored for at least 2 hours after the end of the transfusion. PRBC bags should be stored in the refrigerator at 4 °C, whilst bags of therapeutic plasma and platelet concentrates are kept at room temperature.

The delivery form must be completed correctly at the patient's bedside and a copy filed in the transfusion records.

The delivery form is completed by:
– affixing the labels showing the LBP bag number;
– entering the date and time of the transfusion;
– recording the compliance of the final pre-transfusion control (twice);
– confirming that the identity of the recipient was consistent with the LBP transfused;
– noting the onset of any immediate adverse reaction.

One copy of the completed delivery form is returned to the EFS transfusion site.

Another copy of the completed delivery form is filed in the central database of the health facilities.

The transfusion records must be checked. They must show a copy of the delivery form for each LBP transfused, the result of the immunohaematology tests conducted for the transfusion and, depending on the conduct of the transfusion, any adverse reaction form.

Conclusion

The physician prescribing LBP must systematically evaluate the benefit-to-risk ratio for his/her patient before each transfusion. The justification of LBP, like the transfusion that follows, is subject to strict professional guidelines.

These professional guidelines are now updated by the French National Authority for Health (HAS). The EFS's medico-technical experts are regularly involved in the review and update process. In addition, through national studies on LBP recipients and the means of increasing the issue of LBP, the EFS is contributing to national data on transfusion medicine.

> **Understanding recipients of labile blood products in France**
>
> The use of LBP remains widespread in therapeutic circles. However, as there is no electronic data transfer system that can be used to add patients' medical conditions to their transfusion records, few data are currently available on transfusion indications.
>
> With this in mind, and to meet the demand and expectations of healthcare professionals, the EFS has undertaken to update its information on recipients and transfusion practices in France. To achieve these aims, which are outlined in the objectives and performance contract agreed between the EFS and the State, a nationwide study was conducted on all the EFS's hospitals partners from 21 November to 11 December 2011. It sought to analyze recipients' conditions, transfusion indications and contexts, the type of LBP requested and delivered as well as exchanges between the EFS and ES.
>
> The study looked at one day (24 hours) of delivery, within hospital delivery blood banks and the EFS's delivery sites.
>
> The study date was chosen at random. It used a questionnaire listing the conditions, indications, transfusion contexts, and so on.
>
> In total, 1,660 health facilities were contacted on that date; 4,710 patients and 5,361 prescriptions were examined; 10,763 LBP (8,667 PRBCs, 841 platelet concentrates and 1,255 fresh frozen plasmas) were delivered. The median age of patients was 70 [extremes of 0 to 103 years], and 59% of patients had a history of transfusion known to the EFS. The main disease classes were onco-haematology (18%), oncology (13%), cardiovascular (12%), hepatogastroenterology (11%), traumatology/orthopaedics (10%), non-oncologic haematology and immunology (10%); 32% of admissions were related to surgery and 16% to chemotherapy. Finally, planned transfusion accounted for 52% of cases and life-threatening emergencies 12% of cases.
>
> These results are similar to those of the 2005 study and provide more details on the medical conditions and transfusion contexts. The study opens avenues for further investigation, particularly on LBP practices and indications.

Transfusion medicine: the French model

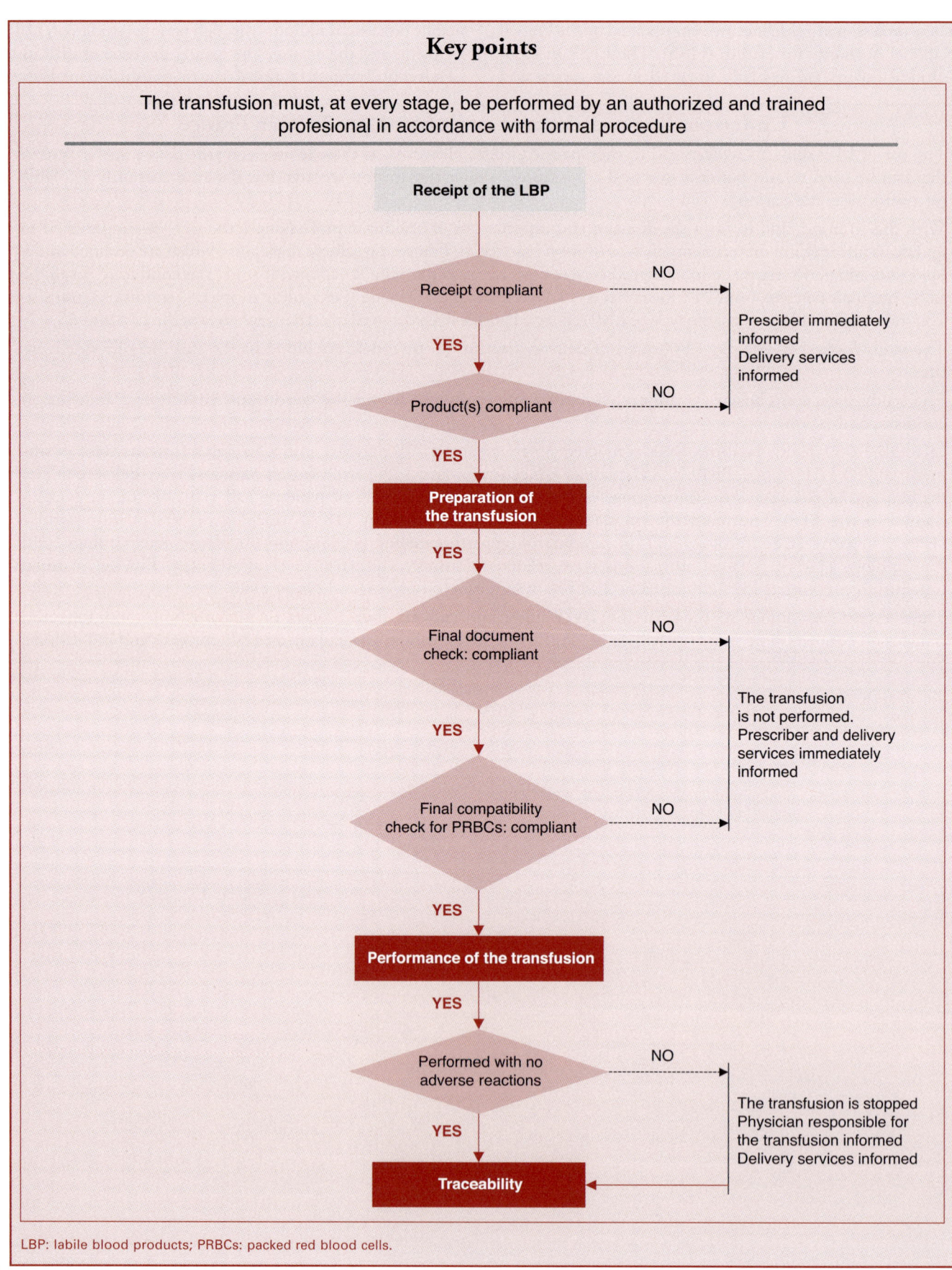

LBP: labile blood products; PRBCs: packed red blood cells.

Part III
Transfusion safety in France

11. Assessment

Stéphane Begue, Anne Chabanel, Magali Sillam

Introduction

Like medicinal products, labile blood products (LBP) are therapeutic preparations whose indications and uses, like those of proprietary medicines, are determined by their characteristics:

- **active principle**, which provides the therapeutic effect required (haemoglobin, platelets, proteins, etc.);
- **presentation** and **form** (concentration, haematocrit, etc.);
- **undesirable compounds** and/or **residual contaminants** (residual leucocytes, chemical compounds used for pathogen attenuation, etc.);
- **storage conditions** (pH, haemolysis, coagulation factor, etc.).

Each of these characteristics offers a therapeutic benefit and guarantee of safety.

Moving the quality of LBP away from optimal values can lead to the risk of inefficacy (insufficient active principle), intolerance (unsuitable presentation or therapeutic form), toxicity, contamination or adverse reaction (cellular or bacterial contaminants, toxic and/or allergenic compounds) or even to all these unwanted situations if stored incorrectly.

The quality control (QC) and assessment of LBP will examine these characteristics, either to determine target values and acceptable limits (assessment) or to ensure compliance with regulatory requirements (QC).

With the exception of visual inspection, these characteristics are measured using standard haematology, biochemistry, haemostasis and microbiology laboratory techniques. The following chapter highlights the role of QC, the practical and methodological approach taken in QC and assessment, as well as the expected benefits of these activities in terms of LBP safety.

Stéphane Begue, stephane.begue@efs.sante.fr
Anne Chabanel, anne.chabanel@efs.sante.fr
Magali Sillam, magali.sillam@efs.sante.fr

Transfusion medicine: the French model

History of the activity

QC really began to develop in the early 1990s following publication of the Act of 4 January 1993, which introduced the requirement to implement a quality assurance system covering all transfusion services and a QC programme for LBP through good transfusion practice. The first Order on the list of authorized LBP and the regulatory criteria they must meet was published in the same period.

For the assessment of LBP, the Act of 4 January 1993 laid the foundations for the regulatory registration of new LBP: "Before distributing a new labile blood product, the establishment preparing it must provide the French Blood Agency with information on its characteristics, preparation, testing, efficacy and safety so that the product can be registered."

In 1996, the French Blood Agency (AFS) created the LBP Committee, which was tasked with authorizing new LBP or new methods of preparing them based on a comprehensive approval application. The information to be provided was detailed in a document entitled "Notice to Applicants". In 2000, this role was transferred to the French Health Products Safety Agency (Afssaps), which maintained the requirements set by the AFS. On 19 November 2010, the Afssaps published an updated version of the Notice to Applicants, determining the content of the application for the assessment of LBP.

Division of the activity across France

All regional establishments have a QC laboratory located, with just one exception, on the same site as the specialized platform preparing LBP.

In 2012, 83 full-time equivalents (FTE/ETP) were allocated to QC, with 81 shared amongst the blood establishments (ETS) and 2 in the head office of the French Blood Establishment (EFS) (Medical Division).

In practical terms, the following amounts of quality controls were performed in 2012:

PRBCs	APC	PPC	Therapeutic plasma			
All parameters	All parameters	All parameters	Proteins	Residual WBC	Factor VIII	Fibrinogen
15,293	6,183	3,296	4,897	6,584	1,174	1,291

PRBCs: packed red blood cells; APC: aphaeresis platelet concentrate; PPC: pooled standard platelet concentrates; WBC: white blood cells.

Mapping of the process

Within vigilance, the QC and assessment of LBP are part of the **"monitoring"** process, which is in turn part of the **"management"** macro-process.

As with all processes in the **"management"** macro-process, QC is conducted cross-functionally in all areas of "production". "QC" is neither upstream nor downstream, but moves in the direction of its main "clients":
- managers of production processes;
- the responsible person and the Chairman of the EFS;
- the regulatory authorities: the French National Agency for the Safety of Medicines and Health Products (ANSM) and Directorate-General for Health (DGS);
- the French Fractionation Laboratory (LFB).

Medico-technical description of "assessment" services

Role of quality control

QC is relevant to LBP and production. The LBP production process, meaning all the coordinated activities transforming raw material into an end product and giving it added value, is the main area covered by QC. This activity, which may not at first thought appear central to transfusion services, has however found its natural place in the donor to recipient chain, bringing all parties measurable indicators of the quality and conformity of products and processes. In providing regular information, safety assurance and monitoring, QC contributes to increasing confidence and shared understanding of LBP quality levels.

For historical reasons, and because the collection, preparation and delivery of LBP remain at the core of transfusion services, here QC primarily means the QC of LBP. Reference is therefore made to LBP-QC, which is the mainstay of the services. The scope of QC is not limited, however, and can be extended to several other activities such as the production of cells, tissues, reagents or advanced therapy medicinal products.

The scope of QC can be defined as all the steps or actions that are taken to obtain evidence of compliance. It covers 5 key aspects, which are: understanding the process (1), sampling (2), laboratory testing (3) and interpreting the results to determine the compliance of the process (4). All these activities are undertaken in a strict regulatory framework (5) which defines both the guidelines to follow and the targets to meet, with QC helping to demonstrate the level of compliance or trigger alerts in the event of deviations (Figure 41).

11. Assessment

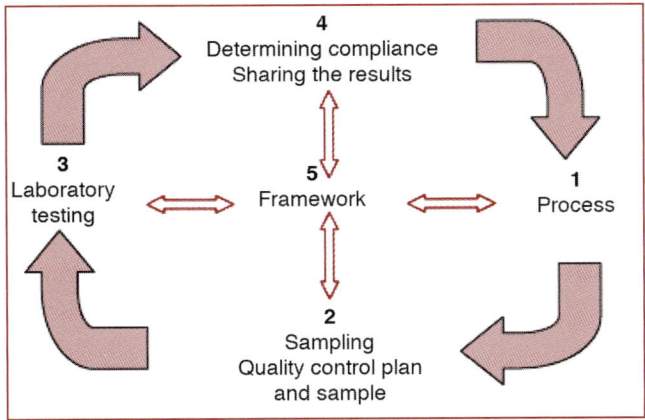

Figure 41. The 5 key elements of Quality control.

QC is expected to determine the compliance of all LBP, but not manage the release of products (see key point 4: determining compliance). To do so, it works within what we call "quality control by sampling". All product monitoring is based on the results of the quality control of a small number of products selected for their representativeness, to which the homogeneity assumption is applied. Generally, between 0.5% and 10% of products are controlled, and so the vast majority of LBP are transfused without being submitted to individual quality control. In this approach, as each unit of LBP has been produced "nominally", *i.e.* without any notable deviation in the production process, the likelihood that all products are compliant if the controlled LBP are compliant is judged to be high.

This **monitoring** is the main service that QC provides.

In specific cases, however, QC may be used to determine the compliance of one or more LBP that are suspected, following an incident, to present a risk of noncompliance. Reference is then made to "confirmation control" (QC confirmation) as quality control will check the individual compliance of each product for which serious non conformity is suspected.

Despite major similarities in their practical implementation, the 2 activities, quality control by sampling and confirmation control, do not provide the same added value: monitoring, vigilance and maintaining confidence for the former, and corrective and restorative action for the latter.

Key point 1: Understanding the process for obtaining labile blood products

Knowing what to control: the labile blood product and its production process

There are many reasons why quality controllers need to understand the production process. The first is simple common sense: they must know how the products are collected and prepared before they can demonstrate their compliance. The second involves an in-depth analysis aiming to identify the main parameters that will build the framework of the process. In this way, their knowledge of the process will help them distinguish between the aspects that have a major impact on the quality or characteristics of LBP and those with only a minor influence. Each LBP has a unique collection and preparation history, reflecting the unique biological characteristics of the donor. All the stages from collection to storage can cause variability in LBP (collection device, volume, transport to the specialized platform, processing time, preparation method, centrifuge, separator, etc.). Therefore, there are several dozen parameters that make each LBP different.

However, transfusion stakeholders spend a great deal of time and energy reducing the effects of variability. Standardizing methods, equipment, medical devices, modes of transport, automated machine programmes, timeframes and many other factors is key not only to limiting variability, but also to achieving common outcomes that can be measured and assessed by all links in the chain. In QC, standardization involves developing procedures that will form the basis of sampling plans and the scope of products for which evidence of compliance is required.

How do controllers develop and maintain their understanding of the production process?

- Contributing to approving new collection or preparation procedures.
- Participating in evaluations and assessments of new procedures with industrial partners.
- Working closely with the services responsible for production procedures (collection, preparation, transport, delivery, etc.) to identify pertinent control points and interpret the results.

Risks associated with incomplete understanding of the production process

Not identifying the various stages in the production process may mean that some products are overlooked. Not fully understanding the procedures may lead to quality controls at an inappropriate point in product preparation, or the failure to quality control parameters which indicate processes' performance.

Finally, an error in defining procedure may render the results impossible to interpret.

> **Not forgetting that**
> Quality controllers are seen by the transfusion community as experts in LBP, procedures and the effects caused by changing production parameters. On that basis, they must be able to communicate impartially on the potential consequences of changes to a procedure, and their awareness of significant changes must prepare them to be on the alert for any event undermining the quality or safety of LBP.

Key point 2: Sampling

Economics are central to the sampling process

Quality controls are based on sampling because:
- due to the quantities produced, it is impossible to control *all* the products;
- doing so would generate little useful information on the process.

There are 2 forms of sampling, one involving the **product** and the other involving the **process**, but they share the same fundamental principle: the sample is **representative**.

This principle assumes that the area sampled (LBP or process) is **homogeneous**.

The concept is similar to the **batch system**, whose primary purpose is to bring together units that are thought to be homogeneous for a given characteristic. Agitation, for example, can help to make LBP homogenous during sampling. For the process, as there is no batch system in place, the issue is much more complex and requires greater knowledge of the history of the products to ensure representative sampling.

Sampling LBP

The sample taken from the product is the part of the LBP that will be sent to the laboratory for testing. Therefore, all the results of QC tests relate to the sample itself. Direct transposition of the results to the blood product bag is not affected by any uncertainty margins over representativeness, which definitively determines the implicit qualities of the sample:
- it must be strictly representative of the product;
- its collection must not involve any risk for the LBP (the operation is transparent and has "not taken place");
- the collection method must be appropriate to the test being conducted, type of LBP, storage procedures and pre-testing processing of the sample.

The different methods for taking samples are:
- non-destructive method: stripping the tubing, using a sample bag, etc.;
- destructive method: if the LBP will in any case be destroyed (*e.g.* if quality control takes place after the expiry date of the PSL).

The sampling or quality control plan

Sampling at process scale, also known as the sampling plan (SP) or quality control plan, must be representative of all the products and by extension the processes from which they result.

This implies that:
- the process is correctly identified (see above);
- the process has been shown to be homogeneous (at least in the parameters assessed by QC);
- within this process, the products taken for quality control are chosen at random.

An SP is defined as:
- an LBP from a clearly determined process: *e.g.* packed red blood cells (PRBCs), SAGM (saline-adenine-glucose-mannitol solution) from delayed whole blood filtration, for a given single-use device (SUD) reference;
- a parameter to monitor (haemoglobin content, residual white blood cells, etc.);
- a required number of quality controls to be performed in a given period*.

*Batch sampling is not required within a specified time, but the concept of batches in transfusion, where production is almost nonstop, is still debated and no consensus has been reached. A certain period of time will then be defined as appropriate for determining evidence of compliance in production. The EFS recently defined this period as a calendar month for the design of SP.

11. Assessment

The main difficulty for an SP, beyond its practical implementation, is calculating the required number of quality controls. When determining this figure, 2 contradictory aims are sought for the number of products involved, which are to:
• provide the most accurate reflection of production possible, which only increases with the number of controls;
• keep costs as low as possible, which means decreasing the number of controls.

The decision does not, however, lie directly with the quality controller. The delicate balance is struck when the EFS's responsible person, based on information from the ANSM, determines the limiting quality levels (LQL), which are the average quality levels below which the process is judged unacceptable (see below).

Calculation of the required number of quality controls

The number of quality controls required will depend on how the parameter is distributed in the product population:
• either the distribution is known (case 1) and not significantly different from "normal" or Gaussian distribution, in which case the percentage of noncompliant LBP in the production can be deduced from the distribution parameters alone (mean and median);
• or the distribution is unknown (case 2), in which case the percentage of noncompliant LBP in the production will be estimated based on the number of noncompliant products seen in a given number of quality controls.

In all cases, the mean, median or number of noncompliant LBP are taken from recent experience of quality controlling (previous or penultimate month).

In case 1, the required number of quality controls will be calculated to obtain a sufficiently accurate estimate of the mean and median of distribution, which will then be used to calculate the percentage of noncompliance with sufficiently low uncertainty (to be acceptable).

In case 2, the required number of quality controls is based on calculating the probability of observing low-occurring events, whose predictive potential is very low given the number of controlled products.

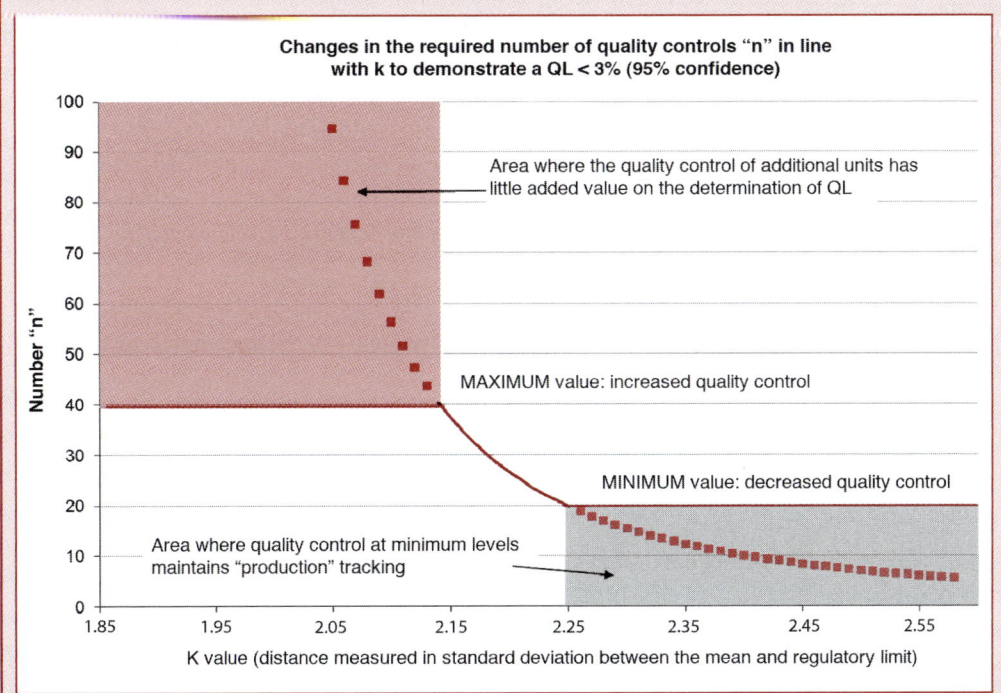

Figure 42. Graphic showing changes in the required number of quality controls in line with recent quality levels in production (expressed by the value k, distance measured in standard deviation between the mean of distribution and regulatory limit).
QL: quality level.

How do quality controllers undertake sampling?

Sampling is the sole responsibility and cornerstone of QC, with any error at this stage having a hidden knock-on effect on the remainder of the process. Managing sampling primarily entails the validation of methods and provision of regular staff training and authorization.

For LBP, specific authorization is required for stripping and sampling from sample bags. This authorization may be based on cross-checks between samplers and/or between different methods (*e.g.* stripping versus destructive).

The per-process SP is redesigned regularly (monthly within the EFS) to reflect recent product quality. The required number of quality controls may be raised if the risk of noncompliance is clarified or demonstrated.

Risks associated with sampling

LBP sampling must reflect the type of tests to be conducted: a sample is not taken by stripping to determine the rate of haemolysis, and tubing is not stripped if it has a luer lock (which represents too much priming volume), etc. Furthermore, LBP sampling is no small matter, as it carries a low but not insignificant risk of losing the LBP though a break in the closed system.

As it interfaces with other activities, LBP sampling is often delegated to the preparation services. If such delegating is possible, it must take place within an extremely strict framework as the quality controller alone remains responsible for the outcome of quality controlling.

The implementation of an SP is also subject to significant risk, such as unrepresentative population, insufficient number of quality controls for the quality levels required, bias in the selection of LBP, etc. Particular vigilance is needed to ensure that the defined SP are implemented in full. The ratio of quality controls performed versus the number planned in the SP is a major activity indicator in QC.

Limiting quality levels: definition according to good transfusion practices (version 2006)

"Any quality-related measurement that must be taken from all LBP, making it possible to define a limiting or acceptable level of compliance. The methodology used by the EFS and the French Armed Forces Blood Transfusion Centre (CTSA) is detailed in guidelines developed at national level by the EFS and the CTSA and sent to the Afssaps for opinion prior to implementation and after amendment."

For all products, LQL determine the maximum proportion (expressed as a percentage and estimated with confidence level ?) of noncompliant LBP that can be considered acceptable due to the limitations of the means of collection, preparation and QC.

Currently, there are 2 regulatory LQL, both involving residual leucocyte contamination:
- for leucocyte-depleted cellular LBP (PRBCs and platelets): LQL = maximum 3%;
- for leucocyte-depleted therapeutic plasma: LQL = maximum 5%.

Production quality levels (QL) must be calculated for comparison against the legal LQL with a 95% confidence level.

The QL for other regulatory parameters are defined in an EFS framework document. They are regularly reviewed to reflect technological advances.

Table XVII. Limiting quality levels applied by the EFS to certain regulatory parameters.		
Parameter	**LQL**	**Established on the basis of...**
Residual leucocytes in cellular LBP	3%	The 3% LQL for the leucocyte depletion of cellular LBP was established on the basis of the average rate of NC in 2,485 routine data items compiled by the LBP group of the SFTS (data from 1997–1998)
Residual leucocytes in therapeutic plasma	5%	LQL established on the basis of aphaeresis plasma results in 2001
Haemoglobin in LD-PRBCs	10%	• Rolling series of 150 data items were analyzed by the ETS to calculate the P-Sup and changes therein in 2005 • Data from the filtration of PRBCs for haemoglobin • Data from the filtration of whole blood for haematocrit
Haematocrit in LD-PRBCs	10%	
Plasma protein (LFB plasma)	10%	2009 data from the NDB were used as the distribution was considered to be normal
Factor VIII	30%	The standard is < 30% of the units quality controlled
Fibrinogen	30%	The standard is < 30% of the units quality controlled
Residual amotosalen in AI-FFP	5%*	On the basis of 699 residual AI results from January to August 2012

*Under development.
LQL: limiting quality levels; LBP: labile blood products; NC: noncompliance; SFTS: French Blood Transfusion Society; P-Sup: upper limit of the confidence interval regarding the proportion of noncompliant units in the production; LD-PRBCs: leucocyte-depleted packed red blood cells; LFB: French Fractionation Laboratory; AI-FFP: amotosalen-inactivated fresh frozen plasma; NDB: national database.

11. Assessment

Key point 3: Laboratory testing

Test results are central to the "quality control" process

QC results are the product of a testing process involving a sample that will have undergone pre-testing processing in most cases. The entire testing process is validated, from conditioning the samples to processing the results. For the majority of tests, the main difficulty is caused by the lack of national or international standards: there are no international reference standards for corpuscular or platelet cell counts, or for determinations of haemostasis factors (such as factor VIII and fibrinogen).

Testing methods have been automated over the last 20 years, which has considerably improved the reliability of results: automated haematology, biochemistry, haemostasis and flow cytometry machines are now common in laboratories.

The list of standard equipment and tests associated with a QC laboratory are shown in Table XVIII.

Table XVIII. Testing conducted on labile blood products by the quality control laboratory and the equipment used.

Tests	Methods	Equipment
Residual WBC	Cytometry (flow or fixed)	Cytometer Automated blood analyzer Automated haemostasis analyzer Automated biochemistry analyzer Anaerobic blood pH meter Spectrophotometer Microscope Rapid haemoglobin reader Laboratory scales Automated culture incubator and chambers centrifuge for 5-50 mL tube, refrigerated Preservatives +2 °C to +8 °C Preservatives -30 °C
Total haemoglobin	Automatic	
Haematocrit		
Platelets		
Proteins: total and extracellular	Spectrophotometer or automated biochemistry analyzer	
Residual platelets	Automatic/microscopy	
Residual red blood cells	Microscopy/automated analyzer	
pH	Blood pH meter	
Free haemoglobin	Automated analyzer	
Volume	Weighing	
Bacteriology	Automated culture incubator/microscope/chambers	
Pathogen attenuation residues (amotosalen, etc.)	High-performance liquid chromatography	
Haemostasis factors (factor VIII, fibrinogen)	Automatic	

How does quality control conduct reliable tests?

The quality requirements of a QC laboratory are not different from those of a testing laboratory.

The testing process can only be managed with qualified and regularly trained staff, high-performance equipment and materials, a structured documentation and results recording system, compliance with good laboratory practice, the validation of all stages in line with established methodological guidelines [International Conference on Harmonisation of Technical Requirements for Registration of Pharmaceuticals for Human Use (ICH), reference documents of the French Certification Committee (Cofrac)], and the implementation of monitoring procedures such as internal quality control (IQC) and external quality assessment (EQA). Obtaining Cofrac certification or similar should be a primary target in order to increase confidence in results.

Special case of subcontracting

Some tests may be consolidated or even subcontracted to specialist laboratories. The requirements for using a remote testing system are: the sample can be stored for long periods and the result is not required for the release of LBP. The cost of testing is an important factor in consolidation by series.

Risks associated with testing

The main risk is providing inaccurate results, which may be caused by human error, defective equipment, misuse of testing kits, inappropriate storage of samples or incorrect processing of the values. These risks can be reduced by managing the aspects referred to above. In LBP-QC, the IQC and EQA management systems are particularly important.

Key point 4: Determining compliance and sharing the results

This stage is of the sole responsibility of quality control

At this stage, QC Managers analyze and interpret the results to ascertain whether quality or regulatory targets have been met. They determine whether the process (for quality control by sampling) or LBP (for confirmation control) is compliant and report their findings to relevant figures. In the event of noncompliance, they alert the establishment's directors.

To fulfil these duties, the QC Manager's position in the EFS must be removed from the processes he/she controls. The separation of judge and judged allows the results to be interpreted impartially and provides unbiased analysis.

Analysis and interpretation

QC results require interpretation that reflects the context and objective of the quality control.

In providing evidence of compliance, quality control provides an answer to a question set by the QC Manager. Will the results be used to grade equipment? Validate a process? Demonstrate the compliance of a routine process? In answering the questions that will be asked by the final recipient, we can see the significant upstream involvement of the sampling strategy in quality control. For example, the quality control strategy is not the same for establishing the overall compliance of factor VIII levels in plasma for fractionation (such as leucocyte-depleted fresh frozen plasma) for all processes as for characterizing factor VIII levels in plasma by origin (type of aphaeresis, machine, device, etc.), *i.e.* with a procedural approach.

The circle of the QC process closes in the conclusion and results submission stage. Results on the process must be provided in a context of continual improvement, making it possible to measure the difference between targets and outcomes, assess the relevance of a quality control – a control is worthless if its value is not recognized – and maintain the vigilance of all parties on quality and safety criteria.

How do quality controllers determine product compliance?

The analysis and interpretation of results is hugely important to:
- identify a deviation, a risk of noncompliance and alert the managers or directors as early as possible;
- facilitate understanding and identification of the root cause(s);
- demonstrate the restitution of results and thereby the effectiveness of corrective measures.

Within the EFS, regional QC Managers are responsible for determining the compliance of LBP prepared in their region.

All the results of regional QC are then compiled in a centralized database (national database), enabling the production of national analyses and summaries. The QC Unit within the Medical Division is responsible for providing these national analyses and summaries, as well as answering all internal and external (authorities, suppliers, etc.) queries on the quality of LBP.

Independence: QC is not responsible for selecting or implementing the corrective measures applied to processes in which a deviation has been identified, which removes self-inspection from the quality circle.

Statistical management of the processes

The "product" of QC is a range of interpreted results. It is presented in the form of **summary tables** with graphics or **control charts** which illustrate trend or dispersion analysis. Insofar as possible, the direct transfer of unprocessed results in the form of lists should be avoided as, when taken out of the context of sampling, they may lead to errors of interpretation and incorrect conclusions by the recipient.

The parameters that are most frequently presented in tables are: the mean, standard deviation (median and interquartile range if the distribution is not normale), minimum value, maximum value, required number of quality controls, number of noncompliant products found, frequency of noncompliance and estimated percentage of noncompliance in production with a given confidence level (generally 95%).

11. Assessment

Table XIX. Example of a summary table: results on packed red blood cells from the whole blood filtration process (2012).

Whole blood filtration	Volume (mL)	Haemoglobin (g/LD-PRBCs)	Haematocrit (%)	Residual leucocytes (× 10⁶/U)		Haemolysis at expiry (%)
Compliance threshold	/	Hb ≥ 40	50 ≤ Ht ≤ 70	WBC ≤ 1		Haemolysis ≤ 0.8
Mean	309	60.1	59.5	1st quartile	3rd quartile	0.43
Standard deviation	20	6.4	3.4	0.034	0.162	0.33
Median	308	60.2	59.6	0.078		0.30
Minimum	207	37.2	38.1	0.005		0.10
Maximum	388	83	74.5	4.8		3.40
Number of quality controls	6,384	6,384	6,384	6,384		852
Number of NC quality controls	/////////	3	29	70		74
% NC	/////////	0.05%	0.45%	1.10%		8.7%
P-sup/QL	/////////	/////////	/////////	1.34%		/////////

LD-PRBCs: leucocyte-depleted packed red blood cells; Ht: haematocrit; WBC: white blood cells; NC: noncompliance; P-sup: upper limit of the confidence interval regarding the proportion of noncompliant units in the production; QL: quality level.

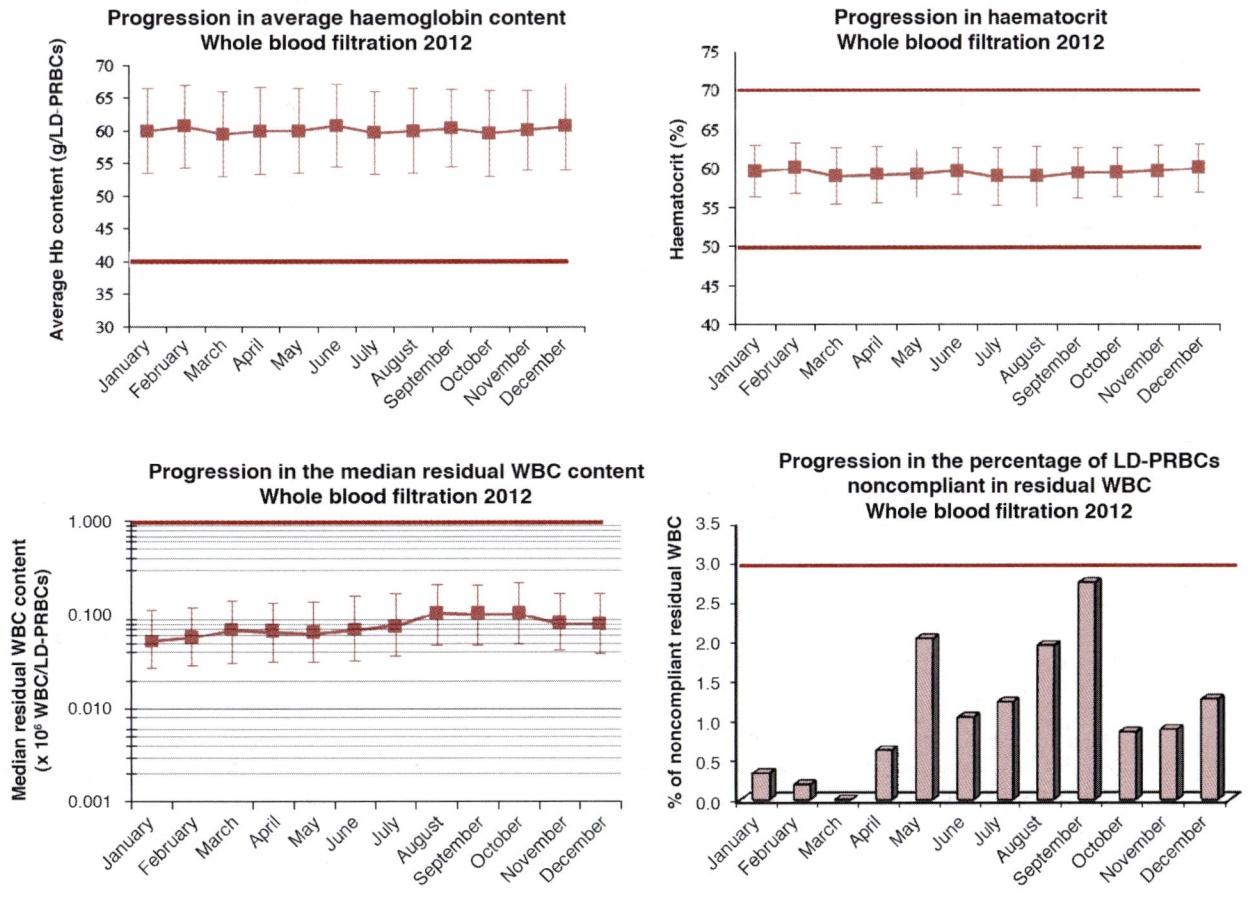

Figure 43. Example of synthesis of Quality control results for labile blood products.
LD-PRBCs: leucocyte-depleted packed red blood cells; Hb: haemoglobin; WBC: white blood cells.

Control charts are used as graphics and, if the sampling strategy allows (regular frequency and required number of quality controls), charts showing averages and errors may be of interest. Presentation and QC result analysis methods are being reviewed within the EFS to ensure full use of the results.

Risks associated with the conclusion and transfer of results
- Insufficient response time between the availability and interpretation of results, and/or transfer to the process manager, particularly in the event of noncompliant LBP or process.
- Presentation of results in an inappropriate format for the final recipient.
- Incorrect use of results.

Key point 5: Guidelines

Guidelines are the matrix around which QC is organized.

Regulatory guidelines are supplemented by the EFS's framework documents and regional work instructions which set out the methods. The quality targets from process and management reviews are made into targets for SP which are also used by the QC Manager to determine compliance.

How?
Guidelines are updated on the basis of regulatory and scientific intelligence, the regular updating of quality targets, and the regular review of methods and procedures.

Risk associated with guidelines
Use of incorrect or outdated guidelines.

Table XX. Characteristics of labile blood products: packed red blood cells.

LD-PRBCs	LD-PC			LD-PC SAGM			Volume reduced	Plasma removed SAGM
	AU	IU	Paediatric	AU	IU	Paediatric	AU IU	AU
Length of storage	21 days	21 days	21 days	42 days	42 days	42 days	1 day	10 days
Volume mL	/	≥ 85 mL	≥ 50 mL	/	≥ 75 + SAGM	≥ 50 + SAGM	*Cf.* origin	/
Haemoglobin (g/U)	≥ 40	22 to 40	% of the product at origin	≥ 40	22 to 40	% of the product at origin	*Cf.* origin	≥ 35
Haematocrit (%)	60 to 80%	60 to 80%	60 to 80%	50 to 70%	50 to 70%	50 to 70%	≥ 70%	40 to 70%
Haemolysis (at expiry)	0.80%	0.80%	0.80%	0.80%	0.80%	0.80%	0.80%	0.80%
Residual leucocytes (/U)	< 1 × 10^6	< 1 × 10^6	< 1 × 10^6	< 1 × 10^6	< 1 × 10^6	< 1 × 10^6	< 1 × 10^6	< 1 × 10^6
Residual proteins (/U)	/	/	/	/	/	/	/	< 0.5 g/U

LD-PRBCs: leucocyte-depleted packed red blood cells; LD-PC: leucocyte-depleted platelet concentrates; SAGM: saline-adenine-glucose-mannitol solution; AU: adult unit; IU: infant's unit.

11. Assessment

Table XXI. Characteristics of packed red blood cells (continued).

Plasma removed LD-PRBCs	Plasma removed SAGM	Non-closed		Cryo-preserved	Cryopreserved SAGM	Irradiated (all)		
	IU	AU	IU	AU / IU	AU / IU	AU before 14 days	IU before 14 days	AU/IU after 14 days
Length of storage	10 days	1 day	1 day	1 day	7 days	*Cf.* origin	28 days	1 day
Volume mL	/	/	/	/	/	*Cf.* origin	*Cf.* origin	*Cf.* origin
Haemoglobin (g/U)	≥ 20	≥ 35	≥ 20	≥ 35	≥ 35	*Cf.* origin	*Cf.* origin	*Cf.* origin
Haematocrit (%)	40 to 70%	50 to 80%	50 to 80%	50 to 80%	40 to 70%	*Cf.* origin	*Cf.* origin	*Cf.* origin
Haemolysis (at expiry)	0.80%	0.80%	0.80%	< 1.2%	< 1.2%	*Cf.* origin	*Cf.* origin	*Cf.* origin
Residual leucocytes (/U)	< 1 × 10^6	< 1 × 10^6	< 1 × 10^6	< 1 × 10^6	< 1 × 10^6	*Cf.* origin	*Cf.* origin	*Cf.* origin
Residual proteins (/U)	< 0.5 g/U	< 0.5 g/U	< 0.5 g/U	/	/	*Cf.* origin	*Cf.* origin	*Cf.* origin
Glycerol (/U)	/	/	/	< 1 g	< 1 g	*Cf.* origin	*Cf.* origin	*Cf.* origin

LD-PRBCs: leucocyte-depleted packed red blood cells; SAGM: saline-adenine-glucose-mannitol solution; AU: adult unit; IU: infant's unit.

Table XXII. Characteristics of platelet concentrates.

Platelet concentrate	PPC		APC			
	Storage solution	Amotosalen	Storage solution	Amotosalen	Paediatric	Plasma removed
Length of storage	5 days	5 days	6 hours	5 days	5 days	5 days
Volume	80 to 600 mL	80 to 600 mL	/	≤ 600 mL	≤ 600 mL	≥ 50 mL
Total quantity of platelets	≥ 1 × 10^{11}	2.2 to 6 × 10^{11}	≥ 1 × 10^{11}	≥ 2 × 10^{11}	2.2 to 6 × 10^{11}	> 0.5 × 10^{11}
Residual leucocytes	< 1 × 10^6	< 1 × 10^6	< 1 × 10^6	< 1 × 10^6	< 1 × 10^6	< 1 × 10^6
pH at expiry	≥ 6.4	≥ 6.4	≥ 6.4	≥ 6.4	≥ 6.4	≥ 6.4
Amotosalen	/	≤ 2 µM	≤ 2 µM	/	≤ 2 µM	/
Residual proteins	/	/	0.5 g/U	/	/	/

PPC: pooled platelet concentrates; APC: aphaeresis platelet concentrate.

Table XXIII. Characteristics of plasma for direct therapeutic use.

Quarantined aphaeresis plasma	Q-FFP quarantine	AI-FFP amotosalen	SD-FFP SD
Length of storage	1 year	1 year	1 year
Volume	≥ 200 mL	≥ 200 mL	≥ 200 mL
Factor VIII	≥ 0.7 IU/mL	≥ 0.5 IU/mL	≥ 0.5 IU/mL
Fibrinogen	/	≥ 2 g/L	≥ 2 g/L
Residual leucocytes	< 10^4/L	< 10^4/L	< 10^4/L
Residual red blood cells	≤ 6.10^9/L	≤ 6.10^9/L	≤ 6.10^9/L
Residual platelets	≤ 25.10^9/L	≤ 25.10^9/L	≤ 25.10^9/L
Inactivating agent	/	≤ 2 µM	Tunb < 2 ppm Triton < 5 ppm

FFP: fresh frozen plasma; Q-FFP: fresh frozen plasma quarantined; AI-FFP: amotosalen-inactivated fresh frozen plasma; SD-FFP: fresh frozen plasma inactivated by solvent/detergent.

> **For amotosalen-pathogen reduced plasma**
> - Factor VIII dosing: after thawing, amotosalen-pathogen reduced plasma (AI-FFP) contains at least 0.5 IU/mL of factor VIII with 70% compliance in the bags tested.
> - Fibrinogen dosing: after thawing, AI-FFP contains at least 2 g/L of fibrinogen with 70% compliance in the bags tested.
>
> The factor VIII and fibrinogen are dosed separately on a sample that is representative of production.
>
> **For quarantined plasma (Q-FFP)**
> Factor VIII levels are checked on a pool of at least 6 units of plasma.

Assessment of labile blood products

The products proposed for inclusion on the list of LBP are assessed by the ANSM via an application whose content is determined by the Director-General of the ANSM. For the assessment of LBP, the ANSM is supported by an expert group (LBP-EG).

In its Notice to Applicants, the ANSM identified 4 situations in which an application for authorization must be submitted (Table XXIV).

For applications in categories **A or B**, the validation is carried out in 3 phases before authorization:
- the first phase does not authorize the use of compliant products;
- the second phase authorizes such use;
- a third phase concerns post-implementation follow-up.

For category **C** applications, tests are conducted in a single phase before authorization.

The quality controls requested by the ANSM cover compliance with LBP characteristics, checking the performance of leucocyte depletion, influence of the preparation methods on LBP quality, and the physicochemical and biological quality of LBP during storage. For a new LBP, toxicological and clinical data may be included at the ANSM's request. The ANSM also considers the protection of donors and recipients. The applications are examined by a group of experts appointed by the Director-General.

Data on the quality of LBP may vary if changes are made to the collection, preparation or storage process.

Eight causes of significant change have been identified:
- new filter or new leucocyte depletion;

Table XXIV. Categories of ANSM authorization applications.

Category of the application	Category A	Category B	Category C	Category D
Entry level	New LBP, not already listed	Major amendment to a listed LBP	Non-major amendment to a listed LBP	Minor amendment to a listed LBP
Phase 1: extensive validation of the process	30 LBP unsuitable for therapeutic use	30 LBP unsuitable for therapeutic use	15 LBP unsuitable for therapeutic use	No
Phase 2: operational validation of the process in routine practice	2 × 100 LBP suitable for therapeutic use in 2 ETS	2 × 100 LBP suitable for therapeutic use in 2 ETS	No	No
Phase 3: quality monitoring of the LBP	Results of QC every 4 months for one year	Results of QC every 4 months for one year	No	No
Content of the application: data on the quality of the LBP				
Composition	Yes	Yes	Yes	No
Data on collection	Yes	Yes	Where appropriate	Where appropriate
Data on preparation	Yes	Yes	Where appropriate	Where appropriate
Data on quality control	Yes	Yes	Yes	No
Data on stability (storage)	Yes	Yes	Yes	No
Non-clinical data	Yes	Where appropriate	No	No
Clinical data	Yes	Where appropriate	No	No

ANSM: French National Agency for the Safety of Medicines and Health Products; LBP: labile blood product; ETS: blood establishment.

11. Assessment

- new SUD;
- new automated preparation machine;
- new anticoagulant;
- new storage solution;
- extension to the length of storage;
- new automated aphaeresis machine;
- new pathogen reduction technique.

A list of data to provide accompanies each one (Table XXV).

Table XXV. List of data to provide in an application for packed red blood cells in category A or B for three standard situations (for the full list, see the Notice for Applicants).

Parameter	New filter or leucocyte depletion	New automated aphaeresis machine	New pathogen reduction technique
Number (end products)	30	30	30
Quality of the LBP: compliant characteristics			
Volume	x	x	x
Haemoglobin	x	x	x
Haematocrit	x	x	x
Residual leucocytes	x	x	x
Residual "added components"			x
Quality of the LBP: performance of leucocyte depletion			
Residual leucocytes prior to filtration	x		
Leucocyte depletion	x		
Loss of haemoglobin	x		
Loss of volume	x		
Haemolysis	x		
Quality of the LBP: when stored			
Haemoglobin content	x	x	x
Haematocrit	x	x	x
Potassium	x	x	x
Lactate	x	x	x
Sodium	Optional	Optional	x
pCO$_2$	Optional	Optional	x
pO$_2$	Optional	Optional	x
pH	x	x	x
Glucose	x	x	x
Haemolysis	x	x	x
ATP or 2-3 DPG or % spherocytes	x	x	x
Aphaeresis procedure			
Collection time		x	
Aphaeresis donor			
Blood pressure before/after donating		x	
Pulse before/after donating		x	
CBC before/after donating		x	
Adverse reactions		x	
Safety			
Bacteriological control at D7	x	x	x
Pathogen elimination/attenuation			x

LBP: labile blood product; DPG: diphosphoglycerate; CBC: complete blood count.

For any other change, which may not be detailed in the Notice to Applicants, an application entitled "request for scientific opinion" is first submitted to the ANSM to obtain its opinion on the category of application to submit and the list of data to provide.

External quality controls undertaken by the ANSM

These quality controls form part of the Agency's remit. As well as a strictly normative assessment of the quality and characteristics of LBP, the controls include the temperature on arrival and during transportation to the ANSM, labelling and the physicochemical, biological and microbiological analyses of LBP. Approximately 700 LBP are quality controlled by the ANSM each year during regular campaigns.

The anomalies identified during the quality controls are classified as "major" or "minor". The most common major anomaly is bacterial contamination of an LBP, which triggers an in-depth investigation involving LBP from the same donation, the donor and the recipients. The most common minor anomaly is an individual factor VIII level of less than 0.5 IU/mL in plasma, which requires, in addition to information on the blood group, further details of the preparation of the LBP and perhaps the recall of the donor at the discretion of the ETS.

Conclusion

QC within the EFS is an area that is changing fast. New preparation processes, such as the automated manufacture of pools of standard platelet concentrates (P-SD-PC) or separation of whole blood, pathogen reduction and the needs expressed by LBP users are constantly increasing the demands on characteristics required from products. If we are to implement advanced automation processes, we need to be increasingly efficient over the characteristics of whole blood, buffy coats (haematocrit, platelet content, volume), platelet concentrates (platelet concentration, plasma/storage solution ratio) and plasma (volume, haemostasis factor levels).

QC must rise to the challenge set by these new requirements. Harmonization of the methods, standardization of the equipment and techniques, technological surveillance, stronger national management and the creation of specialized laboratories are just some of the areas of improvement that should be explored without delay in order to meet, or even exceed, the expectations of internal and external clients.

12. Monitoring

**Rémi Courbil,
Anne Fialaire-Legendre,
Saadia Jbilou, Françoise Maire,
David Narbey, Nicolas Ribon,
Emmanuel Terme**

Vigilance is based on the monitoring, management and analysis of any adverse reactions, incidents and alerts.

On a national level, the Vigilance Unit in the French Blood Establishment's (EFS) Medical Division manages and coordinates all forms of vigilance: haemovigilance, biovigilance, pharmacovigilance, medical devices vigilance, reagent vigilance, identity vigilance and software vigilance. Each one is overseen by a specialist who ensures that adverse reactions and incidents are addressed, leading to the implementation of corrective measures and national initiatives. Following analysis, measures may also be implemented in the short (alert), medium (root cause analysis) and long term (introduction of new practices).

At regional level, a consultant in each area is appointed in the seventeen blood establishments (ETS).

Vigilance is integral to every stage in the transfusion chain, from the donor to the recipient of labile blood products (LBP) (Figure 44).

Medico-technical description of "monitoring" services

Haemovigilance
History

Haemovigilance was created in France with the Act of 4 January 1993, which laid the foundations of the newly organized blood transfusion system. This major restructuring was the result of the French Government's drive to improve transfusion safety in the early 1990s.

Following the human immunodeficiency virus (HIV) epidemic and the inconsistent management by the various independent transfusion structures that then covered the country, the authorities struggled to identify patients who had been transfused between 1980 and 1985 to offer them HIV testing in 1992. To prevent

Rémi Courbil, remi.courbil@efs.sante.fr
Anne Fialaire-Legendre, anne.fialairelegendre@efs.sante.fr
Saadia Jbilou, saadia.jbilou@efs.sante.fr
Françoise Maire, francoise.maire@efs.sante.fr
David Narbey, david.narbey@efs.sante.fr
Nicolas Ribon, nicolas.ribon@efs.sante.fr
Emmanuel Terme, emmanuel.terme@efs.sante.fr

Transfusion medicine: the French model

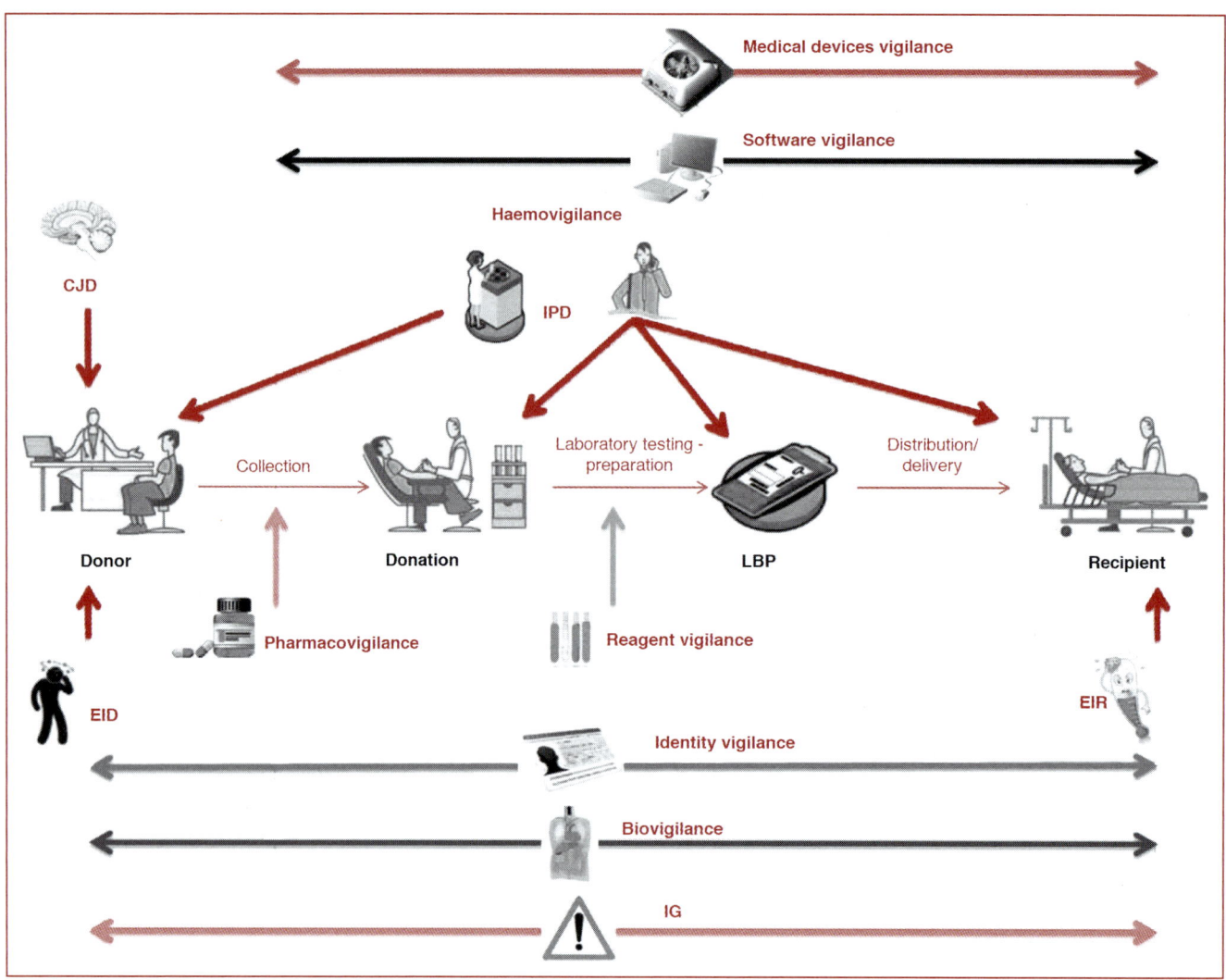

Figure 44. Vigilances involved in the transfusion chain.
IPD: post-donation information; QBD: donation testing; LBP: labile blood product; CJD: Creutzfeldt–Jakob disease; EID: adverse reaction in a donor; IG: serious incident; EIR: adverse reaction in a recipient.

similar health crises in the future, which receive much media coverage, a specific national body, the French Blood Agency, was formed in 1994 and given the task of standardizing the operation of the current system via the introduction of good practice and overseeing its implementation. The agency was also responsible for managing health reports and alerts. This was based primarily on monitoring LBP recipients. Upstream investigations relied on complete traceability of LBP, from the blood donor to the patient and vice versa. For that reason, all health facilities were required to select a single LBP supplier and the ETS were required to keep records of the ultimate destination of every LBP they delivered, *i.e.* was it transfused, and if so to whom, or did it expire or was it damaged and destroyed.

At the same time the various structures were brought together in regional clusters, unifying the statutes of different structures, concluding in the creation of the EFS in 1998, a central government agency (*établissement public de l'État*) formed by 17 ETS which has a monopoly over the collection and distribution of LBP. A separate organisation, the French Health Products Safety Agency (Afssaps), which has since been renamed the French National Agency for the Safety of Medicines and Health Products (ANSM), was then responsible for regulating and inspecting these services. It was also given responsibility for health reports and alerts.

Definition

Haemovigilance is understood to mean "all monitoring procedures organized from the collection of blood and blood components to the follow-up of recipients, with the aim of recording, evaluating and preventing the unexpected or adverse reactions resulting from the therapeutic use of LBP, as well as the serious or unexpected

12. Monitoring

incidents occurring in donors. Haemovigilance also includes the epidemiological follow-up of donors." (Act of 9 August 2004).

Organisation (Figure 45)

The requirement to report any unexpected or adverse reactions due, or likely to be due, to the transfusion of an LBP is binding on all physicians, pharmacists, dentists, midwives and nurses. More broadly, any healthcare professional who observes a serious incident (IG) in the transfusion chain, a serious adverse reaction in a blood donor (EIGD) or an adverse reaction in an LBP recipient (EIR) must report it to the **Haemovigilance Officer** (CHV) appointed by each **ETS and ES** (health facility) using LBP. The latter can also have a **Transfusion Safety and Haemovigilance Committee** (CSTH), which cooperates with and assists the CHV at local level. This network of hospital CHV is led by a **Regional Haemovigilance Coordinator (CRH)** within each Regional Health Agency (ARS), who reports to the ANSM.

The Haemovigilance Officers at each distribution site share information with the Haemovigilance Officers of the ETS delivering the LBP. The latter are the points of contact in the EFS's Medical Division.

A secure remote notification system, e-Fit, is used for both data exchange and quick, easy communication between all the officers, coordinators and respective authorities. Currently, the system manages 4 types of notifications: recipient adverse reaction reports (**FEIR**), serious incident reports (**FIG**), post-donation information (**IPD**) and donor serious adverse reaction reports (**FEIGD**).

Adverse reactions in recipients (EIR)

• **Regulation and definition**

Decree 2006-99 of 1 February 2006 clearly set out the requirement that certain health professionals declare an EIR as soon as it is observed. It states that "any physician, pharmacist, dentist, midwife or nurse who is aware that an LBP has been administered to one of their

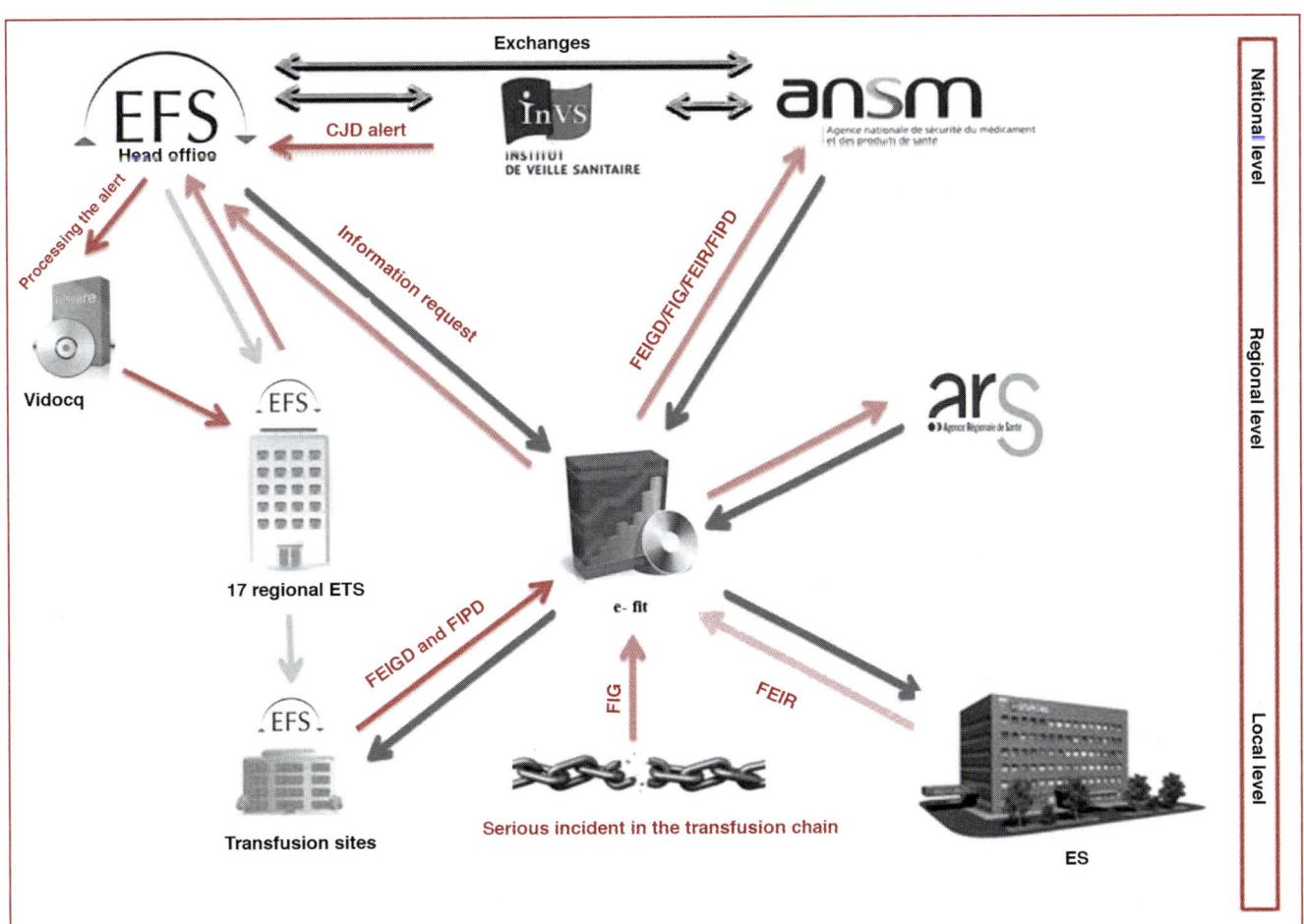

Figure 45. Haemovigilance notification system.
CJD: Creutzfeldt–Jakob disease; ETS: blood establishment; FEIGD: donor serious adverse reaction reports; FIPD: post-donation information report; FIG: serious incident report in the transfusion chain; FEIR: recipient adverse reaction reports; ES: health facility.

patients and who observes an unexpected or adverse reaction due, or likely to be due, to this product, must report it immediately to the CHV of the hospital in which the transfusion took place or, failing this, to the distributing ETS." Article R. 1221-49 of the French Public Health Code (CSP) broadened this requirement to all healthcare professionals, whether the adverse reaction has been observed or is simply suspected, and made the ETS Haemovigilance Officer receiving the report responsible for forwarding the information to the competent CHV.

- **The relevant stages in the transfusion chain**

By definition, an EIR occurs during or after the transfusion of LBP and so affects only the last stage of the transfusion chain (Figure 45). However, its cause may lie in any of the previous stages, in the hospital or the ETS. Distinction is made between the immediate adverse reactions appearing during the transfusion and the following 7 days, and the delayed adverse reactions occurring thereafter.

- **Purpose of notification**

An adverse reaction report form must be completed irrespective of the severity of the reaction. It aims to record the adverse reaction and analyze causality in order to determine the cause and prevent reoccurrence.

The occurrence of an adverse reaction prompts a review of transfusion procedure as a whole, the organisation and operation of the traceability system, and, more broadly, transfusion safety.

The adverse reaction is assessed by the CHV who alert the CSTH or Transfusion Safety and Haemovigilance Subcommittee (SCSTH), pursuant to 4° of Article R. 1221-45 of the CSP. The CSTH or SCSTH can then develop any remedial actions and, through their studies and proposals, contribute to improving the safety of transfused patients. They may also ask the Regional Haemovigilance Coordinator to conduct an investigation into the circumstances leading to the occurrence of this adverse reaction.

As well as this systemic aspect, the FEIR also adds information to the medical records of the patient in question. For this purpose, the hospital CHV sends the approved FEIR to the physician responsible for the patient's care so that it can be included in his/her medical records and stored pursuant to current regulations.

- **Reporting procedures**

These are specified in the Decision of 5 January 2007, which was published in the *Official Journal* dated 16 February 2007: any healthcare professional who observes or is made aware of an adverse reaction occurring in an LBP recipient reports it to the CHV of the hospital in which the product was administered or, failing this, to the ETS Officer, immediately and within 8 hours. The information can be provided by all the means available locally. Working with the hospital CHV and pursuant to Article R. 1221-45, the CSTH or SCSTH ensure that internal procedures for reporting adverse transfusion reactions are written and approved.

- **Notification procedures**

The Decision of the Director-General of the Afssaps on 5 January 2007 determines the format, content and submission procedures of PSL recipient adverse reaction reports (FEIR). In particular, it defines the severity of the EIR, which is scored from 0 to 4, and the causality, scored from 0 to 3 or unassessable, in line with international scales.

E-FIT, which was created and managed by the Afssaps (now the ANSM) in 2004, is used by ES and ETS Haemovigilance Officers, who are identified in the system and hold a healthcare professional card. It is also used by the CRH, the ANSM's haemovigilance consultants to approve notifications, confirm receipt and identify relevant information. The Vigilance Unit of the EFS's Medical Division can consult e-FIT and request further information.

If the ES Haemovigilance Officer does not have access to e-FIT, 2 separate systems, which are likely to change over time, can be used: the protocol and agreement. A guide to completing FEIR is available online from the ANSM, which also provides induction training to officers. Where appropriate, technical reports or additional forms for certain types of EIR or any other useful document may be added to the notification. These notifications must be made to the ANSM and the CRH of the region in question within 15 working days, with information provided as quickly as possible in the event of an issue undermining transfusion safety. The EFS and the French Armed Forces Blood Transfusion Centre (CTSA) each receive the relevant reports.

A "reported" adverse reaction form is created in e-FIT by one of the CHV within 48 working hours of the reaction occurring and is validated by all the CHV involved within 7 working days. The adverse reaction form is said to be "reported" when the reaction presents at least one of the following characteristics:

– involves, or is likely to involve, the safety of at least one other recipient, irrespective of the grade;

– is grade 2, 3 or 4, with the exception of grade 2 adverse reactions with the presence of irregular anti erythrocyte antibodies;

– relates to diagnostics: suspected bacterial incident, irrespective of the grade;

– relates to diagnostics: ABO incompatibility, irrespective of the grade.

12. Monitoring

The CRH, ANSM, EFS and CTSA simultaneously receive the form as soon as it is created in e-FIT. If the issue undermines transfusion safety, the CRH is alerted by one of the CHV as quickly as possible. All the parties involved in the haemovigilance network oversee the FEIR throughout the process.

If e-FIT is unavailable, a replacement procedure is explicitly provided for in the decision of 5 January 2007. The notification timeframes remain unchanged, particularly for "reported" FEIR, which must be sent to their recipients by any available means (fax, email or post). The data recorded using the replacement procedures is entered into e-FIT by the CHV of the hospital in question as soon as the system becomes available.

All FEIR, "reported" or otherwise, are analyzed daily by the EFS's Medical Division which, with its overview, is able to distinguish between new and reoccurring risks, adding an epidemiological dimension to the health intelligence it provides (Table XXVI).

Table XXVI. Changes in EIR indicators.					
EIR – high causality assessment 2. 3 per 100,000 LBP delivered		Indicators 2009	Indicators 2010	Indicators 2011	Indicators 2012
Seroconversion recipients (HIV, HCV, HBV)		0.00	0.00	0.00	0.00
Seroconversion recipients (other)	grades 3, 4	0.00	0.00	0.03	0.03
	grades 2, 3, 4		0.00	0.03	0.09
ABO accidents involving the EFS		0.00	0.00	0.00	0.00
Serious EIR	grades 3, 4	6.89	3.64	2.32	2.67
	grades 2, 3, 4		11.09	10.28	9.51
TTBI	grades 3, 4	0.20	0.03	0.13	0.13
	grades 2, 3, 4		0.07	0.13	0.19
TRALI	grades 3, 4	0.78	0.46	0.35	0.66
	grades 2, 3, 4		0.00	0.74	1.00
Allergy Platelets	grades 3, 4	13.39	3.63	3.10	5.02
	grades 2, 3, 4		19.22	20.67	15.06
Allergy Plasma	grades 3, 4	3.51	5.25	3.97	3.11
	grades 2, 3, 4		9.19	9.0	8.54

Severity 2: severe; severity 3: life-threatening; severity 4: death.
Causality 2: probable; causality 3: certain.
EIR: adverse reaction in a recipient; LBP: labile blood product; HIV: human immunodeficiency virus; HCV: hepatitis C virus; HBV: hepatitis B virus; EFS: French Blood Establishment; TTBI: transfusion-transmitted bacterial infection; TRALI: transfusion-related acute lung injury.

Serious adverse reaction in blood donors (EIGD)

• **Regulation**

Article 3 of Decree 2006-99 of 1 February 2006 requires "the reporting and notification of any serious adverse reaction occurring in a blood donor." The format, content and submission procedures of the FEIGD were defined by Decision of the Director-General of the Afssaps on 1 June 2010.

• **Definition**

Point 1 in Annex I of the aforementioned Decision of 1 June 2010 states:

"An *adverse reaction* in a blood donor is defined as the harmful reaction occurring in a blood donor and linked, or likely to be linked, to the collection of blood."

"A *serious adverse reaction* is an adverse reaction which is fatal, life-threatening, disabling, incapacitating, or which results in or prolongs hospitalization. In particular, an adverse reaction shall be considered serious when it necessitates, or should have necessitated, medical management."

• **Purpose of notification**

Donor safety is a major concern for the EFS and the ANSM. Notifications aim to characterize the EIGD, evaluate the causal relationship with the donation and identify their cause so that appropriate preventive measures (donor selection, organisation of blood collection, etc.) can be taken.

• **Reporting and notification procedures**

Four grades of severity were defined in Annexe II of the Decision of 1 June 2010:
– grade 1: minimal;
– grade 2: moderate;
– grade 3: severe;
– grade 4: death of the donor in the 7 days following the donation.

Transfusion medicine: the French model

All adverse reactions in donors (EID), irrespective of their grade, are recorded in the ETS blood management software. Only grade 2 to 4 reactions must be notified to the regulatory authority.

This notification is made using e-FIT. As with other notifications, the CRH concerned, ANSM, central EFS units and CTSA receive the notifications relevant to them.

Any healthcare professional who observes or is made aware of an EIGD must report it to the hospital CHV, or to the representative appointed for that purpose, immediately and within 8 hours.

The CHV has 14 days to carry out an investigation and notify grade 2 and 3 EIGD in e-FIT. He/she must do so immediately if the reaction has been fatal (grade 4) or is life-threatening to the donor.

He/she may be required to enter additional information on any cardiovascular events or similar, which will be analyzed by the EFS and the ANSM's working groups.

The level of causality must also be shown in the notification:
– causality 0: unlikely;
– causality 1: possible;
– causality 2: probable;
– causality 3: certain;
– UA causality: unassessable.

A replacement procedure must be used if e-FIT is unavailable to report the EIGD requiring immediate notification (Table XXVII).

Table XXVII. Changes in EIGD indicators.					
EIGD – Causality 1, 2, 3 or UA per 100,000 donations	Indicators 2009	Indicators 2010		Indicators 2011	Indicators 2012
	16.69	Jan-July 21.10	Aug-Dec 72.03	133.4	132.34

Causality 1: possible; causality 2: probable; causality 3: certain; causality UA: unassessable.
EIGD: serious adverse reaction in a donor.

Serious incident in the transfusion chain

• Regulation

Decree 2006-99 of 1 February 2006, which transposes European directives on haemovigilance, introduced in Article 3 "the reporting and notification of any serious incident (IG)." The Decision of 7 May 2007 determining the format, content and submission procedures of IG reports was published in the *Official Journal* dated 10 May 2007. The text reiterates that this notification is mandatory and specifies the means of doing so, which centre on existing haemovigilance networks.

• Definition

An IG is an incident relating to blood collection, donation testing or the preparation, storage, distribution, delivery and use of LBP, which may be due to accident or error. It is likely to affect the quality or safety of the products and to cause a serious adverse event, that is, an adverse event which is fatal, life-threatening, disabling, incapacitating, or which results in or prolongs hospitalization.

• The relevant stages in the transfusion chain

IG can occur at any stage in the transfusion chain (Figure 44), in both the ETS and ES. Other stages in the care process, such as transportation (of products, testing tubes, patients, etc.) or laboratory services (clinical immunohaematology, etc.) can contribute directly or indirectly to the occurrence of IG in the transfusion chain. Note that staff members may be involved at all these stages.

• Purpose of notification

IG reveal a dysfunction in the chain which has, *a priori*, been identified in time, but could otherwise have caused an EIR or a EIGD. A FIG must be completed. It is used to record information on the IG and identify possible causes with the aim of preventing reoccurrence. The dysfunction should be halted by removing it from the transfusion chain and reporting it to the CHV.

IG in the transfusion chain are notified in line with the assessment of severity, frequency and other criteria judged relevant by the CHV, in consultation with healthcare professionals, particularly the time at which the incident occurred, the number of previous stages in which it could have been detected, and its exceptional or recurrent nature. Its occurrence leads to an assessment of the various stages in the transfusion chain to determine which are defective and why. It also leads to a review of the organisation and operation of the traceability system and, more broadly, transfusion safety. Priority should be given to serious or potentially serious adverse reactions, narrowly avoided incidents or accidents, or unemotive reactions that can be used as examples. A frequent reaction may lead to a systemic analysis even if it is not considered serious.

These investigations are carried out by the CHV of the ETS and the ES in which the incident took place, or 1 of the two. The purpose is to implement preventive measures.

- **Notification procedures**

In 2007, the scope of e-FIT was enlarged to include IG in the transfusion chain.

The ANSM and CRH receive the notifications. The EFS and CTSA each receive notifications relevant to them.

The CHV notifying the IG has a maximum of fourteen days to complete the investigations and enter the FIG into e-FIT. Notification is immediate if the incident is fatal (recipient or donor), if transfusion safety or the supply of LBP is undermined, if the IG has been made public or if the CHV in the notifying establishment deems it necessary.

The CRH immediately informs the Director-Generals of the ARS and the ANSM, as well as the EFS or CTSA, of any issue that may compromise transfusion safety.

- **Reporting procedures and notification**

Any healthcare professional who observes or is made aware of an IG in the transfusion chain reports it to the CHV of the ETS or the ES in which the incident was detected, immediately and within 8 hours. The information can be provided by all the means available locally.

The notification procedures are the same as those for EIGD and EIR.

The notifier is responsible for amending the report or providing additional documents (root cause analysis, etc.). Any changes are immediately and automatically detailed in an email which is sent to the various parties.

If e-FIT is unavailable, the same replacement procedure as for EIR and EIGD is used. All IG involving an ETS are transferred by the EFS's Medical Division to the EFS's medical experts for information and opinion. Every week, the IG occurring at national level are reviewed by the EFS's Safety Risk Committee for the implementation of an action plan (Table XXVIII).

Table XXVIII. Changes in IG indicators.				
IG involving the EFS – per 100,000 LBP delivered	Indicators 2009	Indicators 2010	Indicators 2011	Indicators 2012
	2.57	4.80	4.74	8.63

IG: serious incident; EFS: French Blood Establishment; LBP: labile blood product.

Post-donation information (IPD)

- **Regulation**

No regulatory text offers a clear and precise definition of IPD. However, the regulations surrounding its notification have gradually been tightened:
- the Decree of 24 January 1994 on haemovigilance guidelines encourages the use of all information to prevent "the occurrence of any unexpected or adverse reaction resulting from the therapeutic use of LBP";
- European directive 2004/33/EC on technical requirements for blood and blood components recommends that donors are asked to inform the EFS of "any subsequent event that may render any prior donation unsuitable for transfusion";
- the Decree of February 2006 on the EFS and haemovigilance makes the notification of "any information that may compromise the quality and safety of LBP" mandatory;
- and the Decision of 6 November 2006 defining the principle of good transfusion practice outlines the requirement to give donors a document after donating which makes them aware of "the need to inform the EFS as quickly as possible of any reasons for changing his/her answers in the pre-donation medical interview, any signs of ill health and any information that he/she believes it would be useful to provide."

- **Definition**

IPD is defined as any information provided to the ETS after a donation which involves the donor and undermines the quality and/or safety of one or more prior donations. IPD covers all donor-related events that may risk the health of the recipient, whether or not the LBP has left the ETS at the time of reporting and whether the risk is confirmed or theoretical. It must be remembered that analysis of this information is always based on the principle of precaution.

- **Notification procedures**

The monitoring and centralization of IPD has been common practice in ETS since 2001. Since April 2002, information that may relate to a potential or confirmed health risk, and whose LBP have left the ETS, has been notified simultaneously to the ANSM, CRH and Vigilance Unit of the EFS's Medical Division.

E-Fit V3 has been used to notify IPD since 23 October 2012 (previously notifications were made by fax and email).

The CHV notifying IPD has 48 hours to 14 days to enter the report form into e-FIT.

This type of reported information must be available for analysis by various parties. This requires detailed clarifications of the donor's clinical symptoms or tests results, which are essential for informed decision-making on the use of LBP, preventing the delivery of unsafe products as well as needless destructions.

The information must be managed reactively on receipt by the ETS. Each ETS has a regional procedure based on the shared IPD management process, which addresses the information's effects not only on the LBP in question but also on future donations for the donor, perhaps leading to a contraindication for that particular donor. This procedure must be clear and fully understood by the professionals involved, with provision made for management in and outside working hours (nights, weekends and public holidays) as reactivity is a fundamental aspect of transfusion safety.

- **Reporting and notification procedures**

The reporting and notification procedures are the same as those for EIR, EIGD and IG.

The information may be obtained from different sources, making it possible to distinguish between:
– *IPD provided directly by the donor* in a telephone call almost immediately after donating. This information may concern the donor alone or in the context of an epidemic. It may also be provided at a later stage after donating: information is sometimes reported during the medical interview at the following donation. In this case, the effects depend on the prior donation;
– *IPD provided by the EFS's donation testing:* this is primarily information on seroconversion, requiring awareness of the risk to the recipient(s) of LBP from the prior donation, if it was collected in the window period for that marker. Therefore, the detection of seroconversion triggers the launch of a downstream investigation aiming to identify and manage the recipient(s) (information, testing, treatment, etc.);
– *IPD provided by an ETS in another region:* the management of IPD should be approached at both regional and national level. Some IPD may involve a donor who is already known in another region and so it must be made available to that region.

- **Purpose of notification**
– *For recipients:* the primary purpose is to block the release, and so prevent transfusion to a patient, of LBP from a donation affected by IPD. If the LBP are still physically in the ETS, their release must be blocked immediately in the computer system and on the premises by informing the department holding the LBP. If the LBP have left the ETS (and been moved to a bank, hospital ward or another ETS), the receiving establishment must be informed as quickly as possible to prevent transfusion. If they have already been transfused to a patient, the prescriber of the LBP must be informed for the purpose of monitoring the patient clinically and biologically and, where appropriate, initiating treatment. This information is generally given by the CHV in the ES concerned.
– *For donors:* if the reporting leads to a contraindication to donation, either temporary or permanent depending on the type of information, this must be recorded in the computer system. The donor must also be informed, in the framework of individual management if necessary.
– *For the collection team:* staff members at the site in question must be told when IPD relates to an epidemic (or to an isolated but particularly contagious agent), so that they can be closely monitored.
– *For the French Fractionation Laboratory (LFB),* which receives plasma for the manufacture of medicinal products derived from blood (MPB). EFS Aquitaine-Limousin (which manufactures fresh frozen plasma pathogen reduced by solvent/detergent) and pharmaceutical companies that use "non therapeutic" donations (for medical research, quality control or the manufacture of laboratory reagents) should also be informed so that they can take the appropriate steps, in consultation with the ANSM where appropriate.

IPD is monitored by the Medical Division by category:
– risks of infection, the leading cause of notification: transmissible disease markers, viruses, bacteria, parasites, etc.;
– theoretic risks: history of transfusion, time spent in the British Isles, neoplasia, risk of Creutzfeldt-Jakob disease, etc.;
– miscellaneous risks: vaccination, intake of medicinal products, etc.

Creutzfeldt–Jakob disease (CJD)

- **Definition**

CJD is a prion disease, also known as transmissible subacute spongiform encephalopathies (TSSE). These degenerative neurological disorders are characterized by their rarity, long incubation period and fatal outcome (first cases described by Creutzfeldt in 1920 and Jakob in 1921).

Reflecting the method of transmission, 3 forms have been described:
– *the sporadic form:* although the most common, its origin is unknown and a risk factor able to explain all cases has yet to be identified;
– *the hereditary form:* Gerstmann-Straussler-Scheinker syndrome and fatal familial insomnia. Genetic prion diseases are caused by a mutation in the gene coding prion protein (PrP). The mutation is thought to transform normal PrP (PrPc) into the abnormal form

(PrPres). Several mutations have been identified, resulting in the 3 different forms of the disease;
– *and the acquired form:* transmitted by the external environment:
  - kuru: a disease found in the Fore tribe of Papua New Guinea, who were known to practice cannibalism as a funeral rite,
  - iatrogenic form: accidentally transmitted to the patient in a medical or surgical procedure (by the transplantation of cornea or dura mater or the administration of growth hormones obtained from the pituitary glands of humans),
  - and the new variant (v-CJD), which results from the transmission to humans of bovine spongiform encephalopathy.

• **Purpose of notification**

The purpose of notification is to prevent any risk of transmitting the disease by blood transfusion.

• **Notification procedures**

Suspected CJD and other human TSSE have been included on the list of notifiable diseases since September 1996. Epidemiological monitoring is currently coordinated by the French Institute for Public Health Surveillance (InVS) and organized around the notification of the cases by clinicians to the Inserm-U708 unit, either directly or by requesting tests to detect 14-3-3 protein in cerebrospinal fluid. Each suspicion is monitored until a diagnosis is made with high probability or certainty (compiling and validating information on suspicions, classification in line with the form, epidemiological description and monitoring the outcome of the case). The ARS and/or Inserm inform the InVS of any patient who may be a blood donor, which in turn informs the Vigilance Unit in the EFS's Medical Division and the CTSA for the conduct of transfusion investigations.

• **Reporting procedures and notification**

Downstream investigations are launched by the Medical Division, which disseminates information to all seventeen regional CHV via Vidocq (the EFS's secure haemovigilance management software) which was introduced in all ETS on 21 June 2004. [This tool provides assistance and support in managing transfusion investigations, one of the key roles of the EFS's CHV. It is used to process and share secure information on donors and recipients who travel across the country. The CHV and Medical Division can consult the entire database. Each user has full access to the upstream and downstream investigations created in his/her establishment.]

The donor and recipient records held by the 17 ETS are then searched.

If the patient is not a known blood donor or LBP recipient, the investigation is closed (the ANSM is informed in an initial and final letter).

If the patient is a known blood donor, an LBP traceability search is performed, the prescriber is informed for the recipient's records, and if necessary the LFB is told.

If the patient is a known recipient, a search is also performed.

• **Risk**

The risk of transmitting CJD through blood transfusion is considered to be theoretical.

For v-CJD, the risk of transmission by blood transfusion is evaluated to be likely.

Precautionary measures have been taken in France to prevent the transmission of CJD by blood transfusion:
– *introduction of contraindications to blood donation for prospective donors:*
  - treated with extracted growth hormone (in 1992),
  - with a family history of degenerative neurological disorders (in 1993),
  - treated with pituitary extracted growth hormone and placental glucocerebrosidase (in 1994),
  - with a history of neurosurgery (in 1995),
  - with a history of transfusion or organ, tissue and cell transplantation (in 1997),
  - who resided in the British Isles for a total of one year or more between 1980 and 1996 (in 2001);
– *introduction of measures for LBP:*
  - withdrawal and destruction of MPB containing plasma from a donor who later developed CJD, has a family history of CJD or was treated with extracted growth hormone (in 1994). (The EFS has records of the products it distributes and so can identify patients who have received an LBP from a donor with a confirmed or suspected case of the disease),
  - search and traceability of recipients of LBP from donations by these donors (in 1995),
  - leucocyte depletion of packed red blood cells and platelet concentrates (in 1998),
  - introduction of nanofiltration by the LFB (in 2000–2004),
  - leucocyte depletion of plasma (in 2001);
– *introduction of measures for recipients exposed to v-CJD:*
  - informing recipients of LBP from donations by these donors,
  - no individual information for recipients of MPB manufactured using plasma from donations by these donors,
  - informing haemophiliac patients who have received MPB manufactured using plasma from donations by these donors,
  - information for healthcare professionals and the general public.

Biovigilance

Definition

Biovigilance, which was created in 2003 (Decree 2003-1206 of 12 December 2003), ensures the safety of organs, tissues and cells of human and animal origin, as well as milk, which are used for therapeutic purposes and related therapeutic preparations. It monitors incidents, and risks of incidents, involving these health products and adverse reactions resulting from their use.

For the EFS, the health products covered by biovigilance are:

- the human organs, tissues and derivatives used for therapeutic purposes in man, whether in routine practice or a clinical trial;
- the tissues and cells used as raw material for incorporation into a medical device or medicinal product (advanced therapy medicinal product);
- the cell therapy preparations used in routine practice;
- medical devices incorporating human tissues and blood derivatives;
- all related therapeutic products.

Purpose

Biovigilance includes:

- the reporting and notification of any incident and adverse reaction which may be due to a product covered by biovigilance, used or unused, or to the activities relating to this product, including collection, preparation, delivery, import, export, transplantation, etc.;
- the compilation, storage and accessibility of information on incidents, risks of incidents, adverse reactions or activities relating to products;
- the assessment and use of this information to prevent the occurrence of any new incidents or adverse reactions;
- the compilation of information on patients, living donors and recipients who have, or may have, been exposed to the adverse reaction or effects of the incident, and monitoring them;
- the conduct of all studies or investigations on incidents or risks of incidents and adverse reactions linked to the aforementioned activities.

In relation to incidents in the transplantation chain, biovigilance does not cover all the nonconformities managed as part of the establishment's continuous quality improvement. Only incidents involving an approved and so distributed or potentially distributable end product, as well as incidents involving an unapproved product but causing a missed opportunity for a potential recipient, risk of shortage or risk to the donor, should be notified.

Healthcare professionals

Similarly to other forms of vigilance, which are already regulated, healthcare professionals (physicians, pharmacists, dentists, clinical biologists, midwifes and nurses) play a fundamental role in the national biovigilance system. They are authorized to prescribe and administer health products and to monitor patients.

Biovigilance is reliant on these healthcare professionals immediately reporting any incident and adverse reaction.

Healthcare professionals must forward all information on incidents and adverse reactions to the Local Biovigilance Officer (CLB) in their area or the ANSM's Biovigilance Unit. They must also retain all documents on the incident or adverse reaction reported to add, where possible, to the information they have provided and cooperate with CLB or the ANSM's Biovigilance Unit in subsequent investigations.

- **The ANSM is the competent authority in biovigilance**

Its primary role is to ensure that reporting and notification requirements are implemented and met as quickly as possible.

The ANSM:

- ensures the safety of the organs, tissues, cells and products of human origin which are used for therapeutic purposes, as well as related therapeutic preparations;
- oversees the implementation of the national biovigilance system;
- sets the directions of biovigilance and ensures that the various partners in the networks follow established procedure;
- leads and coordinates the initiatives of the various parties.

- **Other establishments**

To implement the national biovigilance system and ensure its correct operation, the ANSM works with a network of establishments which includes:

- the French Biomedicine Agency (ABM) which, through regulation services and interregional representatives, provides invaluable local support, particularly in organ transplantation;
- the EFS and the CTSA, which contribute to the biovigilance system primarily through their establishments. A CLB must be appointed in each ETS whenever manufacturing, processing, preparation, storage, distribution, delivery, import or export (meaning a tissue or cell bank) services are provided, or whenever the biological products covered by biovigilance are donated or collected;
- ES, and any other public or private structure providing the following services:

12. Monitoring

- donation or collection of the biological products covered by biovigilance,
- manufacturing, processing, preparation, storage, distribution, delivery, import or export of these products. This includes tissue or cell banks, and the cell therapy laboratories and biotechnology companies that carry out one or more stages in the processing of the human body materials collected for therapeutic use,
- managing transplants of the products covered by biovigilance.

All the aforementioned establishments must appoint a Biovigilance Officer.

• **The Local Biovigilance Officer**

Local Biovigilance Officers act as an interface between healthcare professionals (collection and transplant teams, hospitals, etc.), the ANSM and ABM. In particular, they are responsible for:

- implementing procedures for reporting incidents or adverse reactions, withdrawing or recalling products and exchanging information between sites, ES collection or transplant staff and subcontractors, which are written with all the partners involved;
- compiling all information on incidents and adverse reactions which is brought to their attention;
- notifying the ANSM of any incident or adverse reaction;
- where appropriate, immediately informing the CLB of the ABM and other CLB;
- where appropriate, providing a copy of notifications to officers in other areas of vigilance.

They make the necessary inquiries in biovigilance investigations and conduct any study requested by the ANSM. These investigations aim to assess the risk of reoccurrence and the effects of incidents or adverse reactions, perhaps leading to preventive measures for the other products in stock. They report any issue that may compromise the correct operation of the biovigilance system to the ANSM. At the ANSM's request, they inform the other parties in the national system of the steps taken following the occurrence of incidents or adverse reactions.

If the CLB is responsible for "bank" services, he/she has access to:

- data ensuring product traceability, from release by the manufacturer to use by the ES, which link the batch of therapeutic preparations manufactured to the product of human origin with which it was in contact, ensuring the quality and reliability of the data compiled;
- the biological samples that were used to screen for markers of infection in the donor or the materials taken for further analysis;

He/she submits an annual biovigilance summary report to the ANSM.

In practice

- Biovigilance notifications are made using a reporting form and procedures determined by the ANSM.
- Biovigilance investigations should be coordinated by one person: the "notifying" CLB is the first point of contact of the ANSM's Biovigilance Unit.
- The tissue bank or cell therapy unit that released the product is the only structure able to confirm if other patients are involved.
- Irrespective of the notification system used, it is essential that the CLB in the ES and the tissue bank or cell therapy unit are systematically informed of any incident or adverse reaction, as each has its role to play in biovigilance investigation.

Development of biovigilance following 10 years of implementation

The results are mixed, with an increase in the quantity and quality of incident and adverse reaction notifications recorded alongside a decrease in local resources. However, no fall in the quality or safety of products and practices has been observed. The creation of the ANSM, which aims to reposition the patient at the centre of the health system, suggests that significant changes will be made to vigilance systems in the future. One of the first changes is the creation of a Monitoring Division, which provides assistance in network coordination, and harmonization of vigilance management systems. The management of biovigilance and haemovigilance may also be merged. The National Biovigilance Committee is being replaced by a technical committee and joint vigilance working groups. Therefore, a new chapter is beginning in biovigilance after 10 years of use.

Pharmacovigilance
History

Before the second half of the twentieth century, adverse reactions to medicinal products were observed but did not lead to any coordinated action. It was only in the

1960s that health authorities were shocked into action by the thalidomide scandal. It led the World Health Organisation (WHO) to consider the means of identifying and monitoring adverse reactions to medicinal products, resulting in the introduction of an international pharmacovigilance programme in 1968.

In France, pharmacovigilance developed in the mid-1970s in response to bismuth encephalopathy. In 1984, a Decree made the notification of unexpected or toxic adverse reactions by physicians, dentists and midwives mandatory. It was extended to pharmacists in with the adoption of 2 decrees in 1995: the first on the general organisation of pharmacovigilance and the second on MPB pharmacovigilance. Note that only minor amendments were made to the regulations thereafter.

Risk

Adverse reactions to medicinal products are common, representing the 4th cause of death in industrialized countries. It appears impossible to prevent them altogether due to man's genetic diversity, insufficient consideration of pre-existing medical conditions and interactions with xenobiotics such as other medicinal products, food and contaminants in the environment.

The clinical trials conducted prior to the marketing of medicinal products are still unable to study medicinal product risk in sufficient detail. They are too short, too narrow, not representative of the population (children, elderly, pregnant women, etc.) and include over-simple medical situations. In addition, the trend for granting marketing authorizations (MA) at an increasingly early stage is reducing analysis before commercialisation. This is why the monitoring of marketed products is important in allowing the authorities to take preventive or radical measures if the benefit-to-risk ratio is unfavourable.

MPB must be monitored particularly closely in a traceability system due in large part to viral safety issues.

Definition

Pharmacovigilance aims to monitor the risk of adverse reactions resulting from the use of the medicines and products for human use outlined in Article 5121-1 of the CSP. Pharmacovigilance is provided for MPB and other medicinal products of human origin subject to the specific guidelines applicable to these products, pursuant to 14° of Article L. 5121-20 of the CSP. It is based on monitoring the medicinal products and preventing the risk of adverse reactions resulting from their use. An adverse reaction includes harmful and unintended reactions involving a medicinal product, whether or not it is used as specified in the MA, including misuse, abuse, overdose and professional exposure, or resulting from medication errors. It also entails monitoring medicinal products after marketing to ensure therapeutic safety. For this, the product's benefit-to-risk ratio is constantly assessed.

There are, therefore, several aims: detecting adverse reactions, determining risk (prevalence, incidence, etc.), comparing risk within the same pharmacological family, preventing medicinal product risk, informing healthcare professionals and the general public, and increasing pharmacological knowledge of the product to ensure correct use. Pharmacovigilance also makes it possible to identify new therapeutic indications based on detection of an adverse reaction to medicinal products that are already marketed. Finally, the latest addition to pharmacovigilance is managing health hazards, at both national (with the ANSM) and, following the "Hospital, Patients, Health and Communities" Act, regional level: regional pharmacovigilance centres (CRPV) are set to develop their action in close partnership with the ARS.

Organisation (Figure 46)

In France, pharmacovigilance is organized locally based on the network of 31 CRPV responsible for compiling, validating and assessing adverse reactions to medicinal products, as well as bringing healthcare professionals and, since 10 June 2011, patients information on related issues. Alongside this system, pharmaceutical companies are also required to provide pharmacovigilance for their medicinal products. Reports of adverse reactions occurring within a country are sent to the authorities at national (in France, the ANSM), European [European Medicines Agency (EMA)] and international level (WHO).

- **Upstream alerts**

Physicians, dentists, midwives and pharmacists are required to report any adverse reaction that may be caused by a medicinal product to the CRPV by post or email using a CERFA form or plain paper. However, any adverse effect that may be due to a medicine or product may be reported by any healthcare professional.

As well as general pharmacovigilance requirements, special rules apply to MPB. The traceability of these medicinal products should be particularly thorough and a partnership should be formed with the EFS for the rapid identification of:

- blood donations from which a batch of medicinal products has been manufactured;
- batches of medicinal products that have been manufactured from specific blood donations;
- batches from which the medicinal products administered to a patient originate;
- patients who have received medicinal products from these batches.

In addition, all adverse reactions must be notified immediately for the implementation of measures that may concern all patients potentially exposed to the risk of infection by one or more batches of a given product.

12. Monitoring

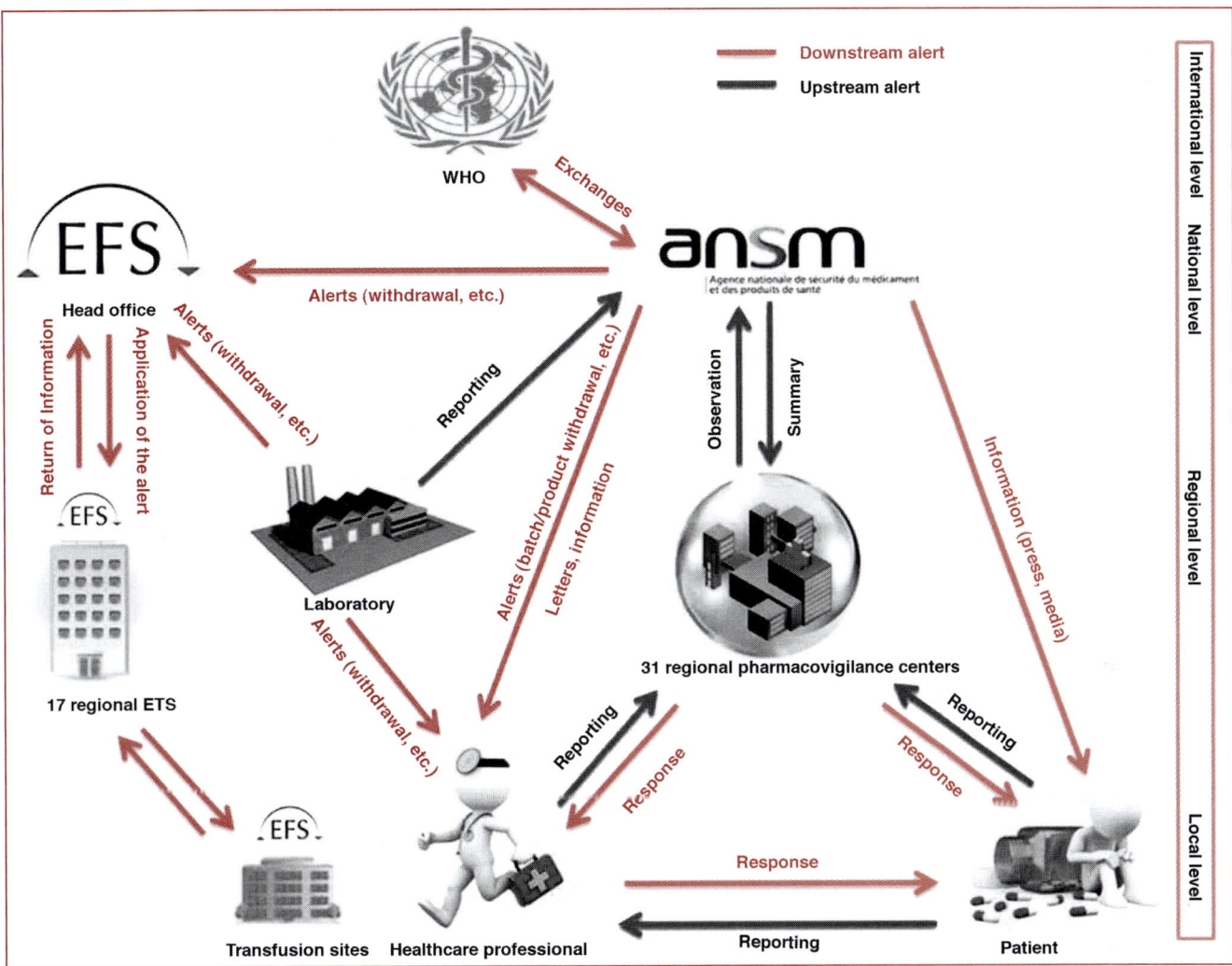

Figure 46. Pharmacovigilance notification system within the EFS.
ETS: blood establishment; WHO: World Health Organisation.

• **Downstream alerts**

As quickly as possible, an external body (the ANSM, a laboratory, etc.) transfers an incident or adverse reaction report downstream to the person authorized to take immediate steps (withdrawal of batches, medicinal product lines, preparations, etc.).

These alerts are sent by fax, post or email and managed by the establishment's Pharmacovigilance Officer.

Similarly, the health authorities may order a precautionary recall of MPB, or the recall may be justified by information on a donor which has been revealed by a subsequent donation. Products may also be recalled if there is a confirmed risk to health; this step would be taken if there was a risk of using the medicinal product.

France has developed the main concepts and played a leading role in pharmacovigilance, with English-language journals translating French articles and the French term "pharmacovigilance" being adopted by other languages. According to the EMA, the Afssaps was one of the mainstays in the construction of the European system, along with Sweden, the UK, the Netherlands and Germany. This was the first official monitoring system to be developed in France. It has become an essential part of health safety. Pharmacovigilance is much more than an activity of monitoring. It sits quite naturally in a wider process of preventing and assessing medicinal product risk in everyday medical practice, respecting the *primum non nocere* principle held dear by Hippocrates.

Medical devices vigilance

History

The importance of medical devices vigilance was recognized by Decree 96-32 of 15 January 1996, relative to vigilance over medical devices and which determines the roles of local officers. Medical devices are essential tools for collecting all the products used to prepare LBP. They come into contact with both donors and recipients of LBP.

Purpose

Medical devices vigilance aims to prevent the occurrence or reoccurrence of serious incidents, or risks of serious incidents, linked to the use of medical devices with the implementation of all necessary corrective and/or preventive actions.

Organisation

Distinction must be made between 2 levels in French organisation: local and national.

At local level, all ETS appoint a Medical Devices Vigilance Officer, who coordinates the services within the ETS. They receive and analyze all reports on the use of medical devices in their region.

They are required to notify the ANSM immediately of any serious incident, or risk of serious incidents, causing, or likely to cause, death or ill-health in a donor, patient or user.

Reports are sent to the regulatory authority using a CERFA form.

The information is also provided to the distributor and/or manufacturer and Medical Division of the EFS. The latter forwards it to all the ETS without delay and works with the ANSM to supplement any interim measures implemented locally if necessary.

At national level, the ANSM assesses the incident reports referred to it, which it receives centrally. The assessment is carried out by an internal team, possibly with external expertise.

Minor incidents undergo statistical processing to detect any deviations.

Major and critical incidents are detailed in a final report similar to the European MEDDEV, which the manufacturer must provide to the ANSM within 60 days. This report must contain an analysis of the causes and outline corrective measures with timeframes for implementation. Critical incident reports must always include an initial assessment allowing any interim measures to be taken immediately.

All the data generated by this vigilance is incorporated into the monitoring of regional ETS contracts and follow-up meetings on the national contracts supplying most of the medical devices used by the EFS and/or the CTSA.

Reagent vigilance
Definition

Reagent vigilance involves monitoring the incidents, or risks of incidents, resulting from use of *in vitro* diagnostic medical devices (IVDD) (automated machines, reagents, software and tubes used in immunohaematology, serology or histocompatibility testing), which may have harmful effects on health.

The failure, noncompliant characteristics or impaired performance of the IVDD must be assessed against the expected results, known interferences and acknowledged limitations of the method, as indicated in its user manual.

It often involves indirect incidents, or risks of indirect incidents, *i.e.* the clinical consequences of inaccurate test results.

Notification

Incidents may be notified to the ANSM by clinical biologists within the EFS (through Local Reagent Vigilance Officers présent in the ETS), healthcare professionals or IVDD manufacturers.

When contacted, the ANSM may fulfil various roles:
– it conducts any studies, investigations and assessments relevant to the reports;
– it may request external expertise from independent bodies;
– it oversees the implementation of the corrective action decided;
– where appropriate, it takes public health measures such as suspending manufacture or import.

Identity vigilance
Definition

Identity vigilance is a system of monitoring and managing the risks and errors linked to patient identification. It covers the patient's entire care pathway, irrespective of "status".

This health vigilance is not prescribed in law.

Origin

In 2009, the annual haemovigilance report of the Afssaps (since renamed the ANSM) found that over half of FIG notifications involved errors in patient identification. This problem was then made a priority, leading to the creation of a national EFS unit in 2010: the Identity Vigilance Competence Centre.

Risk

Poor management of patient identification is an obvious potential risk due to the huge volume of records and large number of anomalies on the databases. Examples include treatment for the wrong patient; error in medicinal product administration; surgery with inaccurate anaesthesia records; mistaken intervention; reversed figures, identity theft, etc. Most of these risks stem from inaccurate data entry into identity records, duplicates (surname, forename, name prefix, date of birth, sex, etc.) and inconsistencies (sex/title).

Organisation
The Identity Vigilance Competence Centre is formed by a Director, Deputy Director, IT Developer and seventeen Regional Officers.

Purpose
The purpose of identity vigilance is to increase the reliability of patient (or donor) identification and the related documents and so to increase the quality of patient management.

To do this, the Identity Vigilance Competence Centre aims to:
- identify critical points and ways to manage patient identification throughout the care pathway;
- implement an EFS identification charter with procedures standardizing data entry (letters, number of characters, etc.) and so preventing the creation of duplicates;
- introduce identification updating procedures (corrections, change of civil status, etc.) for use by authorized personnel;
- raise awareness amongst patients, highlighting the importance of identification;
- make each party accountable (clerks in hospital admissions, ward secretaries, medical staff, laboratory technicians, physicians, database managers, etc.).

Following a report inventorying the identity records (donors/patients) in the databases of the seventeen ETS in 2010, the Identity Vigilance Competence Centre developed an identification management strategy:
- data cleansing: inactivating but not removing data that are not required by law, detecting and correcting anomalies, and monitoring;
- identity management with daily monitoring via a web portal providing access to the results of data queries (portal vigilance);
- communication (prevention);
- development of a donor charter and a patient charter, which were introduced in July 2011 (the donor charter is mandatory and the patient charter is highly recommended).

Software vigilance
Definition
Software vigilance is the vigilance applied to technologies that are not medical devices and the devices used for non-medical purposes in medical testing laboratories, which may have harmful effects on health.

History
Software vigilance was introduced with Decree 2011-1448 of 7 November 2011 on the vigilance provided over the health products mentioned in paragraphs 18 and 19 of Article L. 5311-1 of the CSP (this is the implementing decree of Article 3 of the Order of 13 January 2010 on laboratory services, amending certain articles of the CSP).

Reporting procedures
All healthcare professionals who use these softwares are required to report incidents that may have harmful effects on health to the ANSM immediately, whether they relate to noncompliant characteristics or impaired performance, or to inadequate labelling and instructions for use.

In the assessment of information on a reported incident, manufacturers, developers, distributors and users are required, when requested by the ANSM, to provide information on the design, manufacture, storage, distribution, availability, update and use of these products. The ANSM records, assesses and uses the information sent to it, particularly through studies or investigations on quality and safety, and may order suspensions or withdrawals.

Conclusion

The French monitoring system covers all the critical points in the transfusion chain. It is now necessary to develop and coordinate all the components for maximum effectiveness.

Not all areas of vigilance are as fully integrated (pharmacovigilance) or mature (software vigilance) as haemovigilance. Furthermore, the successive implementation of different forms of vigilance has given the monitoring system a disparate organisation that is unable to manage the frequent interactions required by the complexity of the transfusion chain. This is why it soon become apparent that the different forms needed to be brought together in a single national unit in the EFS Medical Division. The adaptation of this module at regional level is currently being considered.

13. Improvement

Emeline Bizot-Touzard, Éric Hergon, Wided Sghaier

Quality- and process-driven management within the EFS

Most companies strive to optimize their performance. To achieve the best results, all organisations, irrespective of their size, number of sites, area of activity, resources and maturity, need to establish an effective management system. Though first developed in private companies, the implementation of management systems to improve operational efficiencies has gradually been extended to public bodies.

The French Blood Establishment (EFS) has introduced this type of system since it was founded in 2000 and each regional establishment has been ISO 9001 certified since 2006. National multisite certification was achieved in 2012. It provides a governance tool standardizing regional practices as well as improving the EFS's operational quality and efficiency.

In this chapter, we will examine the quality- and process-driven management system, followed by continuous process verification and improvement.

The quality-driven management system

A quality-driven management system encompasses all the steps involved in developing and implementing the policies and targets needed to manage and improve an organisation. Its introduction is the result of a clear strategic choice made by the establishment. It generates continuous progress in results and performance.

An effective system is underpinned by 8 quality management principles on which the quality management system standards of the ISO 9000 series are based:
- **customer focus:** organisations depend on their customers and therefore should understand current and future customer needs, should meet customer requirements and strive to exceed customer expectations;

Emeline Bizot-Touzard, emeline.bizot-touzard@efs.sante.fr
Éric Hergon, eric.hergon@efs.sante.fr
Wided Sghaier, wided.sghaier@efs.sante.fr

13. Improvement

- **leadership:** leaders establish unity of purpose and direction of the organisation. They should create and maintain the internal environment in which people can become fully involved in achieving the organisation's objectives;
- **involvement of people:** people at all levels are the essence of an organisation and their full involvement enables their abilities to be used for the organisation's benefit;
- **process approach:** a desired result is achieved more efficiently when activities and related resources are managed as a process;
- **system approach to management:** identifying, understanding and managing interrelated processes as a system contributes to the organisation's effectiveness and efficiency in achieving its objectives. This principle clarifies the company's operation and removes some sources of dysfunction;
- **continuous improvement:** continuous improvement of the organisation's overall performance should be a permanent objective of the organisation. This involves analysis of dysfunctions, customer feedback, target-setting and evaluation of results. It is often represented by Deming's wheel: plan– do– check– act (PDCA);
- **factual approach to decision-making:** effective decisions are based on the analysis of data and information. Indicators and dashboards can be used to illustrate important information, providing a quick and easy-to-understand overview of the system and facilitating decision-making;
- **mutually beneficial supplier relationships:** an organisation and its suppliers are interdependent and a mutually beneficial relationship enhances the ability of both to create value.

The process approach is central to these 8 principles as the other 7 can be applied directly in process management. Processes are therefore at the heart of companies that wish to develop the quality of their products and services and manage their performance.

Process-driven management

Process-driven management aims to implement continuous improvement that is standalone (logical grouping of activities), effective (managed with sufficient authority) and relevant (process targets based on the general targets).

What is process?

Process is a series of operations or activities undertaken by stakeholders, and using the resources, in line with pre-established standards and methods to achieve a purpose or result. On this basis, process is always shaped around a beneficiary or beneficiary system, whether internal or external.

More broadly, standard ISO 9000:2005[1] describes process as a "set of interrelated or interacting activities which transforms inputs into outputs." The purpose of process is to create a value chain to ensure that customer needs are being met, using the inputs identified. The customers and inputs may be internal or external to the company, depending on the process.

Process may include activities performed by different departments and different sites. They may be cross-functional, creating interfaces between the departments in question. These links remain decisive in improving the product or service provided to the beneficiary.

The input of process activity or process itself is a product needed to perform the activity and obtain the required output. The outputs may be inputs from another process or another activity in the same process. This input is "consumed" by the resources, such as members of the organisation, applying the process in line with methods and specifications devised to obtain the output that will be provided to the end client or "next customer": another process or activity in the process.

Therefore, process can be illustrated as shown in Figure 47.

Any activity may be represented in the form of process and this principle applies to all types of organisation. The company itself is a "macro-process", formed by the processes it needs to function correctly, of which there are 2 types:

- **main processes** are the very foundations of the company. Their introduction, analysis and improvement result directly from the strategic decisions taken by the senior managers. The number of main processes is generally limited to facilitate their management. It is customary to identify a dozen, which can then be tracked. These processes are said to be "complex" because they entail numerous functions and involve a large part of the company, which is typically shown in an organisation chart;
- **"simple" processes** are subsets of the main processes. They generally involve fewer stages and are implemented within departments or subdivisions.

Process-driven management
- **Methodology**

Process-driven management stems from comprehensive analysis of the activities enabling an organisation to fulfil its objectives. It can be used to describe an organisation or activity methodically and so to adapt the company's operation to a given situation. It employs continuous

---

1. BS EN ISO 9000:2005 Quality management systems – Fundamentals and vocabulary.

improvement methods and determines the organisation's workflows. The main features of the system are:
– clarification of the roles and responsibilities,
– understanding and meeting customer needs,
– considering process in terms of added value,
– measuring dysfunctions objectively,
– informing and mobilizing people at all levels,
– staff adopting the methods and tools for improving process quality at all levels,
– measuring the efficacy of changes.

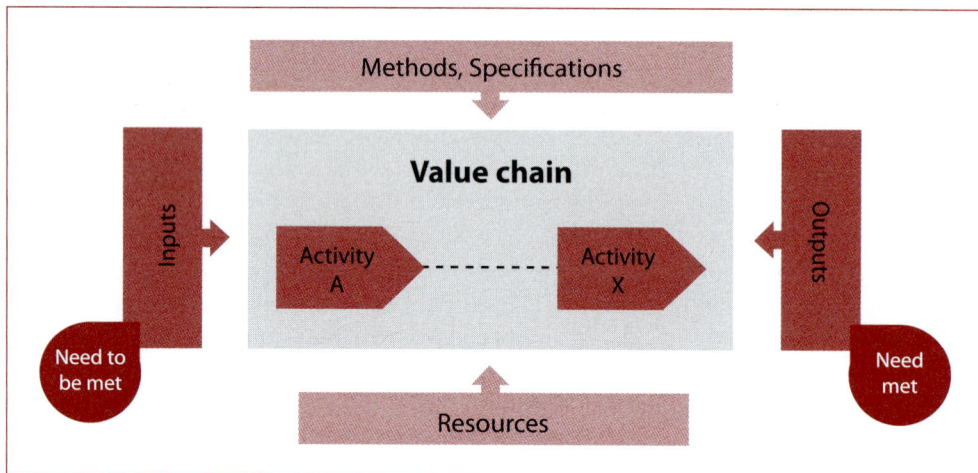

Figure 47. Schematisation of process.

It aims to implement a management system that is:
– standalone, with the logical grouping of activities,
– effective, as managed with sufficient authority,
– relevant, with the introduction of process targets based on the company's general targets.

• **Benefits of process-driven management**

Process-driven management provides a matrix view of company activity rather than analyzing each department's activities individually[2].

It can be used to examine process itself, understand its purpose, the tasks and operations within it as well as the expectations of stakeholders. Knowledge of process and objective assessment of dysfunctions provides a clear view of each component in process.

As the management is comprehensive and systemic, it breaks down barriers between departments, encouraging internal communication between the various actors in process.

This demonstrates the importance of incorporating process management into the company.

Typology of the processes

According to standard ISO 9001:2008[3], "Processes needed for the quality management system [...] include processes for management activities, provision of resources, product realization and measurement, analysis and improvement." Four process typologies can be described:

- **management processes**, which primarily ensure that the decisions taken and procedures implemented are consistent with objectives;
- **production processes**, which cover the activities involved in producing the product, from detecting customer needs to product delivery, ensuring customer satisfaction;
- **support processes** (or resources), which cover all the activities that contribute to the operation of other processes in terms of resources (human resources, information systems, working environment, etc.);
- **measurement processes**, which cover the activities making it possible to analyze the results of other processes against pre-established targets (customer satisfaction, product quality, etc.). If activity tracking generates the data needed for management, the measurement process can be incorporated into the management process.

It is interesting to note that process output data vary with the typologies. The different types of process and outputs can be shown in the Table XXIX:

Table XXIX. Typology of processes and outputs.	
Typology	**Outputs**
Management processes	Policy, strategy, decision-making
Production processes	Product, service
Support processes	Resources
Measurement processes	Indicators, measurements

---
2. Standard FD X 50-176.
3. BS EN ISO 9001: 2008: Quality management systems – Requirements.

13. Improvement

Implementation of process-driven management
Identification of key processes

The contribution made by each process to target achievement, revenue, customer satisfaction, sustainable performance and risk management can be used to identify the company's key processes. They reflect its vision and success factors. However, they are not selected on a permanent basis and should be reassessed in line with developments and policy changes in the company.

Process mapping

Mapping is the presentation of all the company's processes. It involves a visual and graphic illustration of the links between various key processes. It provides a synthetic view of the steps taken in the company to fulfil its objectives and identifies interactions between processes.

There is no "standard" presentation of process mapping. It must be unique to the company and reflect its culture. However, as an exemple, the Figure 48 shows a possible illustration of process mapping.

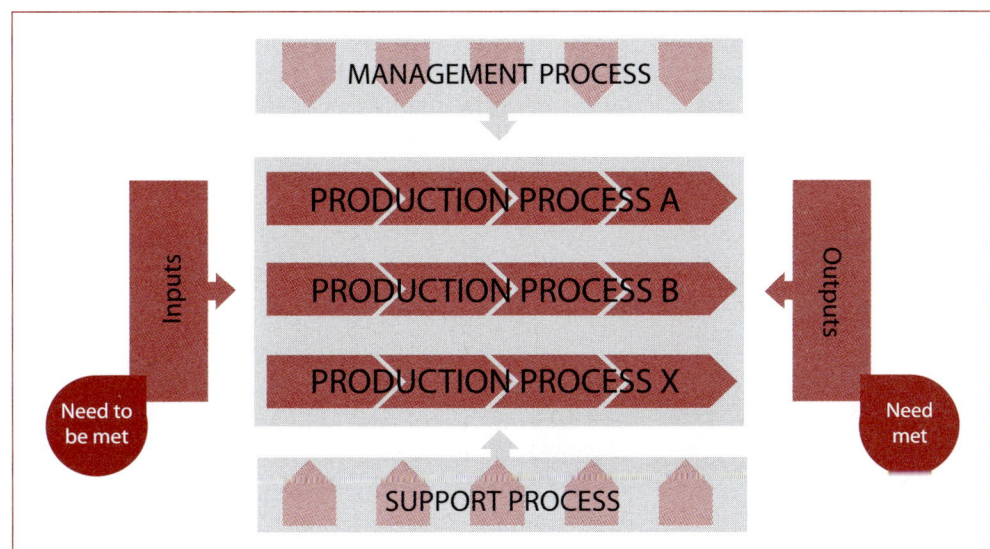

Figure 48. Example of processes mapping.

In complex structures, mapping may be supplemented by specific descriptions of each key process. This more detailed description of activities can then be used to identify their particularities in terms of targets, purposes, resources, stakeholders and management teams.

Process-driven management

Conventional hierarchies do not apply to the process approach as this management system involves many different parties from various departments. With this in mind, it is vital to identify a leader for each process and to implement decision-making and regulation frameworks for all the organisation's processes.

The aim is not to duplicate the management structure or recreate the organisation already in place. Process management must be cross-functional.

- **Process management**

The leader, who has acknowledged expertise in the activity covered by the process, has an overview of its processes and interactions with the organisation's other activities. He/she is appointed and supported by the senior managers.

His/her duties include:

– developing process to increase customer satisfaction;
– measuring target achievement (activity, processes and performance indicators);
– addressing dysfunctions (nonconformities identified by audits, inspections and vigilances);
– identifying avenues for improvement (corrective and preventive actions);
– escalating results to the senior managers.

- **Decision-making and regulation frameworks for process-driven management**

It is recommended that the senior managers regularly assess the "health" and maturity of the processes. To do so, they carry out periodic reviews with a standard agenda covering the points mentioned above and detailed in a report or decision record.

They also organize an annual review of processes leading to:

– a general activity report,
– assessment of target achievement,
– suggested avenues for improvement.

Once summarized, these aspects are the inputs of management review.

Transfusion medicine: the French model

Process optimization

Following the launch, design and initial implementation of the approach, the management system enters into an improvement phase. The system works and processes are managed but improvement, progress and optimization are still possible. Often the detection of dysfunctions triggers a change in how a process operates. Optimization remains a proactive step targeting continual improvement through prevention. It is an ongoing initiative that must involve all process stakeholders.

Stages in process optimization

There are several stages in process optimization. They are based on the main project management phases, incorporate the principles of continual improvement and can be illustrated by one diagram (Figure 49):

Using the PDCA method, each phase provides results making it possible to move to the following stage.

Table XXX shows the contribution made by each optimization phase.

Process optimization resources

Identifying process optimization opportunities may not be easy. Continual improvement methods and tools, which have largely been adopted from quality management, are still essential in securing progress. Knowledge of their effect and use is essential for implementation. They can be used to resolve, in groups or individually, issues on which it is possible to compile objective statistical data.

There are several resources but the most important are shown in Table XXXI:

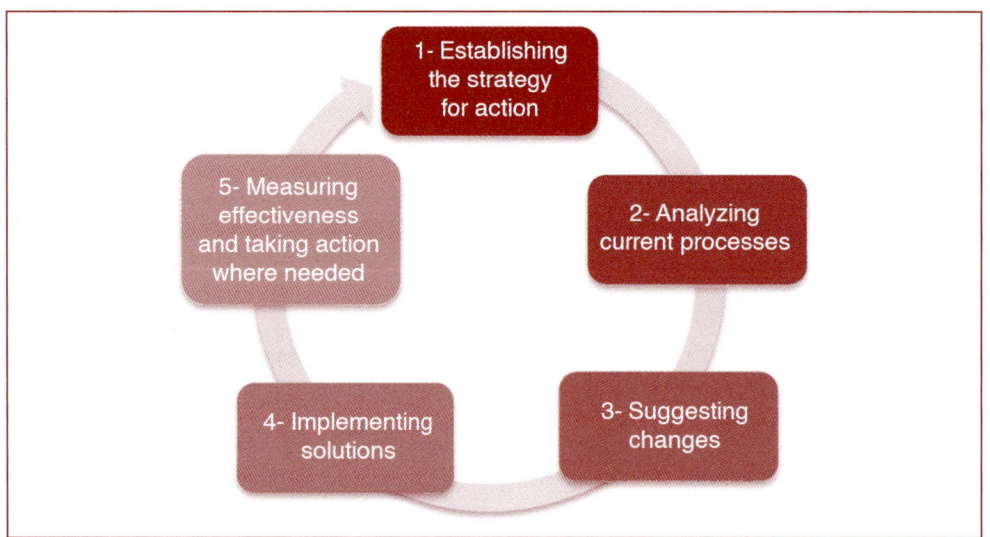

Figure 49. Phases in process optimization.

PDCA	Phase		Results expected
	\multicolumn{2}{l	}{Table XXX. Results expected following process optimization.}	
PLAN	1	Establishing the strategy for action	Identification of all or part of the process to optimize using the policies, strategic objectives and potential for progress *versus* the dysfunctions observed
DO	2	Analyzing current processes	Assessment of the organisation's activity and identification of causes of non-performance as well as avenues for improvement Objective data obtained Justification for a reorganisation of the workflows and process optimization
DO	3	Suggesting changes	Clarifications on the changes needed to optimize the processes and make them more effective and efficient (*e.g.* simplifying current processes or significant changes)
DO	4	Implementing solutions	Development of resources that will rectify the current situation and follow the senior managers' strategic directions as closely as possible
CHECK	5	Measuring effectiveness and taking action where needed	Verification of the effectiveness of the optimization initiatives developed Initiatives amended if necessary

13. Improvement

	Table XXXI. Comparison of the tools and methods of process optimization.		
Type	**Name**	**Action**	**Benefit**
TOOL	Analysis of dysfunctions	Compilation and classification of the dysfunctions observed in a given period	Identification of a priority area for optimization in view of the anomalies detected
	Feedback	Analysis of an event or exercise to understand the causes and the mechanisms leading to innovations or dysfunctions	Capitalization on experience-based learning to draw lessons for the future
	"Cause-effect" or Ishikawa diagram or 5M methods	Diagram visualizing the problem and potential causes by family: Men, Machine, Method, Material and Management	Classification and visualization of all the potential causes of a given problem
METHOD	Benchmarking	Observation and comparison of the resources used by other services or activities, internal or external	Identification of tried-and-tested avenues for improvement that can be adapted to the process under study
	Lean management	Range of management techniques aiming to reduce waste and loss within an organisation	Simplified processes removing activities that provide no added value
	Process reengineering	Analysis and radical redevelopment of a work process. This applies generally to an organisation's key processes	Comprehensive reorganisation of all or part of the organisation's processes in the pursuit of maximum efficacy and efficiency

Auditing and improving the quality-driven management system

The compliance of the management system must be checked periodically. Quality auditing is a useful tool in this area. The fundamentals of quality auditing will be summarized here.

An audit is a methodical and independent review to determine if quality-related activities and results are consistent with process, if process is being implemented effectively and if process is fit for purpose.

A quality audit aims to assess the system's compliance with specified requirements, determine the effectiveness of the quality system in place and its ability to fulfil objectives, give the auditee the opportunity to improve its system and finally to meet regulatory requirements.

An audit should be a thorough and unbiased inspection, providing an overview of the situation and impartial findings. It leads to progress in the quality management system.

The audit is conducted by one or more auditors. These auditors must be independent from the persons with direct responsibility for the audited sector. They must be able to validate a system against a frame of reference, without being influenced by preconceived ideas. Auditors must be familiar with the quality system guidelines and competent in interview and investigation techniques. Several different auditors should provide identical findings in a given process.

The Audit Manager is responsible for the conduct of the audit. He/she must be involved in selecting the auditors, preparing the audit plan, representing the auditors in dealing with the auditee's senior managers, decision making and presenting the audit report.

Auditors must be authorized to conduct quality audits. They are required to prepare the audit, compile and analyze evidence, record observations, and produce and distribute the audit report.

However, they must also meet the requirements that prompted the audit, conduct the audit in cooperation with staff in the audited process, maintain the confidentiality of information provided to them and act with high ethical standards. For this they need personal qualities such as impartiality, good observation, effective note-taking and recording, and strong interpersonal skills (communication, openness, confidence and diplomacy). They must also have the technical knowledge needed to understand the process audited.

The audit has several stages: preparation, implementation, the summary meeting and the report.

The preparation stage involves defining the purpose and scope of the audit, identifying the persons responsible for the audited process, determining the dates, time and length of the audit, building a relationship of trust with the auditee, understanding the frames of reference through examining documents and developing the audit plan.

The implementation stage includes the opening meeting and then the collection of evidence. The opening meeting involves introducing the audit team members to the auditee's senior managers, reiterating the purpose and scope of the audit, presenting the methods that will be used to conduct the audit, identifying the resources needed, confirming the date and time of the closing meeting and, finally, clarifying any points in the audit plan that are unclear.

The collection of evidence involves verifying compliance in all areas, ensuring that procedures are followed and up to date, identifying any sources of noncompliance and documenting each finding with tangible proof.

The summary meeting is held with the audit team and the auditee's senior managers. It aims to present the audit findings and an indication of the system's propensity to meet the stated objectives.

The audit report assesses the level of compliance with applicable standards, related documents and predefined process aims.

An improvement plan is then produced based on the deviations found and is implemented by the auditee. Evidence of improvement and the effectiveness of the actions taken should be verified.

Comprehensive risk management within the EFS

The implementation of a comprehensive risk management policy that addresses the many different risk factors and expectations of interested parties is now essential. A cross-functional approach is needed to cover the complexity of organisations and reduce the potential for accidents, ensuring relevant strategic choices in the future. In this context, the EFS introduced a comprehensive risk management programme based on preliminary risk analysis (PRA) in 2010. The aim was to adopt a harmonized method at national level (single establishment) providing reliable risk analysis per process.

The programme makes it possible to:
- obtain a comprehensive overview of risks within the EFS;
- manage risks insofar as possible;
- provide the EFS's directors with a decision-making tool;
- identify and then share good practice.

The PRA method has been adapted to the EFS's needs. It takes into account all the hazards that the establishment may face in its roles (medical, technical, financial, strategic, management-related, etc.). PRA is used to identify, assess, rank and manage the resulting risks.

The PRA programme is implemented in 2 phases (Figure 50):
- system PRA, which includes the following 2 stages:
  – defining the scope of analysis and formally recording the process/subprocesses to be examined,
- mapping hazardous situations;
- scenario PRA, which has 3 stages:
  – analyzing risk scenario,
- managing the risks and residual risks,
- mapping the risks.

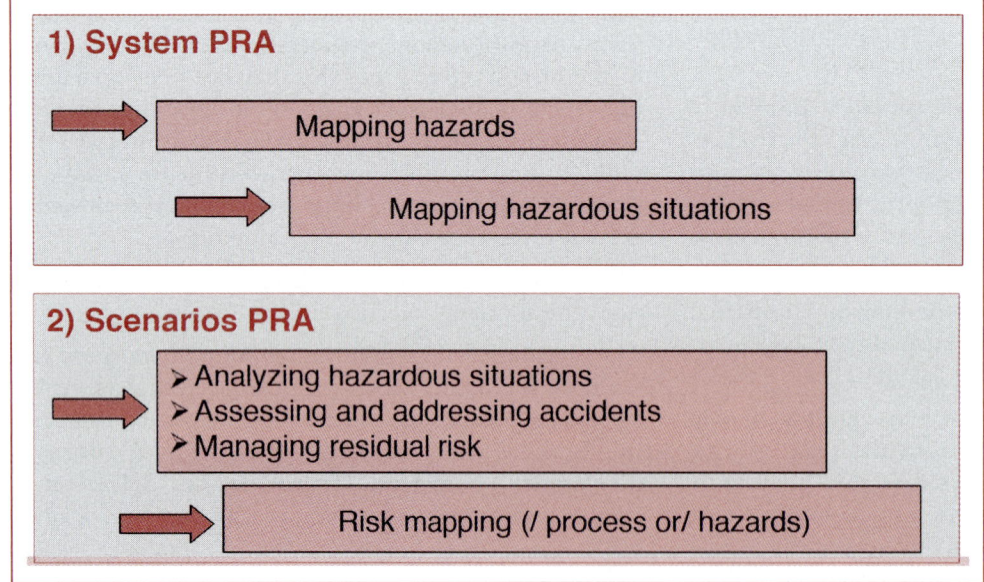

Figure 50. The stages of process PRA (according to Desroches, 2009).

Details of the stages
Step 0: Mapping generic hazards
This stage precedes the formation of PRA working groups. It involves listing generic hazards, specific hazards, hazardous incidents and hazardous conditions. This list applies to all the EFS's processes.

The generic hazards cover the EFS's structure and environment. They are divided into 4 main categories:

13. Improvement

hazards outside the company and internal hazards linked to management, technical resources or production.

The EFS has listed the following generic hazards: medico-technical, strategic, legal, financial, regulatory, ethical, social and environmental, and relating to management (organisation, human resources, human factors and projects), information systems, image, physical safety, commercial matters and logistics.

The list was approved with all the EFS's senior figures: the Chairman, Managing Directors, directors in the head office and directors of regional blood establishments.

Table XXXII provides an extract from the mapping of hazards faced by the EFS.

Step 1: Forming the national working group

A national working group with "business" and "method" experts is formed for each process that is to be analyzed. It must have at least 6 members. Every result is reached by consensus amongst the experts.

The aim of the working group is to:
- describe the various stages in process/subprocesses;
- identify hazardous situations (hazards/process stages cross-matching);

Generic hazards	Specific hazards	Hazardous incident or component
Medico-technical	Process	Error or accident (human factor)
		Error or omission in medical information
		Emergence of an uncontrolled or poorly controlled immunological or biological risk
		Poor management of donor relations
		Refreshments not stored in accordance with food safety regulations
	Products	Quality defect in the products delivered to the health centres
		Safety defect in the products (positive marker, soiled bag, etc.)
Logistics	Transport	Traffic accident
		Failure to maintain vehicles
		Transport provider strike
		Failure to meet packaging and transport regulations
		Delivery issue (delay, incorrect recipient, etc.)
	Equipment and supplies	Quality defect (failure to meet specifications)
		Equipment breakdown (not IT)
		Failure to inspect and maintain equipment
		Poor stock management (*e.g.* stockout or overstocking)
		Supply failure
	Premises	Inappropriate specifications for premises (size, temperature, lighting, maintenance, etc.)
		Insufficient security in premises
		Failure to store hazardous products
		Failure to maintain premises, including specific areas (*e.g.* classified facilities, cold rooms, cleanrooms, etc.)
Information system	Software	Incompatible software
		Software not maintained
	IT equipment	Defective IT equipment (PC, printer, etc.)
	Processed data	Failure in the information system (unavailability of the network infrastructure or telephone system, loss of data, etc.)

Table XXXII. Extract from EFS hazards mapping.

- define the severity scale specific to the process under study;
- analyze risk scenarios (causes, feared events, effects, etc.);
- contribute to determining action to reduce risk and manage residual risk.

Step 2: Defining the scope of analysis and describing the processes

The processes are described separately or collectively, in terms of functions or stages (activities, tasks), and broken down into 2 or 3 subcategories.

It is important to determine an adequate level of accuracy to facilitate the programme whilst maintaining feasibility. The subcategories must make it possible to identify the areas of the system that are likely to be affected by hazards without creating an overcomplicated model that is difficult to use.

Step 3: Mapping hazardous situations

Hazard/system interactions are factors generating hazardous situations, which are created by the sensitivity or vulnerability of the system's components and the level of hazard to which they are exposed (Desroches, 2009).

A hazardous situation is defined as a stage in the system (process) that entails dangers or threats. It is unstable but reversible. The feared event occurs when an underlying cause exposes a vulnerable component of the system to hazards, triggering an incident. The feared event, underlying cause and trigger form the basis of a scenario (Figure 51).

The intersection between hazards and stages makes it possible to prioritize the analysis of hazardous situations. Priority is assessed using a three-level scoring system (1, 2 or 10) and reflects the stages' vulnerability to hazards (Table XXXIII).

The hazardous situations scored as 1, meaning the most vulnerable, are analyzed in the following steps.

The hazardous situations scored as 2 or 10 are not analyzed immediately by the national working group.

Table XXXIV shows an example of the mapping of hazardous situations.

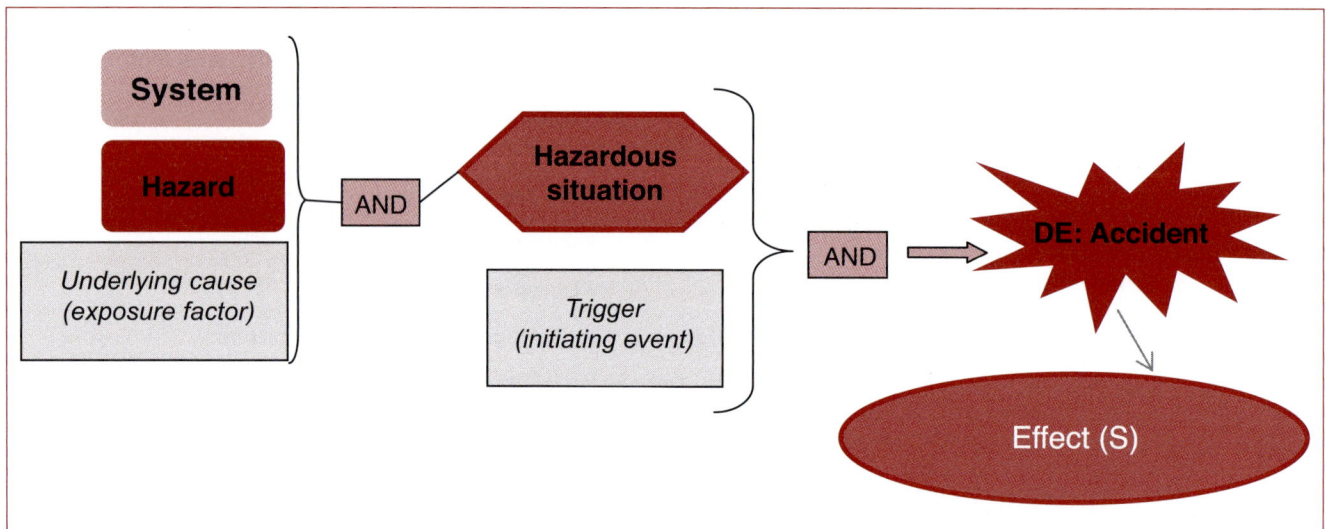

Figure 51. Illustration of a risk scenario [Desroches].
DE: dreaded event; S: severity.

Table XXXIII. Scoring of hazardous situations.		
	Hazard/process interaction	Analysis, assessment and action
1	High to very high	Immediate
2	Low to moderate	At a later stage
10	High to very high	Dependent on another authority or project
	No interaction	None

13. Improvement

Table XXXIV. Extract from hazardous situation mapping.

141	248	192	Recruiting	Welcoming prospective donors						
Generic hazards	Specific hazards	Hazardous incident or component	Recruiting	Welcoming the prospective donor	Identifying the prospective donor	Creating or updating the records in the system	Linking the donation and donor	Producing the collection form (FP)	Sending the information forms, collection form and written questionnaires	Giving explanations and answering questions
Logistics	Transport	Traffic accident	2				2			
		Transport provider strike	2				2			
		Failure to meet packaging and transport regulations	2				2			
		Delivery to the incorrect recipient	2				2			
		Delay in delivery	2				2			
	Equipment and supplies	Quality defect	2				2			
		Failure to maintain equipment	2				2			
		Supply failure	2				1			
	Premises	Inappropriate specifications for premises (size, temperature, lighting, maintenance, etc.)	2				2			
Medico-technical (operations)	Recipients	Error or mistake	1		1		1			
		Failure to provide medical informations								
		Emergence or re-emergence of a transmissible disease	10							
	Products	Quality defect in the products or services delivered by the health facilities	1						1	
		Safety defect in the products								
	Donors	Poor management of donor relations	1				1			
		Error or mistake affecting the donor	1		1		1		1	
		Incorrect medical information provided								

Step 4: Analysis of hazardous situations by the working group

Scenario PRA is based on the mapping of hazardous situations. The inputs are the mapping, severity scale, probability scale and risk acceptance criteria. The outputs are the mapping of initial and residual risks in the form of diagrams and risk management action plans.

The decision-making and probability scales are generic scales applicable to all analyses. Both scales have been approved by the EFS's senior figures.

The severity scale is adapted to the process being analyzed.

• **Severity scale**

Analysis of risk scenarios is based on a five-level severity scale (S1 to S5) grading the effects, whether they impact on performance (S1 to S3) or safety (S4 and S5) (Figures 52 and 53).

• **Probability scale**

The probability of risk scenarios is determined using a generic scale with 5 levels (P1 to P5), which is applicable to all processes (Table XXXV).

Probability can be assessed in terms of periodicity (*i.e.* within a certain period of time) or frequency (*i.e.* number of occurrences).

• **Criticality matrix**

Decisions are guided by criticality (Table XXXVI) defined by a three-level scale and the related risk acceptance criteria (Figure 54).

The risk acceptance criteria, which are based on the severity and probability scales, make it possible to visualize 3 criticalities, C1, C2 and C3, for initial and residual risks. The criteria are also used to systematize decisions related to risk severity/probability.

• **Analysis of risk scenarios**

Risk scenarios are analyzed using a table (Figure 55), which serves as a framework for the system.

For each of the hazardous situations identified in stage 3, the national working group analyzes the **causes** and **the feared event** and identifies the risk reduction methods already in place at national level as well as the **effects**.

Table XXXV. Generic probability scale (EFS).

Probability category	Definition	Periodicity	Frequency/Likelihood	Definition
P1	Impossible to improbable	5 years < T		Less than once in 5 years
P2	Remote	1 year < T ≤ 5 years		Between once in 5 years and once a year
P3	Occasional	1 month < T ≤ 1 year		Between once a year and once a month
P4	Probable	1 day < T ≤ 1 month		Between once a month and once a day
P5	Frequent	T ≤ 1 day		More than once a day

Table XXXVI. Decision-making scale.

Criticality	Level of risk	Decisions and actions
C1	Acceptable as it is	No action is taken
C2	Tolerable if managed	Risk management measures implemented and tracking organized
C3	Unacceptable	The risk is addressed and risk reduction action is taken, failing which all or part of the activity is invalidated

Severity category	Definition	Subindex	Description of the effects
S1	Minor	10	No impact on the performance or safety of the activity
		11	
		12	
		13	
		14	
		15	
S2	Significant	20	Decline in system performance with no impact on safety
		21	
		22	
		23	
		24	
		25	
S3	Serious	30	Major decline or failure in system performance with no impact on safety
		31	
		32	
		33	
		34	
		35	
S4	Critical	40	Decline in system safety or integrity
		41	
		42	
		43	
		44	
		45	
S5	Catastrophic	50	Major decline or failure in safety or system loss
		51	
		52	
		53	
		54	
		55	

Performance
Safety
No impact
Activity loss
Activity failure
Safety loss
Safety failure

Figure 52. Generic severity scale.

Step 5: Regional adoption of national PRA (assessment of risk scenarios)

The analysis performed by the national working group is sent to the Process Managers in regional blood establishments and the centralized services, which should self-assess their levels of risk management, providing details of the methods already in place at regional level (Figure 56).

Severity category	Definition	Subindex	Description of the effects
S1	Minor	10	No impact on the performance or safety of the activity
		11	Delay in the delivery of products or services
		12	Needless expenditure with no major impact on the budget
		13	Minor failure not affecting product quality or use
		14	
		15	
S2	Significant	20	Decline in system performance with no impact on safety
		21	Delay in the delivery of products to the LFB
		22	Minor and temporary decline in brand image with no loss of image and/or clients
		23	Moderate dissatisfaction – no donor retention
		24	Delay in management (of donors or recipients)
		25	Temporary drop in stocks of PSL (products destroyed – products not collected – insufficient donor recruitment)
S3	Serious	30	Major decline or failure in system performance with no impact on safety
		31	Minor harm to the donor, recipient or staff (haematoma, fainting, discomfort, anaemia, pain, etc.)
		32	Marked decline in brand image
		33	Significant dissatisfaction – no donor retention
		34	Insufficient donor follow-up (missed opportunity for the donor)
		35	Significant drop in stocks of blood products (threshold level) (many products destroyed – products not collected)
S4	Critical	40	Decline in system safety or integrity
		41	Temporary invalidity or reversible harm to the health of the donor, recipient or staff (severe anaemia, fracture, intolerance to the donation, injury, etc.)
		42	Temporary suspension in activity
		43	Redundancy scheme
		44	Significant drop in stocks of blood products (critical level)
		45	
S5	Catastrophic	50	Major decline or failure in safety or system loss
		51	Permanent invalidity or irreversible harm to the health of the donor, recipient or staff (contamination, etc.)
		52	Definitive stoppage in activity or closure of the establishment
		53	Death
		54	Stockout of blood products (< critical level)
		55	

Figure 53. Severity scale specific to the aphaeresis donor process.
LFB: French Fractionation Laboratory; LBP: Labile blood products.

		Severity				
		1	2	3	4	5
Probability	5	2	3	3	3	3
	4	1	2	3	3	3
	3	1	2	2	3	3
	2	1	1	2	2	3
	1	1	1	1	2	2

Figure 54. Criticality matrix.

Step 6: Determining risk reduction initiatives, assessing residual criticality and identifying residual risk management measures

The responses of regional blood establishments are weighted and consolidated at national level.

The objectives are to:

- obtain a national overview of the level of risk management;
- determine risk reduction initiatives. These are approved and then recorded in the risk reduction plan;
- assess residual criticality;
- define residual risk management measures for the risk scenario scored as C2 in residual criticality. These are approved and then recorded in the safety parameters (Figure 57).

The results of PRA are shown in the form of risk mapping by subprocess and by hazard (Figure 58).

The finalized PRA (analysis of risk scenarios, risk reduction plans and safety parameters) is approved and distributed for implementation.

The effectiveness of the actions is verified and residual risk is reassessed, where necessary.

The PRA is reviewed periodically and/or in the event of substantial changes to the activity.

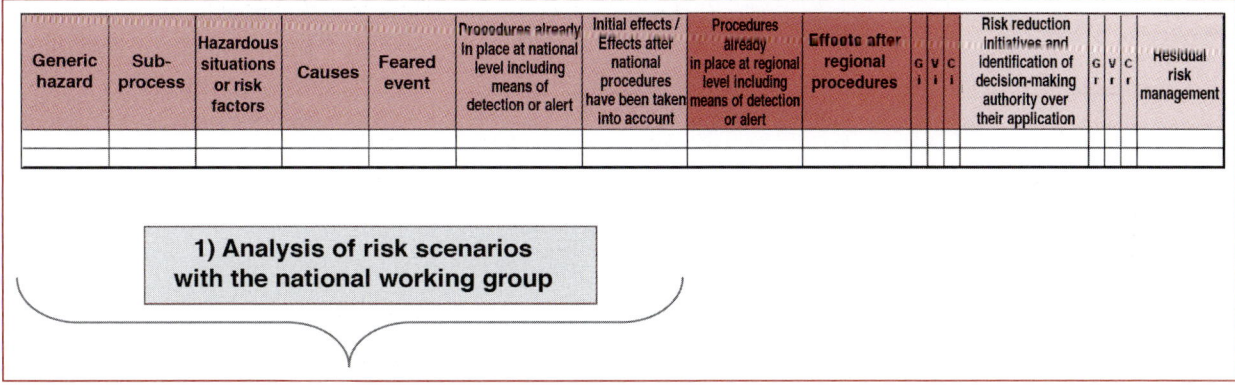

Figure 55. PRA of scenario risk (focus on the initial national risk).

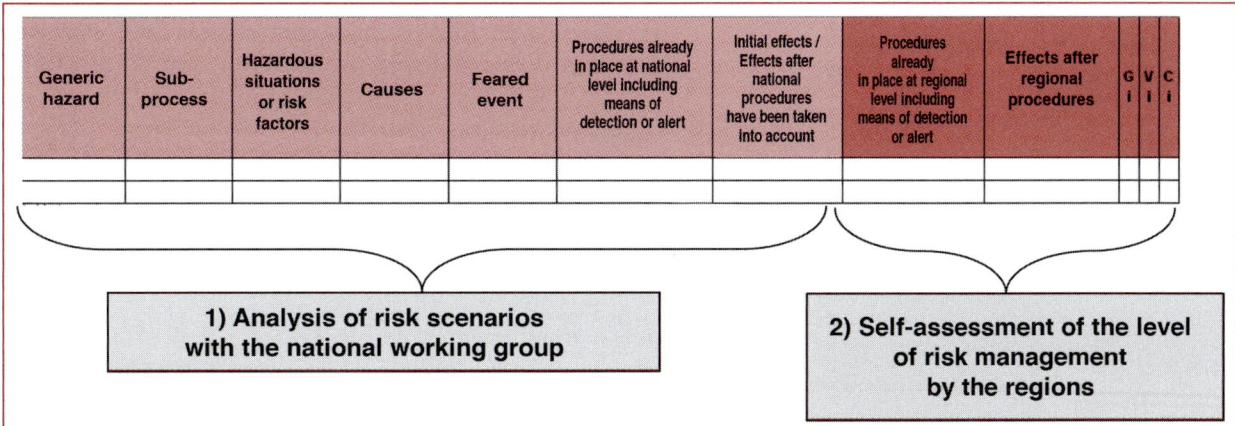

Figure 56. PRA of scenario risk (focus on the initial regional risk).

Transfusion medicine: the French model

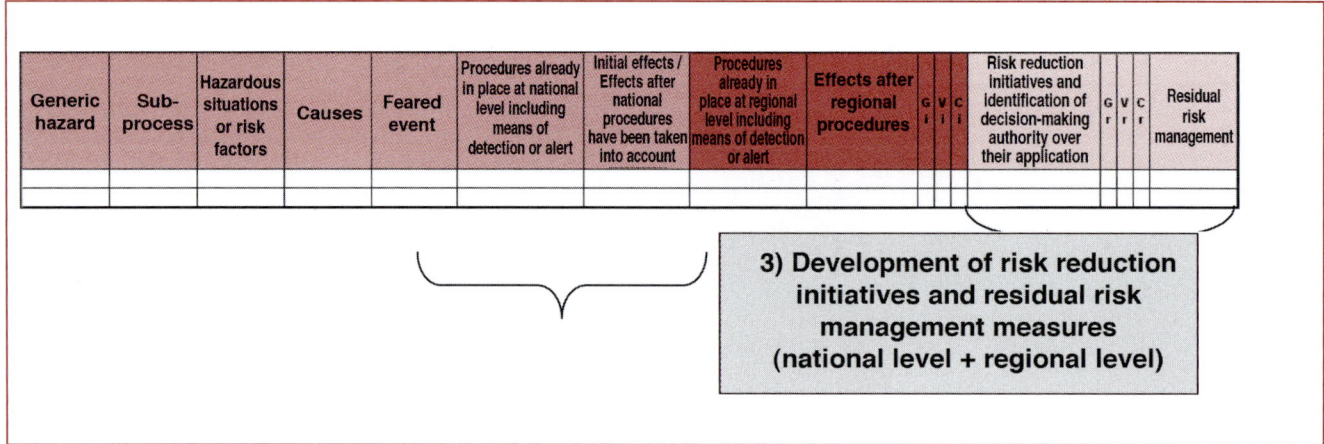

Figure 57. PRA of scenario risk (focus on residual risk).

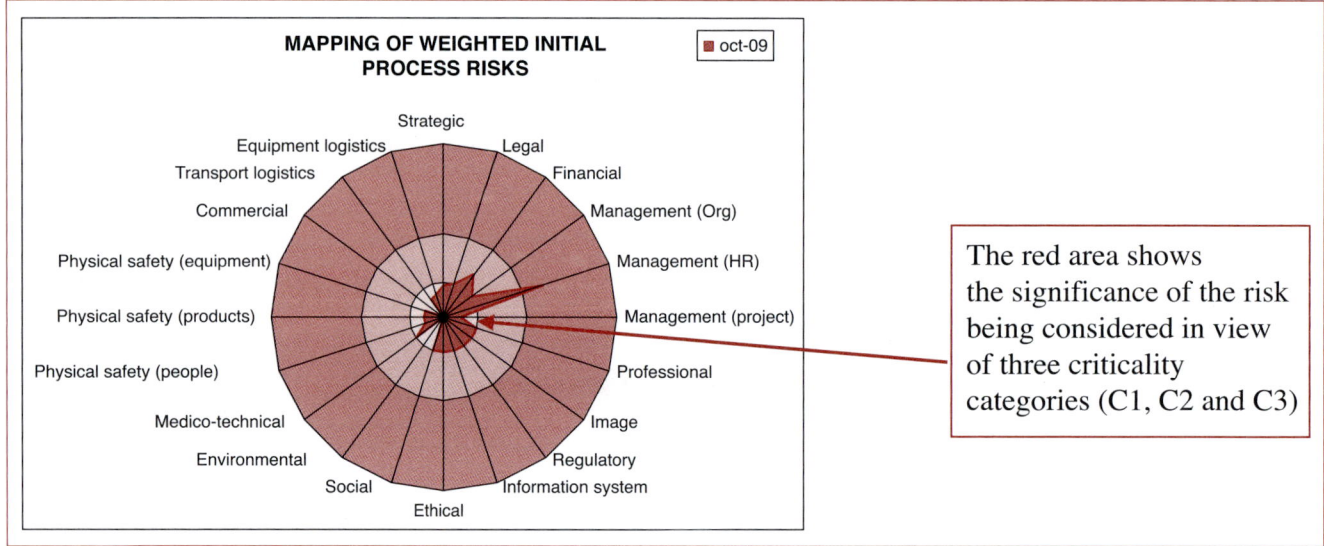

Figure 58. Example of risk mapping by hazard (radar chart).
Org: organisation; HR: human resources.

Conclusion

To conclude, the PRA method has several benefits:
- inductive and systematic analysis;
- semi-quantitative, easy to use method;
- risk management concepts incorporated into the working groups;
- a comprehensive view of the risks, incorporating all types of hazard (policy-related, strategic, regulatory, operational, financial, etc.);
- harmonization of practices through the dissemination of risk reduction initiatives.

However, PRA is only applicable at level local, within a process, and not the establishment as a whole (the overall system and its environment). To obtain a multi-level risk management programme (local and nation-wide), PRA must be supplemented by a method applicable at national level, which is why the EFS is committed to comprehensive risk assessment through identification of the establishment's vulnerabilities.

Part IV
Research within the EFS and the future of transfusion medicine

14. Research within the EFS and the future of transfusion medicine

Pr. Pierre Tiberghien

Research is a strategic priority for the French Blood Establishment (EFS) and is fully incorporated into its activities and goals, enabling it to contribute to scientific and medical advances and to prepare for the future. This involves allocating greater resources to research, working more closely with universities, State-funded science and technology research centres (EPST)[1], hospitals and industry partners in management and coordination, increasing the support for major national and international projects that are of strategic interest for the EFS and pursuing scientific excellence.

Research: a strategic focus for the EFS

Research, which is inseparable from the establishment's medical and technical activities and part of its regulatory remit[2], is a prerequisite for any scientific, medical and technological advance improving the quality and safety of the public services it provides.

Research is at the interface of life, health, human and engineering sciences, central to ongoing concerns over the quality and appropriate use of the blood products prepared from over 10,000 daily donations, a source of medical and technical progress and a tool for anticipating tomorrow's transfusion practices and increasing the prestige of public services. Research is a priority for the EFS.

This research drive, which is being developed with universities, EPST, health facilities and industry contacts, has a very unique position in an establishment such as

---

1. *Établissements publics à caractère scientifique et technologique*, such as the French National Institute of Health and Medical Research (Inserm) or the French National Centre for Scientific Research (CNRS).
2. The EFS's research unit was recently endorsed by the Act on 22 March 2011, which confirmed its role in research and knowledge dissemination in transfusion and related areas.

Pr. Pierre Tiberghien, pierre.tiberghien@efs.sante.fr

Transfusion medicine: the French model

the EFS. As a provider of public transfusion services, the EFS is the vehicle for donors' generosity and the guardian of their safety, the body responsible for self-sufficiency in labile blood products (LBP), a specialist in the production of LBP and cell therapy products which must meet the highest quality standards, an expert in immunological and microbiological risk and, finally, a key partner for health facilities in delivering the right product to the right patient. For all these reasons, the EFS needs to have access to medical, biological and technical research that reflects the significant social and ethical, as well as industrial and pharmaceutical, aspects of its activities. In practice, research within the EFS forms part of a continuum between basic, applied and clinical research.

The EFS has particular responsibility in transfusion medicine, in terms of both research and training. This clinical-biological area, which stands at the intersection of several other specialist fields, not least haematology and immunology, needs to be supported and developed given the high stakes involved in transfusion and its move towards cell therapy and regenerative medicine. Without claiming any exclusivity, the EFS, which includes numerous academics[3], is a major contributor to research and training in this area.

With its upstream processes, which have a strong research element, and downstream applications, which are more closely related to the services provided by an *établissement public industriel* (industrial public establishment) the EFS has the potential to develop innovation. It can then be shared externally in technology transfers, as well as internally, improving the public services.

The EFS's research drive

The EFS's research activities are divided amongst twenty laboratories in thirteen regional establishments, as shown on the map in Figure 59. Most have contractual relationships with universities and EPST, such as the French National Institute of Health and Medical Research (Inserm) and the French National Centre for Scientific Research (CNRS), which should be strengthened and increased[4]. As an associate member of the French National Alliance for Life Sciences and Health (Aviesan) since 2010, the EFS contributes to strategic thinking and scientific coordination within the alliance whilst developing closer relations with other members.

---

3. In 2013, the EFS employed 20 academics, including 14 university lecturers.
4. Currently, 60% of all EFS teams are contracted with EPST or universities, with the target of increasing this figure to 80% in 2014.

In 2012, 152 full-time equivalent (FTE) researchers, engineers and technicians were employed by the EFS for research purposes, and the research budget totalled €21 million, of which €14 million was its own funds, or 1.66% of its turnover.

Research management within the EFS

The 2010-2013 objectives and performance contract (COP) highlighted the dynamism of the EFS's research policy, which has extended its expertise into new activities, such as cell and tissue engineering. Yet it appeared that research within the EFS was insufficiently focused on the establishment's mandate, inconsistently certified and badly coordinated with other parties.

As a result, the EFS has acquired additional research methodology and management tools over the last 3 years. It has also accelerated the restructuring of its teams in line with universities and EPST, and within Aviesan, and increased the development of its research and innovation activities, creating a specific division in 2010[5]. Alongside this, and again in the framework of its COP, the EFS agreed to increase the (self-financed) research budget significantly, with a 1.35 to 2% rise in turnover targeted over 3 years.

The EFS's scientific strategy is devised and implemented by the Scientific Division, which has over time been given additional resources and optimized management tools. These tools include the introduction of annual EFS calls for proposals with a significant budget[6], the creation and development of national projects in priority

---

5. The roles of the Scientific Development Division stand at the confluence of 3 major fields:
- science, for identifying and understanding the innovations and inventions released by the EFS;
- law, for using industrial property to protect innovations and inventions and safeguard the EFS's interests in dealings with academic and industrial third parties;
- finance, for estimating the potential value of innovative technologies to prepare and deliver technology transfers to industry and ensure the best financial return for the EFS in licence agreements.

As an example of the EFS's development activities, the patent portfolio grew from 13 patent families in July 2010 to 30 patent families, including 91 applications underway in January 2013 (versus 23 applications in July 2010).

6. An initial call for research proposals with a budget of €1.7 million over 2 years was launched in 2010. Following an independent external assessment and internal evaluation of their compatibility with the EFS's roles and scientific aims, 14 projects were financed, involving eleven blood establishments (ETS). This was followed by a second call for proposals in 2011, with a budget of €2.5 million over 2 years. Finally, a third €3 million call for tender is supporting 9 proposals in 2013, with 10 projects about to mature and an investment fund available in twelve EFS regions if necessary.

14. Research within the EFS and the future of transfusion medicine

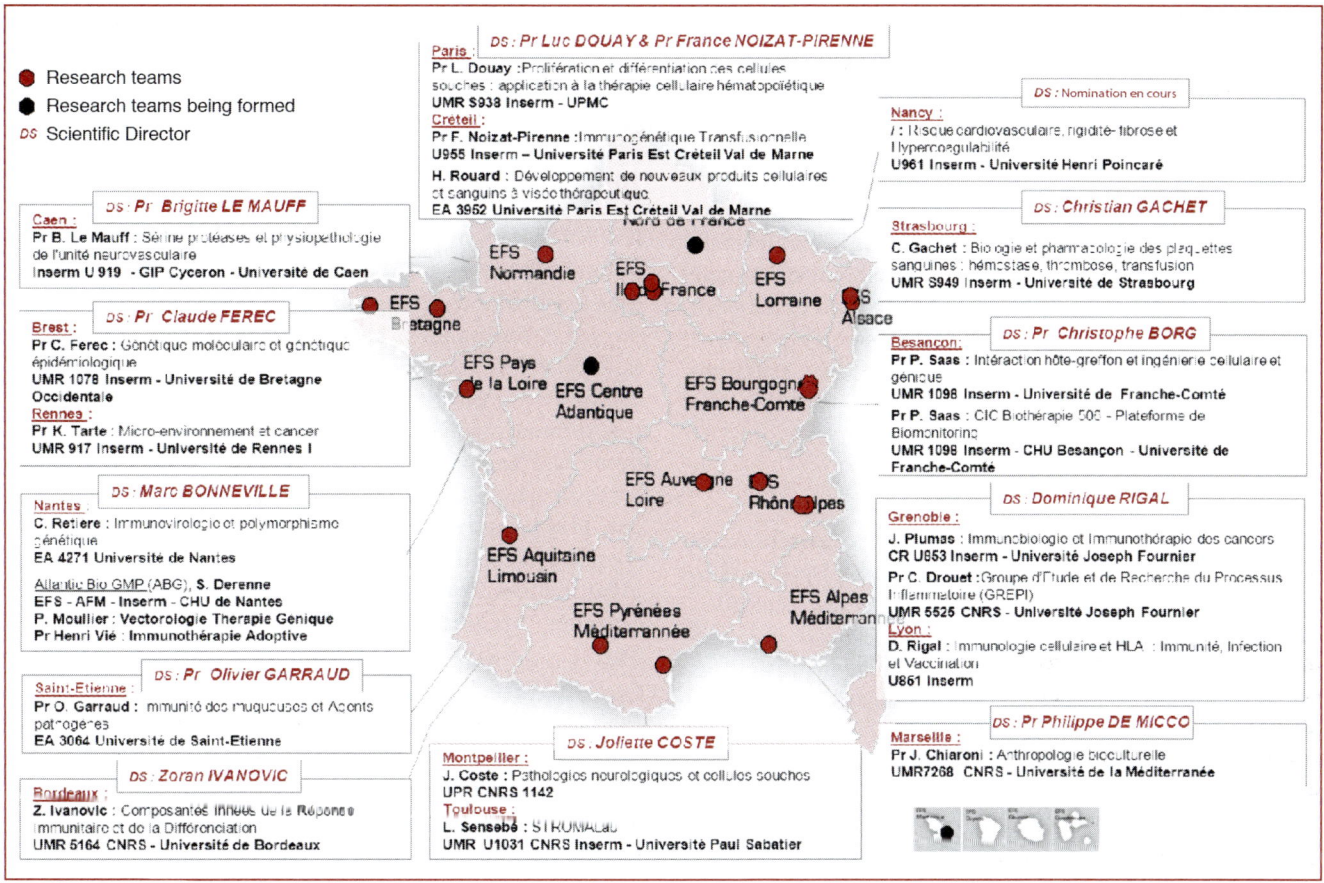

Figure 59. Map of the EFS's research teams.
ATMP: advanced therapy medicinal products.

areas, underpinned by strategic partnerships wherever necessary, the tracking of relevant indicators and, finally, the ongoing review of research activities with the French Evaluation Agency for Research and Higher Education (AERES)[7].

The implementation of an internal call for proposals scheme allows us to allocate greater financial resources to projects that are reviewed twice: externally and independently for scientific quality and internally for compatibility with the EFS's roles and scientific priorities. In this way, the areas of science that relate closely to the EFS's "core" purposes receive priority funding. These can be divided into 6 major themes:
- donation: medical and social aspects;
- blood components: characterization, collection and preparation;
- microbiological and immunological risks (host-product interactions);
- transfusion medicine,
- products resulting from cell and tissue engineering, cell therapy and regenerative medicine;
- epidemiology, public health and health economics.

Alongside this internal funding scheme, and depending on the coverage of priority areas, the EFS may organize thematic calls for proposals open to teams outside the EFS.

Co-funding (French National Research Agency, European Union, etc.) is also encouraged: it follows an independent assessment and highly competitive selection of projects conducted within the establishment, guaranteeing their quality. The EFS is involved in several major projects selected in the framework of the "Investissements d'Avenir" ("Future Investments") funding scheme, particularly in the areas of infectious disease, cell therapy and gene therapy.

Despite its academic recognition [subsection 47.01 of the French National University Council (CNU): "haematology and transfusion"], transfusion is not sufficiently incorporated into university programmes. In a context of critical medical demographics, the need for

---

7. An independent administrative authority formed in 2007, the AERES is tasked with evaluating higher education and research institutes, research bodies, research units, higher training and qualifications, as well as approving their staff appraisal procedures (http://www.aeres-evaluation.fr/). The AERES will shortly evaluate the EFS as a research institute, with a self-inspection scheduled for 2013 and an inspection in 2014.

professional-qualification training is growing and the transfusion sector is set to become more attractive. To meet these needs, the EFS has instigated the creation of a Transfusion and Cellular Medicine University Institute (IUMTC). This institute will be affiliated with a university and linked to other higher education institutes providing transfusion-related training via an agreement signed by the establishments. In this framework, the EFS and University Paris-Est-Créteil Val-de-Marne (UPEC) have recently taken steps towards an agreement in principle with the signing of a framework agreement and the implementation of the first joint teaching programmes.

The major strategic focuses

The EFS is involved in **a broad range of research activities, including basic, mechanistic and physiopathological, and clinical research**. To give a few examples, the studies currently being conducted within the EFS include those focused on platelets, haemostasis and inflammation, the genetics of blood groups, determinants of alloimmunization and host-product interactions, ensuring the safety of blood products in view of transmissible agents, regenerative medicine and cell therapy.

Several EFS teams are contributing to the development of new **cell therapy** products in tissue repair (Toulouse, Créteil) and antitumor (Grenoble, Besançon) or anti-infection immunity (Nantes). Gene transfer tools are being used to develop innovative approaches in **gene therapy** (Nantes), obtain red blood cells expressing new blood group antigens (Marseille) or produce safe T lymphocytes (Besançon). The activation and adhesion of **platelets** and their role in coagulation, thrombosis and immunity are being studied in man and in experimental models (Strasbourg, Saint-Étienne). The potential of **stem cells** in transplantation (Bordeaux), regenerative medicine (Toulouse, Rennes) and transfusion (Créteil) is being actively explored. In **microbiology**, the EFS is involved in characterizing and detecting **emerging pathogens** (Marseille). **Prion** research is yielding important findings in both diagnostics and transfusion risk assessment (Montpellier, Lille). In relation to these risks, the contribution of various **pathogen reduction** methods in LBP is being actively explored (Strasbourg, Grenoble). Significant expertise in **genetic epidemiology** (Brest) is being used in studies on iron overloads and donations via blood letting. In **immunology**, several EFS teams are participating in studies to further understanding of the **immune relationships** between recipients and the blood products or transplants they receive and so reduce the risk of adverse effects, **transfusion deadlock** or **rejection** (Créteil, Nantes and Besançon). In **donation**, the **immunogenetic** characteristics of recently emigrated populations and their effects on blood donation and transfusion are being studied (Marseille, Créteil). Finally, and in another major area, **cardiovascular risk factors** in blood donors (Besançon) and the **prevention of fainting** (Grenoble) are being explored in clinical investigations with our partners in health facilities.

Inflammation and transfusion

A TRALI (Transfusion-Related Acute Lung Injury) is a pulmonary oedema caused in part by the presence, in the transfused blood product, of antibodies directed against the HLA molecules present in the recipient. The risk of a TRALI has been significantly reduced in recent years by the rejection of plasma or platelet donations from at-risk donors, namely women with children or who have developed anti-HLA antibodies. Yet risk factors remain, some of which can be managed, such as the presence of anti-HNA antibodies in the blood product. Others are more problematic, such as the presence of a pre-existing inflammatory condition in the recipient, but this may promote "personalized" transfusion practices.

This demonstration that an LBP, typically plasma or platelets, could cause an acute inflammatory response, in this case pulmonary distress, led to the realization that LBP could be associated with systemic adverse reactions. These reactions could be inflammatory and responsible for morbidity/mortality, which can be difficult to associate with transfusion, particularly for serious polysymptomatic conditions.

Several experimental models in rodents and the first clinical studies in man suggest that factors resulting from transfusion (or already present in the blood product) can cause a range of harmful effects. They may appear in the short or medium term and can be worsened by the length of storage of LBP with, as a possible commonality, localized or systemic microvascular lesions[8].

This area of research, which could be described as emerging, is certainly one of the most important in transfusion. It is being addressed by several EFS research

---

8. Various factors have been identified, such as haemolysis *in vivo* leading to the production of free heme stimulating danger signal receptors such as TL4, excessive iron release, reduced bioavailability of the nitric acid or loss of expression of the Duffy blood group molecule on the red blood cells transfused. Finally, lipid mediators or the microparticles present (or produced in excess) in the LBP could also contribute to these harmful effects. The advancing knowledge put forward to explain the inflammatory risk linked to the product and/or patient receiving packed red blood cells also applies to patients receiving platelet concentrates. Platelets release significant quantities of inflammation mediators spontaneously during storage, which would constitute a micro-aggression, and this production appears increased in the presence of cell stress factors; stressed and aged platelets release microparticles and undergo oxidation in the lipid membranes, which could also be one of the physiopathological components of TRALI and acute febrile non-haemolytic reactions.

teams, particularly the changing role of platelets or red blood cells in line with collection and storage conditions in inflammation (Saint-Étienne, Besançon), determinants and effects of alloimmunization (Créteil) and the role of mediators such as microparticles (Besançon). Alongside this, the EFS is involved in an international clinical trial on the effects of the length of storage of packed red blood cells (ABLE, described below). Finally, in this same area, the EFS is going to great lengths, firstly, to increase the accessibility and analysis of data on the mid- and long-term effects (efficacy and adverse reactions) of LBP and, secondly, to promote transfusion support and more generally the appropriate use of LBP[9].

Cell and tissue engineering, transplantation, immunotherapy and regenerative medicine

Drawing on its expertise in the production, collecting and testing of cell products, whether red blood cells or hematopoietic transplants, and aware that today's cell therapy will most likely become tomorrow's transfusion therapy, the EFS has invested significantly in the areas of cell and tissue engineering. It manages and makes available to patients the majority of therapy and cell engineering platforms in France, both for routine activities and innovation. In 2012, over half of stem cell transplants were prepared on an EFS platform. The EFS also makes an essential contribution to the network of placental blood, producing over 80% of the placental blood transplants prepared in France (3,700 in 2011).

In this framework, 6 EFS platforms have been identified and supported (Atlantic Bio GMP[10] in Nantes, Besançon, Bordeaux, Créteil, Grenoble and Toulouse), which are able, in working closely with research teams, to develop new cell therapy products in the new regulatory context of advanced therapy medicinal products.

The EFS is developing several projects in this area. In relation to haematopoietic stem cells, an EFS/CNRS research team and Bordeaux University Hospital have developed amplification techniques for placental blood transplants, which are currently being assessed in a clinical trial in the hospital. Another area, cell immunotherapy, has seen a number of significant developments. A new antitumoral cell vaccination using immune cells has been finalized by an EFS research team in Grenoble and is about to be assessed in an initial clinical trial (supported by Cancéropôle Lyon-Auvergne-Rhône-Alpes-CLARA). In Besançon and Nantes, coordinated efforts to produce immune cells (T lymphocytes or natural killer cells) that are able to fight infections or cancers are ongoing. These immune cells, which may be genetically modified for safety reasons or for antigen targeting, are undergoing clinical assessment.

Stem cells offer considerable prospects in medicine in general, particularly for transfusion medicine. In the framework of a clinical trial sponsored by the EFS (Créteil/Pierre and Marie Curie University), an EFS team has recently shown that it is possible to produce red blood cells *ex vivo* from human hematopoietic stem cells and that these cells administered *in vivo* have similar properties to red blood cells from a donor. These studies, which are examining the production of red blood cells from stem cells, today from bone marrow, tomorrow from induced pluripotent stem cells, are continuing within a programme of cooperation supported by the public-sector bank supporting innovation OSEO. The possibility of producing other formed elements of blood, including platelets, is also being explored within the EFS, particularly in Strasbourg.

The EFS has also taken steps to structure and support its research into the therapeutic potential of mesenchymal stem cells, particularly in cardiovascular medicine, orthopaedics and immunology. The regeneration of damaged tissue in age-related degeneration and chronic inflammatory diseases is currently a major medical issue. Mesenchymal stem cells are adult progenitor cells that can be isolated from bone marrow and fatty tissue. They are the best response to these conditions due to their differentiation potential and their trophic and immunological properties. These research activities, which are receiving significant support, particularly at European and regional level, are being concretized by the creation of an integrated research centre focusing on mesenchymal stem cells and their therapeutic uses in Toulouse.

Emerging infectious risks and pathogen reduction

The prevention of infectious risk in transfusion is a major safety issue for the EFS. This risk is being addressed through the proactive monitoring of emerging infectious risks, as well as ongoing investment in pathogen detection and reduction.

---

9. In support of this strategy, several recent studies suggest that "restrictive" transfusion practices on packed red blood cells (use of a haemoglobin cut-off of 7–8 g/100 mL and/or on the basis of clinical signs) should be preferred (Carson *et al. N Engl J Med* 2011; *JAMA* 2013). In general terms, compliance with "good transfusion practice" can be improved. For example, a recent study demonstrated that 34% of platelet transfusions in a prophylactic context in England did not follow good practice guidelines (Estcourt *et al. Vox Sanguinis* 2012).

10. In 2009, the EFS opened Atlantic Bio GMP (ABG) near Nantes, a production platform for advanced therapy medicinal products, in partnership with the French Myopathies Association, Inserm and Nantes Teaching Hospital. Covering 1,330 sq m, it brings the scientific and medical community in France and Europe advanced therapy medicinal products that are compliant with good manufacturing practice, thereby guaranteeing optimal levels of quality and safety. In September 2011, an initial patient with Leber's congenital amaurosis was treated at Nantes Teaching Hospital with a viral vector produced by the ABG. Five of the 9 planned in the trial have since been used.

Transfusion medicine: the French model

Pathogen reduction techniques in LBP are being explored in research, particularly in relation to packed red blood cells and platelets. The reduction of pathogens in platelet concentrate has been introduced in a pilot scheme in France's overseas *départements* and Alsace. Strategic cooperation between the EFS and the company CERUS on the development and assessment of a reduction method for packed red blood cells began in 2010.

As well as efficacy in pathogen reduction, the quantitative and qualitative impacts of these technologies on LBP are essential parameters that need to be evaluated in clinical studies. This is the objective of the EFFIPAP trial (detailed below), which is sponsored by the EFS and aims to evaluate the frequency and severity of haemorrhage following the transfusion of platelets, comparing those which have or have not been treated by pathogen reduction using the Intercept technique[11].

Prion risk remains a concern for the EFS, which warrants ongoing research. In this context, the EFS is extremely attentive to developing knowledge on this subject and is actively contributing to research in the area. The research team on the Montpellier site is heavily involved in the development of prion detection technologies as well as the evaluation of various methods (leucocyte-depletion filters, specific ligands, etc.) to reduce the infectious load of a contaminated blood product. The EFS is also working with an expert prion research team within the French Alternative Energies and Atomic Energy Commission (CEA). The EFS is a founder member of the Alliance Biosecure foundation, whose primary aim is to promote research into prion diseases.

Finally, active scientific and epidemiological monitoring should ensure reactivity in the event of a new emerging pathogen. This was one of the reasons for the EFS's participation as founder member in the Hospitalo-University Institute Mediterranean Infection and in increased cooperation with the French Institute for Public Health Surveillance (InVS) (see below). Mention can be made here of research studies on the hepatitis E virus (emerging in transfusion risk), arboviral risk (Dengue, Chikungunya, etc.) and the contribution of proteomics to bacterial detection in LBP.

Clinical research in transfusion

As with other therapeutic preparations that have been used for many decades, particularly those that are considered to be biological rather than pharmaceutical products, LBP have seldom been examined in control studies and, even today, transfusion is too infrequently the subject of clinical research. Although several randomized trials on transfusion practices (relevance of transfusion thresholds) have recently been published, there are few trials on the efficacy (and adverse reaction in the mid and long term) of LBP in line with their preparation, despite the fact that several million patients are transfused around the world using the 92 million blood donations collected each year (WHO[12] figures). On that basis, and given its particular responsibility in transfusion medicine, the EFS has opted to focus on clinical research on blood transfusion in close cooperation with our clinical partners.

The themes currently developed by the EFS as a matter of priority include the effect of the length of storage of packed red blood cells (ABLE trial[13]), the impact of pathogen reduction methods on the efficacy of platelets (EFFIPAP trial[14]),

---

11. Amotosalen treatment (intercalating agent) followed by UVA radiation.
12. World Health Organization.
13. Packed red blood cells can now be stored for 42 days. This timeframe is based solely on haemolysis and *in vivo* circulation data, and the requirements have remained unchanged for over fifty years. Several studies, most retrospective, suggest that the transfusion of packed red blood cells that have been stored for long periods could be associated with adverse reactions and increased mortality. ABLE (Age of Blood Evaluation – Trial in the Resuscitation of Critically Ill Patients), an international, randomized, double-blind, multicentre clinical trial, aims to examine whether the transfusion of packed red blood cells stored for 7 days or fewer is associated with a significant reduction in mortality in 2,510 critically ill patients in comparison with patients receiving conventionally stored packed red blood cells (a fortnight on average). With the EFS's support, the trial began to recruit patients in France in February 2011 and is currently recruiting in Canada, France, the Netherlands and the UK. It is scheduled to end in April 2014 and is coordinated by Dr J. Lacroix (Montreal, Canada); in France, it is coordinated by the Biotherapy CIC of Besançon University Hospital with 160 patients enrolled thus far.
14. The quantitative and qualitative impact of pathogen reduction using the Intercept™ technique (amotosalen + UVA) on the haemostatic functions of platelets is being widely studied. To date, 5 randomized trials comparing platelets treated by Intercept™ to standard platelets have been published. One of them, HOVON, was prematurely discontinued due to rapid confirmation of a smaller increase in the corrected platelet count increment (CCI) and more importantly a significant increase in bleeding in the Intercept™ treatment arm. The same increase, albeit to a lesser extent, in the incidence of bleeding was also observed in a randomized clinical trial conducted in the United States (SPRINT). Unfortunately, these trials are relatively dissimilar and have all been criticized for different reasons. Furthermore, only one of them was designed around an endpoint on the risk of bleeding, which is a central risk when evaluating platelets. However, a meta-analysis recently conducted by an independent investigator based on the 5 available trials reports that the use of platelets treated by Intercept™ may increase the risk of bleeding in patients whose platelet level is maintained at over 10,000 or 20,000/mm³ through an increase in the number of transfusion episodes.

All these findings have led the EFS to conclude that additional research on the clinical impacts associated with the use of Intercept™-treated platelets is required before any decision on implementing the technology is made. In this context, the EFS decided to sponsor the randomized clinical trial EFFIPAP (Efficacy of Pathogen-Attenuated Platelets), which aims to verify the non-inferiority of platelets treated by Intercept™ with regard to frequency of haemorrhage compared with standard platelets. This trial, which will include 810 patients in 8 French university hospitals over 2 years, is led by the EFS in liaison with the CIC of Grenoble University Hospital and began in February 2013.

the prevention of fainting in blood donation (EVASION trial[15]) and more generally epidemiological research in transfusion. To facilitate these developments, the EFS has made it easier to sponsor clinical trials and built strong cooperation-relationships with the biotherapy clinical investigation centres (CIC) of Besançon and Grenoble University Hospitals.

Research preparing for tomorrow's transfusion

Transfusion that will be more focused on product quality and efficacy

Beyond passing safety concerns (particularly in microbiology), growing attention should be paid to the quality of products in relation to their efficacy *in vivo*. There is a real risk of a subtle decline in the quality of LBP, linked to the progressive introduction of new production methods whose qualitative impacts have not been sufficiently evaluated. On this basis, the ongoing debate on the impact of pathogen attenuation methods is significant[16]. Furthermore, it is interesting to see that current thinking on the packed red blood cells/platelets/plasma ratio to be preferred in the treatment of haemorrhagic shock is leading stakeholders to question the place of whole blood within LBP. Finally, similar to targeted medicinal products in cancer treatment, more personalized "à la carte" transfusion services reflecting patient characteristics are likely to emerge, and so the appropriate preparations should be made for them.

Transfusion incorporating innovation at every link in the production and delivery chain

The procedures for collecting, preparing and testing LBP are being required to incorporate as early as possible technological innovations in areas as varied as automation, the traceability of large numbers through radio-frequency identification (RFID tags) and the "omics" within miniature diagnostic devices. Therefore, following recent developments in microbiology, immunohaematology genomics will see some major changes. Proteomics will also provide new opportunities that should be developed. Finally, delivery and transfusion medicine will not be left behind, with innovations provided by micro-techniques in the final checks before transfusion and the quality and exhaustiveness of paperless data exchanges to the transfusion support services.

Transfusion accepting its move to cellular medicine

Without knowing it, transfusion has been at the heart of cellular medicine for many years. The EFS's successful move into haematopoietic (peripheral stem cell transplants, placental blood) and tissue transplantation (corneas, vessels) demonstrates the benefit of pooling skills in this way, which boosts expertise and efficiency. For tomorrow, regenerative medicine, from the mesenchymal stem cells providing tissue repair to the availability of neo-organs, brings considerable opportunities and responsibilities that transfusion must seize. If it were necessary, the recent demonstration that the production of red blood cells from stem cells was not a pipe dream should remind us that "cultured" red cells may hold the key to transfusion deadlock tomorrow and perhaps to a "Copernican" revolution in transfusion a little further into the future. Furthermore, the EFS must be part of this transfusion revolution.

Underpinned by its expertise and values, the EFS should promote new avenues for research and innovation within public services, and take them through to development. As it is now a pharmaceutical site producing advanced therapy medicinal products, but still and more than ever a public body, the EFS can propose the joint development of new therapeutic solutions upstream to universities and EPST, and downstream to health facilities. This new framework should enable optimized return on investment for all public service stakeholders.

Responsible transfusion aware of its responsibilities as a public service

In the wake of health crises, significant resources were poured into transfusion safety. These brought about exemplary developments in risk management and today transfusion can be proud of the very low level of serious adverse reactions reported by French haemovigilance, which, given the 10,000 LBP produced and transfused every day, is reputed to be one of the most exhaustive in the world. There is, however, a serious risk of focusing on the "known" in the future and neglecting less well known and/or emerging risks (the obscure).

---

15. Fainting accounts for the majority of adverse reactions in whole blood donors, particularly at the first donation, and can also impact on retention and donation numbers in these donors. In a context of prospective follow-up, the incidence of fainting is 1 to 4% irrespective of severity (and in the region of 0.1% for moderate to severe cases). The EVASION trial (evaluation of the efficacy of hydration by isotonic solution with or without muscle exercise in the prevention of fainting in whole blood donation) aims to evaluate if hydration with 500 mL of isotonic drink and muscle exercise during whole blood donation can reduce the incidence of fainting.
16. This is why we thought it important that platelets that had undergone Intercept™ treatment (after additive solution) were compared to untreated platelets in additive solution as well as untreated platelets in plasma (their natural medium) in the EFFIPAP trial.

Therefore, "new" risks should be given all the necessary attention, despite the strong pressure on budgets in the current climate and the considerable resources already allocated to transfusion safety. For this, better management of medico-economic parameters should be encouraged in the future. This will make it possible to transfer resources to managing new risks that are considered more significant than "historic" risks, with no increase in costs[17]. Alongside this, steps should be taken to ensure that investment in public transfusion services is used as efficiently as possible. It is in this framework that transfusion has particular responsibility in the future development of cell and tissue therapies. Tomorrow, donation testing platforms may be used in public health initiatives, *e.g.* in screening programmes for human immunodeficiency virus (HIV) or hepatitis C virus (HCV) in the general population[18], or towards a better use of medical testing to benefit the health of donors[19].

In conclusion, public transfusion services are an incredible platform for research and innovation. From more fundamental upstream research, ideally conducted with universities and EPST, to more applied research directly relevant to its roles and medical advances, the EFS's research activities are enabling the establishment to meet all 3 requirements of public service specified in the "Rolland Act": equality, continuity and flexibility.

---

17. A recent study by our Dutch colleagues is enlightening in this respect, giving a cost per life-year saved of €5.2 million (adjusted for quality) for the addition of NAT testing (HIV, HCV and HBV) to the other tests conducted on donations (Borkent-Raven *et al. Transfusion* 2012). In the same study, systematic HTLV serology is associated with a cost per life-year saved of €45.2 million.

18. It is interesting to compare studies on the cost/benefit of the introduction of NAT testing for LBP (see previous note) to recent studies on systematic hepatitis C screening in the general population in the United States, which here gives a cost per life-year saved of $15,700 to $35,700 (Rein *et al. Ann Internal Med* 2012).

19. As an example, a recent study carried out in Besançon, showed that the realisation of a formula (*vs* the absence of formula), triggered while abnormalities were present in the blood count (realised systematically during blood donation), permits the detection of a significant number of haemopathies: (n = 65 for 57,000 formulas realised within a sample of 700,000 donations, from 167,000 donors) among which 3 acute leukemias, 30 chronic lymphoproliferative syndroms (mainly chronic lymphocytic leukemias) and 20 myeloproliferative syndroms.

15. The cell and tissue therapy within the EFS

Anne Fialaire-Legendre

Cell or tissue therapy involves using isolated or groups of cells (tissues) of autologous, allogenic or xenogenic origin for therapeutic purposes. Cell and tissue engineering is the term given to all the stages needed to make these products available: collection, preparation, testing and storage ahead of use.

Two categories of cells coexist **in cell therapy**: stem cells (haematopoietic and mesenchymal) for regenerative or replacement therapies and immune cells (mononuclear cells producing natural killer T lymphocytes and dendritic cells) for immunotherapy. In haematopoietic stem cell transplantation, the transplant can come from bone marrow, peripheral blood after mobilization by haematopoietic growth factors and placental blood. The donor may be the patient (autologous transplant), a related donor (identical HLA in most cases), an unrelated "phenol-identical" donor (from a register of voluntary bone marrow donors) or an unrelated newborn (placental blood bank). These transplants are used to treat haematological malignancy (85%), haemoglobin disorders, bone marrow aplasia and immune deficiencies. The techniques used for the collection and cryopreservation of cell therapy products are semi-automated or in closed system, supplemented by processing methods such as the selection *ex vivo* of cell population or expansion of haematopoietic progenitors.

Tissue allografts are obtained during collection from a living donor (femur heads, placenta) or a deceased donor as part of multi-organ harvesting (corneas, arteries, valves, skin, larger bones, tendons, ligaments) or non-heart-beating organ donation in the mortuary (corneas, skin). It takes place with the consent of the donor or his/her next of kin. Medical selection prior to collection is carried out by the physicians in the collecting health facilities. The tissues sent to the French Blood Establishment (EFS) are then prepared and packaged for therapeutic use. Between collection and transplantation,

Anne Fialaire-Legendre, anne.fialairelegendre@efs.sante.fr

these allografts are typically kept at low temperatures: storage at +4°C or cryopreservation at -80°C or -175°C (with the exception of corneas, which can be stored at +4°C but in France are organ-culture-stored at +30°C). Other tissues are stored using more experimental techniques: islets of Langerhans, hepatocytes or foetal neuroblasts.

Tissue grafts are irreplaceable in many life-threatening situations, such as the treatment of serious burns victims where skin grafts can be used to cover the wounds and prevent dehydration and infection. This is also the case of allografts of heart valves and large arteries, whose resistance to infection makes them the treatment of choice for replacing infected prosthetics.

History

The earliest transplants were tissue grafts and took place some time ago (1869: first skin graft by Reverdin; 1914: first cornea transplant by Elschwig; and 1951: first arterial allograft in humans by Oudot).

The EFS's core purpose is the production of health products from raw material taken from the human body. The rapid development of cell or tissue therapy has largely been made possible by the knowledge gained through transfusion. Its expertise and proficiency in production traceability and quality tools have made it possible to attain high product quality and safety standards, which are shared in the EFS's cell and tissue therapy network.

Cell collection and separation techniques (aphaeresis), and the automation and development of closed systems, have therefore been directly applied to the collection of haematopoietic stem cells. The same can be said of cryobiology, with the development of cryopreservation techniques for haematopoietic grafts and, by extension, tissue grafts such as vessels.

Finally, the use of cells is associated with known and controlled immunological risks in transfusion medicine, such as alloimmune haemolysis, transplant rejection or graft-versus-host disease. Although the immunological problems caused by tissue grafts are less visible than organ transplant rejection, they remain responsible for graft alterations in the long term, e.g. cell infiltration in the medium, calcifications and aneurysmal dilatation of transplanted aorta.

The quality assurance requirements and issues associated with managing a small number of donors, products and recipients are both considerable and highly specific. Therefore, the expertise and experience acquired through transfusion in a considerably larger area of activity are being used to support the development of cell and tissue therapy.

The EFS's role in cell and tissue therapy

Unlike those in transfusion, activities involving tissues and cells are competitive, and the EFS needs to operate within this system whilst continuing to provide public services that meet ethical, regulatory and quality requirements, with the highest possible safety standards for recipients.

The EFS has been developing cell and tissue engineering activities for over twenty years, with the implementation of a network of cell and tissue engineering platforms shared across the country. It is now a major stakeholder (60% of national activity) in cell and tissue engineering. With its eighteen cell therapy product preparation platforms (essentially haematopoietic stem cells for use in bone marrow transplant), the EFS has become the largest cell therapy structure in France. The EFS is also in the process of restructuring its tissue banks to maintain quality and increased efficiency, moving from 17 to 6 multi-tissue banks and 2 cornea banks involved in research and development with local ophthalmology centres. To maintain local availability and highlight the EFS's expertise and products, partnership and development managers have been appointed and are now contributing to the development of these banks. Finally, the EFS is the largest placental blood bank in the country (80% of activity), with national coverage provided by 6 EFS and 2 hospital banks. All these banks have applied for FACT international accreditation (Foundation for the Accreditation of Cellular Therapy), and 2 have already obtained it. By the end of 2011, 41 of the 58 maternity hospitals involved in collecting allogeneic placental blood in France were linked to EFS banks.

The EFS's 2011/2012 activity data are summarized in Tables XXXVII and XXXVIII.

With its structure, the EFS is now able to incorporate new manufacturing processes and is heavily involved in the clinical development of advanced therapy medicinal products (ATMPs). The "ATMP" sector includes research within or outside the EFS, and the development (compliance with good manufacturing practice), production, quality control and supply of ATMPs to health facilities or institution research teams [French National Institute of Health and Medical Research (Inserm), French National Centre for Scientific Research (CNRS), French National Institute for Agricultural Research (INRA), etc.] whilst protecting intellectual property and promoting these products. Mention can be made here of the production of red blood cells from stem cells or virale vectors in the treatment of Leber's disease. The process "supplying cells and tissues" interfaces upstream with the "therapeutic collection's" activity (in the EFS's medical health centres) and downstream with the departments in charge of transplantations in the health facilities (Figure 60).

15. The cell and tissue therapy within the EFS

Table XXXVII. Cell therapy.							
	HSCs		HSCs BM		MNC	HSCs PB	
Incoming activity							
Origin of the cells	Auto	Allo	Auto	Allo	Allo	Intrafamilial	Non-intrafamilial
2011	2,956	763	9	358	139	79	200
1st six months 2012	1,284	314	2	167	58	42	90
Variation	-13%	-18%	-50%	-7%	-17%	+6%	-10%
Outgoing activity							
Origin of the cells	Auto	Allo	Auto	Allo	Allo	Intrafamilial	Non-intrafamilial
2011	1,737	704	12	358	175	9	184 (124 patients)
1st six months 2012	784	296	1	162	91	0	82 (52 patients)
Variation	-10%	-16%	-83%	0%	+5%	-100%	-11%

HSCs: haematopoietic stem cells; BM: bone marrow; MNC: mononuclear cell; PB: placental blood.

Table XXXVIII. Tissue therapy.				
Incoming tissues	2011		1st six months 2012	
	Incoming	% NC	Incoming	% NC
Corneas	4,758	61%	2,771	NA
Amniotic membranes	694	22%	343	NA
Femur heads and viral-inactivated grafts	2,291	26%	1,052	NA
Transfer	2011		1st six months 2012	
Tissues / Transfer site	Distribution	Other French bank	Distribution	Other French bank
Corneas	1,627	298	932	NA
Amniotic membranes	663	187	269	NA
Femur heads and viral-inactivated grafts	4,649	512	3,003	NA

NC: nonconformity; NA: not available.

Conclusion

Cell and tissue engineering is a considerable challenge for transfusion medicine. Transfusion stakeholders have all the knowledge and skill needed to produce cell and tissue therapy products. The development difficulties do not lie in the techniques specifically used for such products, but in the ability to collect, prepare, test, process, store and distribute a product in a context of good manufacturing practice, vigilance and optimal reactivity towards the donor, recipient, therapeutic indication and biological risks incurred. Therefore, the objective for the EFS is to assert its ambition to prepare any cell and tissue therapy product for any patient. Drawing on its expertise and network, it seems possible to guarantee the efficient development, both in scientific and financial terms, of these new therapeutic approaches whose potential for patients appears considerable. At the same time, the implementation of these synergies guarantees the sustainability of the EFS's activity and expertise, and its development as a major contributor to medical advances.

Transfusion medicine: the French model

Figure 60. Schematisation of the process.

Inputs		Prescription (patient need), collection form related products, cellular and tissue products raw material, related biological samples					
Continuous improvement →	EFS head office	Determines the strategy					
	ETS	Implements the strategy					
		Cellular products			**Tissue products**		
	ETS	Steps	Operators	Management instruments	Steps	Operators	Management instruments
		Receipt of the cellular product	Laboratory technicians and secretaries	Collection and transport documents	Receipt of the tissue product	Laboratory technicians and secretaries	Collection and transport documents
		Processing of the cellular product	Laboratory technicians	Record of processing of the cellular product	Processing of the tissue product (including subcontracting)	Laboratory technicians or subcontractors	Record of processing of the tissue product
		Storage			Storage	Laboratory technicians	
		Validation	Production and QC Manager	Record of validation of the processing of the cellular product	Validation	Production and QC Manager	Record of validation of the tissue product
		Request for cellular product	Clinician/bank	Prescription and verification	Request for tissue product	Clinician/bank	Prescription and verification
		Processing of the cellular product to be distributed	Laboratory technicians	Record of processing of the cellular product	Processing of the tissue product to be distributed	Laboratory technicians	Record of processing of the tissue product
		Distribution of the cellular product		Distribution document and verification that the cellular product has been allocated to the right person	Distribution of the tissue product		Distribution document and verification that the tissue product has been allocated to the right person
		Transport of the cellular product	Transport provider, laboratory technicians	Transport and traceability documents	Transport of the tissue product	Transport provider, laboratory technicians	Transport and traceability documents
		Follow-up	Manager, Transplant Committee, ABM	Activity report, report of the Transplant Committee, letter upon patients exit from aplasia	Follow-up	Manager, Medico-Technical Committee of the Tissue Bank, ABM	Activity report, report of the Medico-Technical Committee, various documents
	EFS head office	Tracks and assesses the activity					
Outputs		Validated cellular and tissue products, distribution form, transport form, record of validation of the product					

EFS: French Blood Establishment; ETS: blood establishment; QC: quality control; ABM: French Biomedicine Agency.

Part V
The EFS's European and international activities

16. The EFS, a European stakeholder in blood transfusion

Yves Charpak, Nina Prunier

The French Blood Establishment (EFS) is the sole national provider of blood transfusion services in France. It covers the entire country, including France's overseas *départements*. It is required to deliver sufficient blood products to meet the needs of the entire population resident in France. It must also meet the needs of its public and private partners, supplying cord blood (French Biomedicine Agency (ABM)], plasma for fractionation [French Fractionation Laboratory (LFB)] and tissue to hospitals. In addition, it provides essential treatment for certain diseases (*e.g.* haemochromatosis).

Its monopoly over blood products, many diverse activities and size mean that it is unique in Europe (and even in the world), closely "watched" and therefore able to influence practices and regulations at European level. Other countries also have sole providers but these are "smaller", whilst others have varied activities but their scope of action is often more limited. It is, therefore, essential that we work with our colleagues in neighbouring countries and share our experiences, as the ethical values that are broadly shared in blood transfusion chains across Europe may be threatened by changing practices elsewhere in the world (paid donations, international trade in products, pressure from industry, etc.).

It must be acknowledged that blood transfusion is evolving quite quickly, Europe included. We must monitor the restrictions and developments in our European neighbours and the work ongoing in international bodies with authority over blood transfusions, an area in which France is an influential stakeholder: supranational mandates and powers are legitimately exercised over blood transfusion and products derived from the human body by various international institutions, with a significant and unavoidable impact on our national practices and regulations.

Yves Charpak, yves.charpak@efs.sante.fr
Nina Prunier, nina.prunier@efs.sante.fr

European and international institutions

The European Union

Since the 1992 Maastricht Treaty, European Union (EU) institutions have had the power to act in public health matters. Although the organization of health systems remains the primary responsibility of EU Member States (in line with the "subsidiarity" principle), the safety of products derived from the human body (blood products, tissues, cells and organs) has special status, as Article 168 of the Treaty on the Functioning of the European Union gives the EU direct powers to adopt standards at European level:

> "[...] the European Parliament and the Council [...] contribute to the achievement of the objectives referred to in this Article through adopting in order to meet common safety concerns:
>
> a) measures setting high standards of quality and safety of organs and substances of human origin, blood and blood derivatives; these measures shall not prevent any Member State from maintaining or introducing more stringent protective measures".

This mandate came into force in the 2000s with the adoption of European directives on blood products (2002), tissues and cells (2004) and organs (2010), and the regulatory means of implementation. It should be said here that the directive on blood products is being revised.

Furthermore, the **European Medicines Agency (EMA)** takes action over medicinal products derived from human blood or human plasma and regulations on "plasma raw material", as well as monitoring these medicinal products (which enter into the framework of a recent European directive restructuring pharmacovigilance). The EFS feels its effect in the acceptability and safety of French plasma for fractionation.

The **European Centre for Disease Control (ECDC)** in the EU is increasingly taking action on European health safety and monitoring emerging diseases that may impact on blood transfusion and other products derived from the human body (tissues and cells).

The EFS is not involved in these bodies directly, but indirectly through its ongoing work with their French representatives, the Directorate-General for Health (DGS), the French National Agency for the Safety of Medicines and Health Products (ANSM) and the French Institute for Public Health Surveillance (InVS), ahead of negotiation meetings in the relevant bodies. The EFS is also involved in working groups prior to meetings of the European authorities.

The Council of Europe

The Strasbourg-based Council of Europe, which brings together the 47 countries of the "European region" and operates outside the EU framework, has been active in blood transfusion since the 1950s. Whilst it is best known for its role in defending human rights and European law, it has over time generated a vast body of treaties that are binding on the States that ratify them. Some of these treaties concern public health and the new problems affecting society, such as bioethics.

Since 2007, the European Committee for Blood Transfusion (CD-P-TS), a steering committee composed of national representatives whose secretariat is led by the **European Direction for the Quality of Medicines and Healthcare (EDQM)**, has been responsible for a work programme on the ethical, organizational and scientific aspects of blood transfusion. In particular, the Committee manages the update and annual publication of the *Guide to the Preparation, Use and Quality Assurance of Blood Components*, a leading guide in Europe and beyond. The European Commission uses it as a basis for its regulatory approach to these topics and funds the Council of Europe's work in the area through its annual public health programme. Discussions are ongoing as to whether all or part of the guide should be made legally binding on Member States by the EU to provide a frame of reference for transfusion quality assurance.

The EDQM also produces production quality monographs for every medicinal product, including those derived from human blood or human plasma, which have regulatory value in the EU and are binding on producers. Some transfusion products, such as the EFS's virus inactivated by solvent/detergent (SD) plasma, are also addressed: *Monograph on human plasma (pooled and treated for virus inactivation)*.

The EFS is a member of the CD-P-TS as France's official representative and EFS experts participate in several working groups preparing the opinions, resolutions, the guide, etc.

Another steering committee covers the EFS's secondary activities involving tissues and cells: like the CD-P-TS, the European Committee on Organ Transplantation (CD-P-TO) makes technical recommendations in this area.

Although the Council of Europe is, in theory, a separate institution to the EU, in practice the 2 organizations maintain a relationship based on cooperation and synergy. The European Commission recognizes the role of the CD-P-TS and EDQM in providing technical expertise and a "toolbox" that is particularly useful for clarifying the detailed implementation of European directives on blood, developing projects and common technical standards, helping less advanced Member States reform their transfusion systems and collecting data on Europe's transfusion services.

The World Health Organization

The World Health Organization (WHO) has issued several resolutions that have been accepted by its Member States, including France, on blood transfusion, voluntary, unpaid donations, national self-sufficiency and plasma-derived medicinal products. The EFS participates in expert groups on these themes and its involvement led the WHO to suggest that France host the tenth World Blood Donor Day (2013). The EFS also oversees "sensitive" projects: a proposal to include red blood cells and whole blood on the list of essential medicinal products is being discussed by a group of international experts, with the potential for tension at international level caused by the need to guarantee the supply of these products to all the world's populations (including, where appropriate, by exchanging blood products amongst countries and changing the status of blood products to "medicinal products"), and the ambition to make all countries self-sufficient...

The European Blood Alliance

The European Blood Alliance (EBA), a private non-profit organization, brings together almost all European non-profit-making blood transfusion service providers, as well as non-European observers that share the same values (Australia and the United States). The EBA monitors European activities at all times and has influence over the aforementioned bodies. The EFS is a member of its Board of Directors and is actively involved in a number of areas, notably providing direct and unwavering support on European regulations and projects.

Role of the EFS

In addition to its formal involvement in these European bodies, the EFS also responds to many of their enquiries and requests throughout the year. In 2012, 30 or so of these exercises enabled the institutions to review transfusion services in Europe and internationally, and, when presented in detailed reports, this information provides vital guidance for shaping the EFS's technical and organizational choices or preparing for future advances. Projects within the EFS on how services are provided in other countries have even led to further studies, through the EBA in particular

Representing and influencing at European level also forms part of an **international benchmark scheme** launched by the EFS a few years ago to create a source of information, learning and adaptation. Two approaches are developed: firstly, the active exchange of information with other transfusion organizations in Europe and around the world and, secondly, the gathering of all forms of information. The aim of the scheme is clearly to question our practices by studying and analyzing the techniques and results of other forms of organization. It should enable the EFS to anticipate necessary changes through better knowledge of its European and international environment, as well as highlight and promote the strengths of the French transfusion model, which may then inspire our foreign counterparts.

Two in-depth benchmarks have been undertaken to date, one with the Netherlands, where a single transfusion service provider coordinates all activities (Sanquin), and the other with Germany, where there are over 100. A benchmark with Italy is ongoing. Each project brings its own set of surprises, revealing similarities where one might have expected differences, but also through the diametrically opposed, but equally efficient, means of solving problems. The aim is to develop strong technical and even scientific cooperation.

Based on all this information, the EFS publishes an internal summary document, *Transfusion Europe*, every year to make an overview of blood transfusion services in neighbouring European countries, supported by facts and figures, as widely available as possible. This ongoing European intelligence has also led to the publication of a newsletter on developments in European policy and the regulation of blood transfusion, completing the scheme. It is widely distributed within the EFS and sent to a number of institutional partners every 2 months. Of course, numerous less formal exchanges also take place between EFS employees and their European (and international) counterparts during meetings and scientific and professional conferences.

In sum:
- Europe plays a decisive role in determining and developing our activities, especially in terms of product quality, safety and use. Most decisions are made within EU institutions, but the Council of Europe is a "technical" antechamber readily used by the European Commission to shape its directives and opinions;
- each blood establishment in Europe plays its role, as permitted by its resources and capabilities, in implementing, evaluating, researching and influencing changes to European directives, be that alone, with its national authorities and/or through the EBA, which provides a forum for debating and defending the interests of "European" public transfusion services;
- French transfusion stakeholders should increase their involvement in all these areas in order to use their influence, play a proactive role in public transfusion services and enable the EFS to anticipate future advances.

17. The EFS's international activities

Leslie Sobaga

As well as fulfilling its primary role in maintaining France's self-sufficiency in labile blood products (LBP) and ensuring optimal quality and safety, the French Blood Establishment (EFS) works in close cooperation with the international community to support the development of transfusion systems in partner countries through technical assistance programmes. Although blood transfusion is essential to raising healthcare standards in any country, the self-sufficiency, quality and safety of LBP cannot be guaranteed everywhere in the world.

Following a presentation of the strategic and methodological approach taken by the EFS's international activities, the main areas of cooperation, some of which were initiated over twenty years ago, will be discussed with examples of the undertakings on different continents illustrating the EFS's work.

Presentation of the EFS's international activities

Overview of the global challenges

Health is an important factor in human development. Improve the health is essential to reduce poverty, which is both a cause and effect of illness. The 2000 Millennium Summit identified 8 Millennium Development Goals (MDGs), 3 of which relate to health (see text box), making it a "global public good" central to development policies. Health is also a factor in economic growth.

Blood transfusion is an essential component of the health system. Healthcare standards in a given country are dependent on the ability of the LBP supply system

Leslie Sobaga, leslie.sobaga@efs.sante.fr

17. The EFS's international activities

> **The Millennium Development Goals (Goals 4, 5 and 6 more specifically on health)**
>
> 1. Eradicating extreme poverty and hunger
> 2. Achieving universal primary education
> 3. Promoting gender equality and empowering women
> 4. **Reducing child mortality rates:** Reduce the under-five mortality rate by two-thirds, between 1990 and 2015
> 5. **Improving maternal health:** A. Reduce the maternal mortality rate by 3 quarters between 1990 and 2015; B. Achieve universal access to reproductive health by 2015
> 6. **Combating HIV/AIDS, malaria, and other diseases:** A. Have halted and begun to reverse the spread of HIV/AIDS by 2015; B. Achieve universal access to treatment for HIV/AIDS for all those who need it by 2010; C. Have halted and begun to reverse the incidence of malaria and other major diseases by 2015
> 7. Ensuring environmental sustainability, and
> 8. Developing a global partnership for development

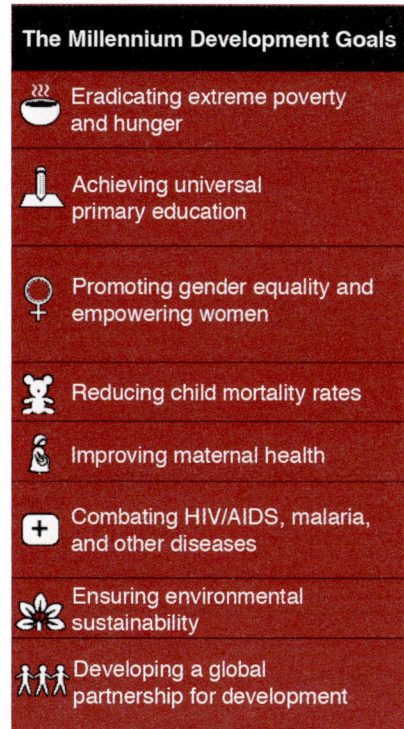

to meet requirements, both quantitative and qualitative. According to the World Health Organization (WHO), nearly 92 million blood donations are collected every year, with almost half of those donations taking place in the high-income countries that are home to 15% of the global population. Annual donations per blood centre are on average 30,000 in high-income countries versus 3,700 in low-income countries. The median blood donation rate in high-income countries is 36.4 donations per 1,000 people, *versus* 11.6 in middle-income countries and 2.8 in low-income countries.

The EFS's commitment to supporting the development of transfusion systems in other countries is therefore consistent with the principles of solidarity (sharing medical advances and expertise), respect for human rights and efficiency (adoption by the country, alignment with national strategy and systems, and focus on results).

The EFS's international strategy

Purposes

Centring primarily on technical assistance and skills transfer, the EFS's international initiatives aim to assist partner countries in developing a safe, efficient and sustainable transfusion system that ensures the self-sufficiency, quality and safety of LBP, as well as improving local health systems and access to healthcare.

They contribute to disseminating the ethical principles that have underpinned the organization of blood transfusion in France since the Act of 21 July 1952 (anonymous, non-remunerated, voluntary donation, not-for-profit).

They also highlight French expertise in blood transfusion services within the international community.

> **Improving maternal health: the facts**[1]
>
> More than 350,000 women die annually from complications during pregnancy or childbirth, almost all of them – 99 percent – in developing countries. The maternal mortality rate is declining only slowly, even though the vast majority of deaths are avoidable. In sub-Saharan Africa, a woman's maternal mortality risk is 1 for 30, compared to 1 for 5,600 in developed regions.
>
> Every year, more than 1 million children are left motherless. Children who have lost their mothers are up to 10 times more likely to die prematurely than those who have not.
>
> Maternal mortality remains unacceptably high. Most maternal deaths could be avoided. More than 80 percent of maternal deaths are caused by haemorrhage, sepsis, unsafe abortion, obstructed labour and hypertensive diseases of pregnancy.

---

1. Source: United Nations (UN).

Transfusion medicine: the French model

Strategic framework

International cooperation is part of the EFS's remit, as defined in the French Public Health Code. It is developed in the strategic framework of the EFS, which is determined by the Chairman, and reflects its social responsibility.

It also forms part of France's policy of cooperation, specifically in the health sector. Working with the Foreign Affairs and Health Ministries, the EFS's international activities stand at the crossroads of France's development and health policies. They cover political issues (global position, local relationship) and are part of the French "health diplomacy".

The EFS's international initiatives are also part of the fight against poverty and exclusion in countries of the North and countries of the South, in line with MDGs 4, 5 and 6 on health.

The EFS's international policy is based on 2 strategic areas of focus:
- steering **international "solidarity" initiatives** towards sustainable, high-stake projects that guarantee close and consistent cooperation with partner countries;
- increasing and strengthening cooperation initiatives through the development of **partnerships** and participation in **international calls for tender**.

In terms of international "solidarity", the aim is to develop and promote long-term cooperation initiatives that elicit a significant structuring effect for the country in question.

The framework document for France's cooperation policy emphasizes the implementation of partnerships with 4 geographical areas:
- *Sub-Saharan Africa*, and with seventeen priority low-income countries (PPP) in particular. The list of PPP adopted by the Inter-Ministerial Committee for International Cooperation and Development (CICID) on 5 June 2009 included Benin, Burkina Faso, Central African Republic, Chad, Comoro Islands, Democratic Republic of the Congo, Ghana, Guinea, Madagascar, Mali, Mauritania, Niger, Senegal, and Togo. Three other countries were added in 2012: Burundi, Djibouti and Rwanda;
- *middle-income Mediterranean countries*, with the Mediterranean region being the second priority area for French development cooperation behind Africa;
- *emerging countries:* major countries with systemic challenges, such as China, India and Brazil; countries with regional challenges, such as Indonesia and South Africa; and, beyond that, all middle-income countries in which the pace of economic and social change is accelerating. Development cooperation with these countries is pursuing 2 fundamental objectives: the move towards a fairer, more manageable growth system and increasing aid to the poorest countries;
- *countries in crisis and in post-crisis*, 6 countries are on the indicative list: Afghanistan, Haiti, Sudan, Yemen, Iraq and the Palestinian Territories.

Supported by an official request from the partner country, cooperation projects developed by the EFS are consistent with these broad outlines.

Regarding the second strategic axe, the aim is to develop partnerships with international organizations and stakeholders in the framework of multilateral projects, competent bodies and working groups (WHO, ISBT[2], AABB[3], European Commission, Council of Europe, etc.).

This also includes interfaces with French stakeholders in public development aid (French Development Agency) and international expertise (such as France Expertise Internationale).

Support for, or synergy with, the international activities of French health and transfusion stakeholders is being developed: partnerships with the French Fractionation Laboratory (LFB), interface with the network of French health agencies (French Biomedicine Agency, ANSM[4], French National Authority for Health in liaison with the Directorate-General for Health), technical consultancy for the activities of the International Relations Committee of the French Federation for Voluntary Blood Donation (FFDSB), links with Rotary International, and so on.

Ways of cooperating with other European transfusion structures are also being considered, which would allow them to potentiate initiatives (introduction of consortiums, training programmes, etc.).

Finally, the EFS monitors European and international calls for tender that are relevant to blood transfusion and is committed to promoting its technical expertise by the creation of consortiums to develop a comprehensive and tailored response to projects that receive substantial funding.

National organization and resources

Supported by all the experts in the EFS's regional establishments and headquarters, the International Affairs Department manages and coordinates the initiatives under the authority of the Chairman. This national coordination contributes to the consistency, efficiency and visibility of the establishment's initiatives. In particular, it draws on the coordinator establishments and experts involved in the implementation and follow-up of the given cooperation.

---

2. ISBT: International Society of Blood Transfusion.
3. AABB: American Association of Blood Banks.
4. ANSM: French National Agency for the Safety of Medicines and Health Products.

17. The EFS's international activities

The operational knowledge of the appointed experts and their ability to adapt to the local context guarantee the quality of the assistance provided to partner countries. This is an advantage in a sector in which independent structures may not always have access to practical expertise or cutting-edge technology.

With its own budget allocated by the EFS's specific economic model (at the crossroads of solidarity, commercial and institutional economics), the International Affairs Department oversees the implementation of the various components of the missions: operational, safety-related, financial, etc. Some missions are also financed by embassies in the case of bilateral cooperation.

Meeting the EFS's commitments (signed agreements, multiannual action plans, etc.) and constant demand from the international community necessitates the ongoing optimization of our organization and the appropriate adaptation of our resources.

Principles and procedures

The implementation of international cooperation and action plans is tailored to the objectives and needs of the partner countries.

> Several criteria are essential in the initial stages of a project:
> - an official request from the country's highest authority, confirmed by the French embassy;
> - a partnership agreement at national level;
> - a commitment to a mid/long-term project, which justifies the transfer of skills.
>
> The aim is therefore to incorporate the framework of support needed to ensure the success of the project into the design of the cooperation programme, whilst following French policy directives and the recommendations and guidelines of the Foreign Affairs Ministry (Figure 61).

An initial assessment is conducted to review the overall state of the country's transfusion system, *i.e.* medico-technical resources, organization, regulation and policy in use. It will then be possible to design and approve the partnership agreement, terms of reference and action plan with the partner. This assessment also provides an opportunity to ensure that resources and practical support are available to local stakeholders.

The project may then employ the **EFS's expertise** in all areas of the transfusion chain and environment, as well as in support activities and cell and tissue engineering:

- expertise in every link in the transfusion chain: promoting donations, collecting blood, preparing LBP, testing donations, delivering/distributing LBP, immunohaematology and vigilance. It is also possible to add the provision of medical care;
- expertise in the transfusion environment and support activities:
  – local organization and infrastructure,
  – legal and regulatory framework (good practices, etc.),
  – management of transfusion structures and activities, quality and regulatory management, continuous improvement methods and tools,
  – management of information systems,
  – financial and accounting management, procurement policy,
  – human resources management,
  – management of premises and equipment,
  – supply, logistics and transport.

The **means of support** vary depending on the objectives and needs of the countries. In particular, they can include technical assistance, consultancy and exchanges of experience:
- assessment of overall expertise (initial review);
- operational missions in the framework of agreed action plans.

These projects aim to determine the impact of transfusion on the health system and to implement an appropriate and realistic LBP supply strategy. A comprehensive action plan is then designed for the length of the cooperation and is based on skills transfer and feedback at the highest level:

– local organization and infrastructure;

– legislation (framework law), standards and good practices;

– central and cross-functional processes.

Support can also rely on:
- organizing and leading training sessions or programmes;
- introducing qualifying training at national level;
- organizing conferences or seminars attended by EFS experts;
- conducting external audits, assistance with conducting internal audits or assessments;
- receiving and training transfusion organization managers in France, receiving delegations or interns within the EFS;
- participating in multilateral projects or working groups (European Commission, WHO, etc.).

Transfusion medicine: the French model

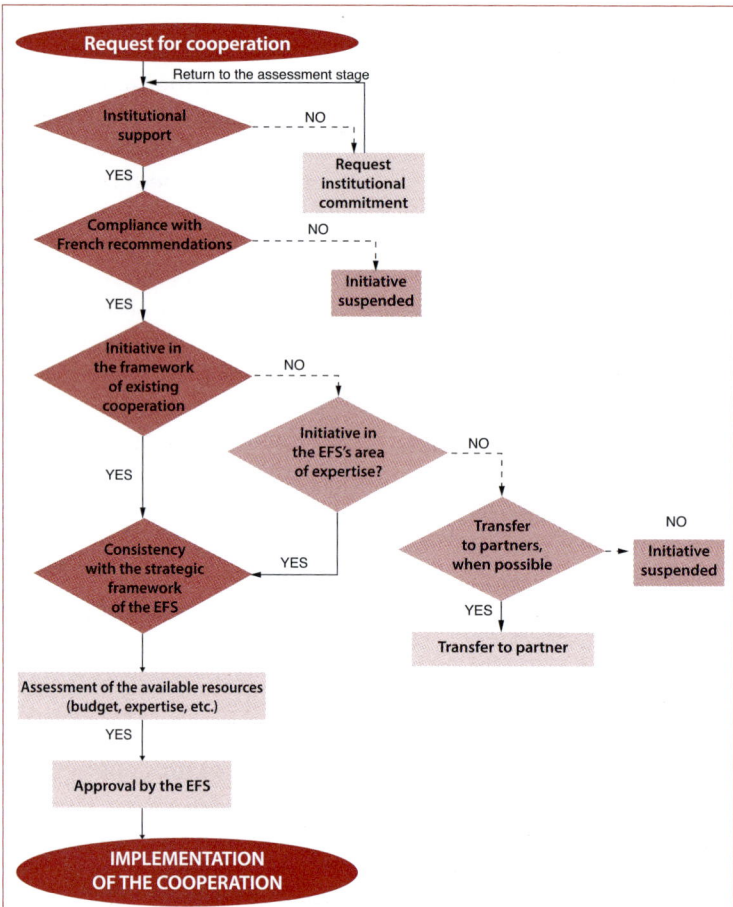

Figure 61. Principles of validation to initiate international actions.
EFS: French Blood Establishment.

The EFS's international cooperation

Overview of the projects
Main initiatives underway in the "sustainable international solidarity" category

In line with the 4 priority geographical areas determined in French cooperation policy, the EFS is pursuing sustainable, high-stake projects, some of which have been ongoing for many years, with Morocco, Chile and Algeria. It could also include the cooperations with Brazil and China (Table XXXIX).

The EFS has also been asked to assess the demand and geopolitical context in countries including Mauritania, Burkina Faso, Argentina, Democratic Republic of the Congo and Cameroon.

Main projects in the "international partnerships and calls for tender" category

The EFS has a longstanding partnership with the WHO, leading to major initiatives linked to the following strategic objectives:
- improving transfusion safety at international level: guaranteeing universal access to safe, high-quality and effective LBP, the safe and appropriate use of these products, and the safety of donors and patients;

The EFS's international cooperation, past and present

Albania, Algeria, Argentina, Benin, Bolivia, Brazil, Burkina Faso, Cameroon, Chile, China, Colombia, Croatia, Cyprus, Guinea, India, Iran, Lebanon, Luxembourg, Macedonia, Madagascar, Mauritania, Mexico, Morocco, Peru, Tajikistan, Thailand, Togo, Tunisia, United Arab Emirates, Uzbekistan, Venezuela, Vietnam, Yemen, etc. (Figure 62).

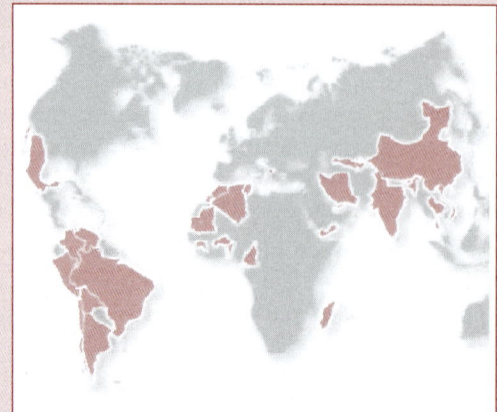

Figure 62. Map of the EFS's international cooperation.

17. The EFS's international activities

Table XXXIX. Initiatives underway in the "sustainable international solidarity" category.

Partner country	Objectives of the project	Partners
MOROCCO	Seminars and training, medico-technical and organizational support, receiving interns. Assisting the implementation of the new national strategy: review, strategies and action plan	Embassy NBTC (Rabat)
CHINA	Zhejiang, Henan and Jiangsu Provinces: assisting the organization of blood transfusion, safety, modern technology	DGOS BTC provinces
CHILE	Cooperation in the framework of the "transfusion medicine" qualification, San San Sebastian University Receiving delegations	Embassy Chilean Health Ministry
BRAZIL	Receiving delegations and technical inspections Participating in congresses France/Brazil transfusion seminars	Embassy Brazilian coordination
TUNISIA	Participating in the master's degree "quality" Medico-technical cooperation with the CTS Supply of corneas	WHO BTC Monastir University of Monastir
BENIN	Cooperation and assistance for the creation of a NBTC	NBTC Embassy, AFD
ALGERIA	Cooperation with the Algerian National Blood Agency: consolidation, creation of a quality control laboratory, quality management system, information system, interns	ANS Embassy

NBTC: National Blood Transfusion Centre; WHO: World Health Organization; DGOS: Directorate-General for Care Provision; BTC: blood transfusion centre; AFD: French Development Agency; ANS: National Blood Agency

- ensuring self-sufficiency in blood and blood products, based on Voluntary Non-Remunerated Blood Donation (VNRBD), pursuant to WHA Resolution 63.12 "Availability, safety and quality of blood products";
- strengthening transfusion systems;
- developing quality systems for optimal transfusion safety.

Cooperation has been developed in the following areas, including in particular:
– participating in World Blood Donor Day. France is the host country in 2013;
– supporting improvements in transfusion systems, particularly in French-speaking African countries: providing technical assistance, developing educational documents and tools, implementing action plans and training, etc.;
– participating in and contributing to working groups and networks, particularly: WHO Global Blood Safety Network, Expert Consensus Statement on achieving self-sufficiency in safe blood and blood products, based on VNRBD, etc.;
– contributing to the Global Database on Blood Safety (GDBS).

This area includes European calls for tender (funding for the instrument for pre-accession assistance), whose selection processes are underway for Turkey (technical assistance for recruiting future donors, two-year action plan).

Key global data (2011)

The EFS is cooperating with over 35 countries, with varying levels of involvement. An assessment has shown that staff involvement in international cooperation, in various areas, represents 280 man-days (Figures 63 to 65).

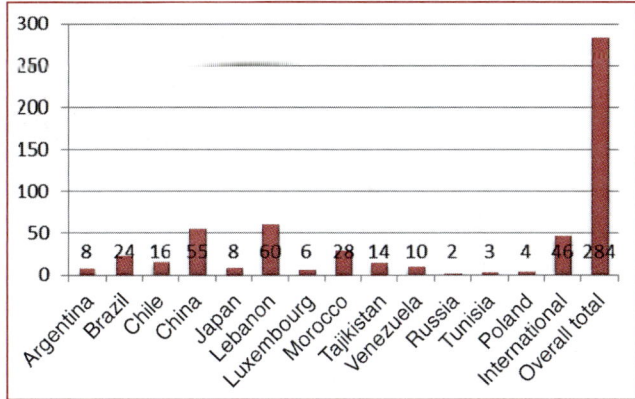

Figure 63. Man-days per country (excluding transport).

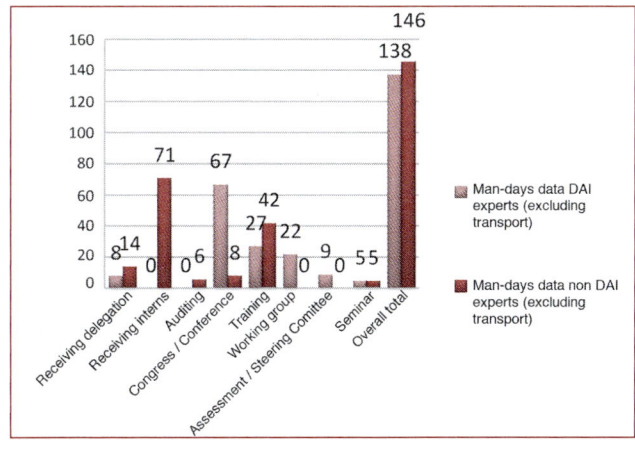

Figure 64. Breakdown of initiatives by category.
DAI: International Affairs Department; COPIL: Steering Committee.

Transfusion medicine: the French model

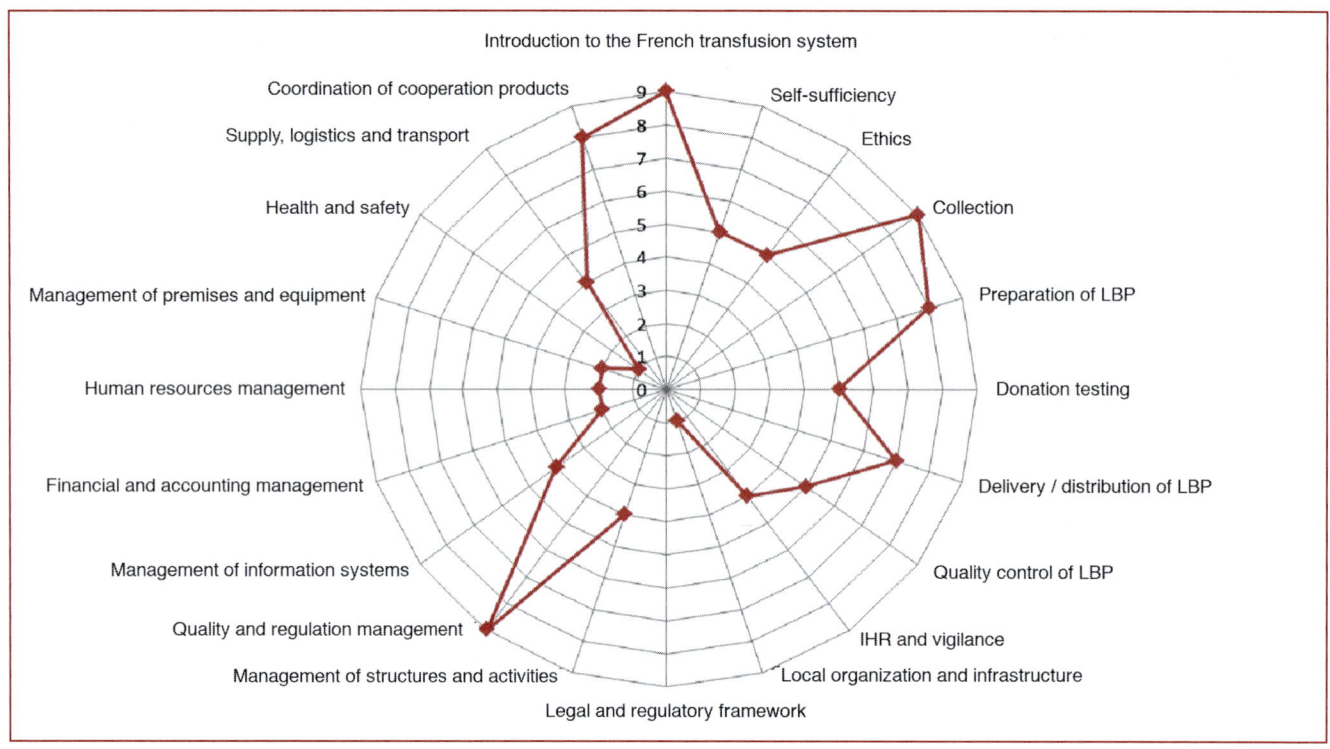

Figure 65. Initiatives by area (number).
LBP: labile blood products; IHR: Immuno-haematology receivers.

Illustrations
Cooperation with Lebanon

Based on rich and longstanding Franco-Lebanese friendship, cooperation in transfusion services was made official by the signing of partnership agreements between the EFS, Lebanese Public Health Ministry and ESA, École Supérieure des Affaires in Beirut (guaranteeing the coordination of EFS/ministry interfaces) in January 2011. The framework put in place over 3 years includes assistance in developing a framework law specific to blood transfusion, drafting blood product standards and good practices guidelines, implementing an information system, and establishing a national haemovigilance, quality management and project management system.

A cooperation protocol between the French and Lebanese Ministries of Health, which was signed in November 2011, ensures the synergy and consistency of the initiatives of health agencies (EFS, ANSM, French National Authority for Health, etc.) involved in the programme, which also includes, in addition to transfusion management, accrediting healthcare facilities, training healthcare professionals, hospital management, registering medicinal products and regulating medical devices.

The Lebanese population is estimated at 4.1 million inhabitants. The country covers a total area of 10,452 sq km and is divided administratively into 8 regions, or mohafazats. Blood transfusion services are divided in the same way as hospital services, which explains their extreme decentralization, as each health facility has its own "blood bank". The Lebanese Red Cross also provides transfusion services with 12 "blood banks" shared amongst the various administrative regions. Blood donors are unpaid volunteers in around 5% of cases and family members and/or paid volunteers in 95% of cases. It is estimated that 120,000 donations are collected each year. Platelet concentrates (approximately 11,000/p.a.) are prepared solely by aphaeresis. Around 85% of collections are made by public and private health facilities and 15% by the Lebanese Red Cross.

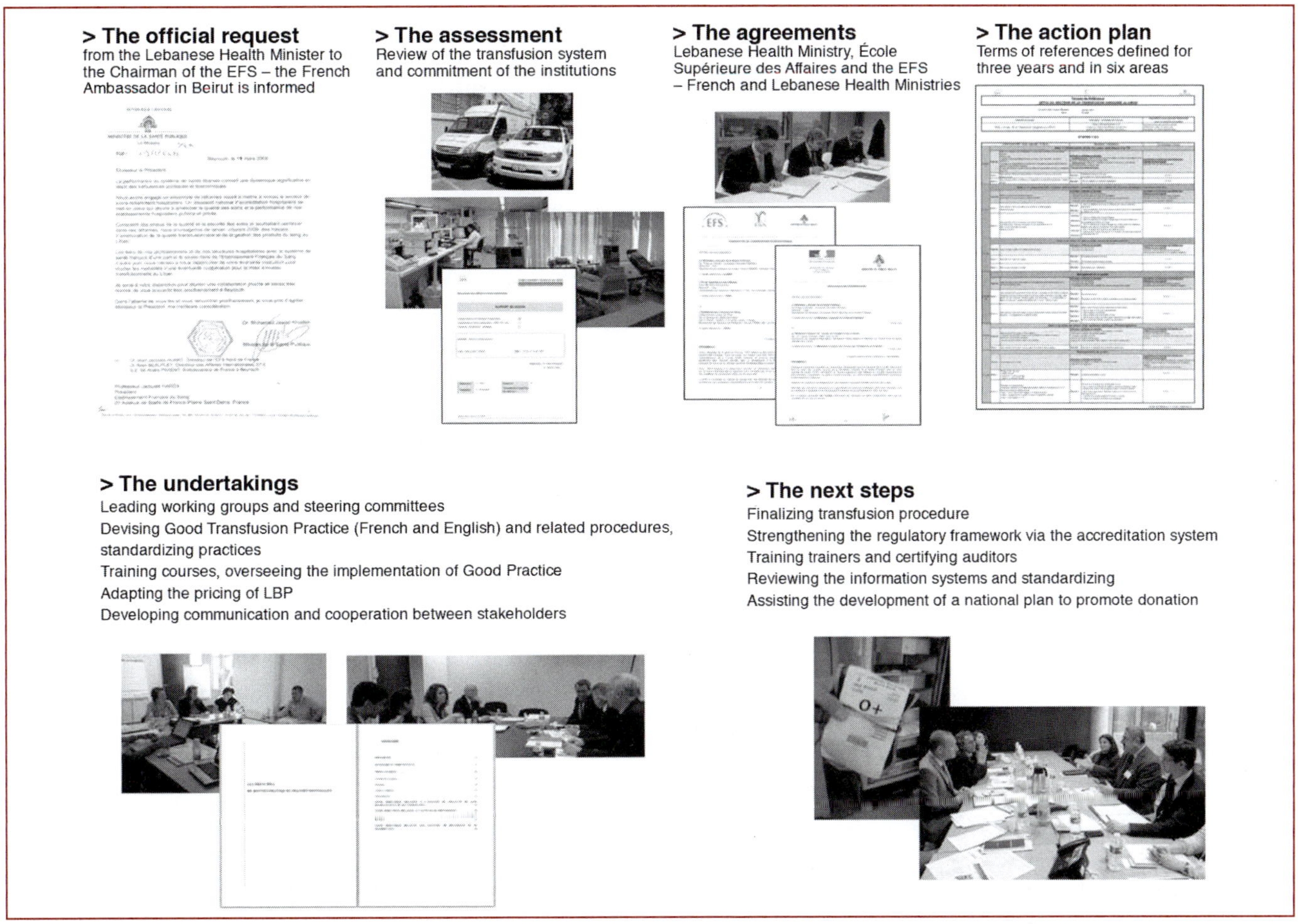

17. The EFS's international activities

> **The official request**
from the Lebanese Health Minister to the Chairman of the EFS – the French Ambassador in Beirut is informed

> **The assessment**
Review of the transfusion system and commitment of the institutions

> **The agreements**
Lebanese Health Ministry, École Supérieure des Affaires and the EFS – French and Lebanese Health Ministries

> **The action plan**
Terms of references defined for three years and in six areas

> **The undertakings**
Leading working groups and steering committees
Devising Good Transfusion Practice (French and English) and related procedures, standardizing practices
Training courses, overseeing the implementation of Good Practice
Adapting the pricing of LBP
Developing communication and cooperation between stakeholders

> **The next steps**
Finalizing transfusion procedure
Strengthening the regulatory framework via the accreditation system
Training trainers and certifying auditors
Reviewing the information systems and standardizing
Assisting the development of a national plan to promote donation

Main steps in the implementation of the Franco-Lebanese cooperation in blood transfusion.
EFS: French Blood Establishment; LBP: labile blood products.
© Photos: EFS.

Cooperation with China

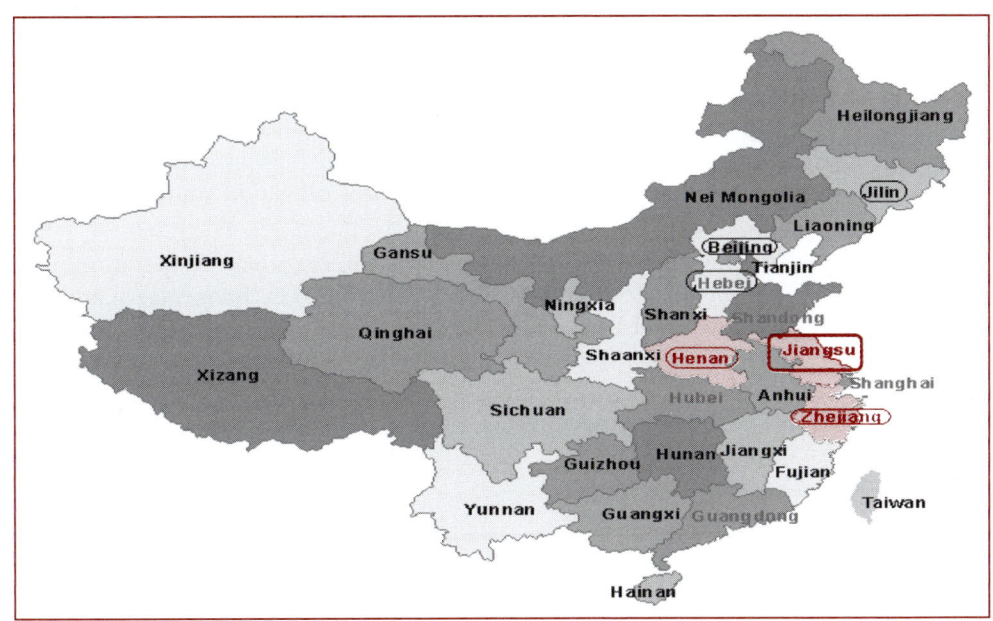

Transfusion medicine: the French model

Between 2004 and 2007, contacts with China largely involved receiving delegations (municipality of Beijing, Jilin Province, Zhejiang Province, Hebei Province, joint WHO-EFS training scheme in Beijing, etc.).

In the framework of cooperation between the French Health Ministry and the Health Ministry in Beijing, the Directorate-General for Care Provision (DGOS) later initiated cooperation with several Chinese provinces. In 2009, the work of the Director-General for Care Provision led to concrete cooperation in line with the declaration of intent signed by the French and Chinese Health Ministers on 11 August 2008.

It was in this context, in liaison with the DGOS, that the EFS received 2 delegations from Henan and Zhejiang Province in March and July 2010 to present the organization of blood transfusion services. The EFS's participation in 2 seminars with managers of transfusion centres in these provinces in 2011, in the cities of Hangzhou and Zhengzhou, made it possible to continue exchanges on the development of transfusion services, the French transfusion system and good practice in a quality environment. In December 2011, EFS Alpes-Méditerranée received a delegation from Zhejiang Province.

Following a rapprochement with the Blood Transfusion Centre (BTC) in Jiangsu Province, again in liaison with the DGOS, the EFS received a manager from the Nanjing centre in 2011 for training on the entire transfusion chain. Following this training, technical cooperation was developed with the BTC in Jiangsu Province. It was formalized on 10 April 2012:
- signing in Nanjing of the partnership agreement between the EFS and the BTC of Jiangsu Province, with the unveiling of the commemorative plaque for the Franco–Chinese blood establishment (ETS), attended by Prof. Jun Sun (Director of the BTC), Xiaoshu Hu, Vice-Director of Jiangsu Health Bureau and Director of Jiangsu Food and Drug Administration, and Emmanuel Lenain, Consul-General of France in Shanghai;
- participation in the Franco–Chinese seminar on the following topics for managers of transfusion centres across the province: quality management system, haemovigilance, and the quality and safety of LBP;
- presentation and exchanges on transfusion in Jiangsu, with visits to the Nanjing and Suzhou centres.

In the framework of the signed agreement, the next steps entail visits and technical exchanges (seminars with specific themes), making it possible to share experience on topics such as self-sufficiency, the safety of LBP and haemovigilance. A delegation led by the director of the BTC in Jiangsu Province will also be received to mark World Blood Donor Day 2013, which France is hosting.

> Jiangsu Province is the fifth largest Chinese province by population and second by total gross domestic product (GDP). In 2011, Jiangsu Province used 1,316,515 units of LBP for a population of 75 million people, which places it in third position amongst the provinces for the use of LBP in China.

Conclusion

Blood transfusion is an essential component in the operation and safety standards of health services. In light of the difficulties faced in various countries, the cooperation and technical assistance projects led by the EFS with partner countries help to support local transfusion systems with procedures adapted to local strategies, organizations and specificities.

As the programmes require structural change and substantial investment, they must be understood and supported at the highest institutional and political levels in the country to ensure their sustainability and long-term success.

The EFS is pursuing ongoing projects by assessing new requirements in specific and changing contexts. It is adapting its methods and resources to constantly changing requirements, in particular by developing the panel of experts involved in the programmes, optimizing the review of its initiatives and harmonizing its work at national level. It is also adapting to growing challenges and debates on blood transfusion on the international stage.

Finally, international cooperation is giving the EFS opportunities to exchange, learn and embrace other solutions and cultures, which are enriching its practices.

Conclusion

The French model is one transfusion medicine model

It is built on history, values and, of course, people.

History because, from donor to recipient, along a chain marked at every stage by solidarity and generosity, the model has allowed each patient to receive the labile blood products they need for nearly a century, facilitating the development of modern medicine and surgery.

Values because the model is underpinned by four founding principles, which are altruism, voluntarism, anonymity and absence of profit. Lawmakers have given a single government agency a monopoly over blood transfusion services, making the French State responsible for **self-sufficiency** in labile blood products, **transfusion safety** and **efficiency** in the management of this rare and precious commodity, human blood.

Finally, the people taking on a variety of different roles with different areas of expertise, united by one shared goal: helping to save lives every day by making an enthusiastic contribution to public health services and participating in this wonderful human adventure.

We believe that the French transfusion medicine model, headed by a single **establishment**, is one of the few to combine high ethical standards and internationally recognized efficiency.

The model is active and under constant development, reflecting scientific findings, technological advances, the experiences of benchmarking and social changes. It should be regularly reviewed and explained.

Dr Alain Beauplet
Dr Rémi Courbil
Mr. Jean-Marc Ouazan

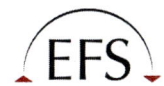

Regulatory references

Joëlle Debeir

Main legislative provisions and national and European regulations on the activities of blood establishments providing labile blood products and medical laboratory analyses

Main European instruments

- Regulation (EC) No 1907/2006 concerning the Registration, Evaluation, Authorisation and Restriction of Chemicals (REACH)
- Council Directive 93/42/EEC (amended) of 14 June 1993 concerning medical devices
- Directive 98/79/EC (amended) of the European Parliament and of the Council on *in vitro* diagnostic medical devices
- Directive 2002/98/EC of the European Parliament and of the Council of 27 January 2003 setting standards of quality and safety for the collection, testing, processing, storage and distribution of human blood and blood components and amending Directive 2001/83/EC
- Commission Directive 2004/33/EC of 22 March 2004 implementing Directive 2002/98/EC of the European Parliament and of the Council as regards certain technical requirements for blood and blood components
- Commission Directive 2005/61/EC of 30 September 2005 implementing Directive 2002/98/EC of the European Parliament and of the Council as regards traceability requirements and notification of serious adverse reactions and events
- Commission Directive 2005/62/EC of 30 September 2005 implementing Directive 2002/98/EC of the European Parliament and of the Council as regards

Joëlle Debeir, joelle.debeir@efs.sante.fr

Community standards and specifications relating to a quality system for blood establishments
- Commission Directive 2003/94/EC of the Commission of 8 October 2003 laying down the principles and guidelines of good manufacturing practice with regard to medicinal products for human use and investigational medicinal products for human use
- Commission Decision of 7 May 2002 on common technical specifications for *in vitro* diagnostic medical devices
- Recommendations and resolutions of the Council of Europe (see *Blood and Blood Components – Safety, Quality, Training and Ethical/Matters Concerning Preparation, Use and Quality Assurance Council of Europe/Resolutions, Recommendations and Convention 1st Edition*)
- *Guide to the Preparation, Use and Quality Assurance of Blood Components*, 16th edition (2010)
- European Pharmacopoeia, 7th edition (7.8) 2013

Main national and European instruments by activity

Provisions applicable to the EFS and ETS	
European Commission Directive	Directive 2002/98/EC of the European Parliament and of the Council of 27 January 2003 setting standards of quality and safety for the collection, testing, processing, storage and distribution of human blood and blood components and amending Directive 2001/83/EC
CSP	Articles L. 1211-1 to L. 1211-9 (ethical principles) Articles L. 1222-1 to L. 1224-3 (EFS/ETS organization and remit) Articles L. 1271-1 to L. 1271-8 (legal provisions) Articles R. 1222-1 to R. 1222-16 (Board of Directors, Chairman, responsible person, Scientific Board, budget and accounts) Articles R. 1223-1 and R. 1223-2 (Governing Board) Articles R. 1223-3 to R. 1223-7-1 (authorization and inspection) Articles D. 1223-21 to D. 1223-27 (appointment of directors) Articles R. 1224-1 to R. 1224-5 (SOTS)
Other instruments*	Order of 3 August 2010 on the procedures for submitting applications for authorization, authorization renewal and amendment of elements of the authorisation of the ETS outlined in Article L. 1223-1 of the CSP Order of 24 December 2009 determining the format and content of the annual ETS activity report provided for in Article R. 1223-8 of the CSP Decision of 6 November 2006 defining the good practices principles provided for in Article L. 1223-3 of the CSP Order of 24 April 2002 implementing the regulation on good transport practices for collections, products and samples derived from human blood Amended Order of 29 May 2009 on the carriage of dangerous goods by road (TMD: Carriage of Dangerous Materials) Amended Order of 12 May 2000 determining the procedures and implementation of the provisions outlined in Articles R. 668-7, R. 668-12 (5o), R. 668-16 and Articles 4 to 7, 9 and 10 of Decree 97-1104 of 26 November 1997 on the qualifications of certain ETS staff members, pursuant to Article L. 667-8 of the CSP BS EN ISO 9001-2008

EFS: French Blood Establishment; ETS: blood establishment; CSP: French Public Health Code; SOTS: plans for the organization of blood transfusion services.
* Main instruments implementing or clarifying the CSP or other standards providing a frame of reference for ETS activities.

Collection	
European Commission Directive (specific annex)	Commission Directive 2004/33/EC of 22 March 2004 implementing Directive 2002/98/EC of the European Parliament and of the Council as regards certain technical requirements for blood and blood components (Text with EEA relevance) European Directive (amended) 93-42 of 14 June 1993 concerning medical devices
CSP	Articles L. 1221-1 to L. 1221-7, L. 1222-1, L. 1222-3 and L. 1223-3, L. 1222-9 (general principles and good practices) Articles D. 1221-1 to D. 1221-4 (volunteerism) Articles R. 1221-5 (selection), R. 1222-17 to R. 1222-22 (staff qualifications) Articles R. 1223-3 to R. 1223-7 (authorization), R. 1223-8, R. 1223-10, R. 1223-13 (activities), R. 1224-1 (SOTS)
Other instruments	Guideline on *Collection* (good practices provided for in Article L. 1223-3 of the CSP) Ministerial orders, technical guidance of the French Blood Agency, decisions of the Director-General of the Afssaps and the ANSM, clarifying and organizing in particular: – blood donor selection criteria (conditions for collection and medical contraindications to donation), pre-donation information documents, medical questionnaires – the conditions for awarding certificates and badges to voluntary blood donors, classification of the schemes

CSP: French Public Health Code; EEA: European Economic Area; SOTS: plans for the organization of blood transfusion services; Afssaps: French Health Products Safety Agency; ANSM: French National Agency for the Safety of Medicines and Health Products.

Regulatory references

Preparation		
Directive European Commission (specific annex)	Commission Directive 2004/33/EC of 22 March 2004 implementing Directive 2002/98/EC of the European Parliament and of the Council as regards certain technical requirements for blood and blood components Directive 2002/98/EC of the European Parliament and of the Council of 27 January 2003 setting standards of quality and safety for the collection, testing, processing, storage and distribution of human blood and blood components and amending Directive 2001/83/EC Commission Implementing Directive 2011/38/EU of 11 April 2011 amending Annex V to Directive 2004/33/EC with regards to maximum pH values for platelets concentrates at the end of the shelf life	
CSP	Articles L. 1221-8 and L. 1221-8-2 (list, characteristics and assessment of LBP) Articles R. 1222-25 to R. 1222-27 (staff qualifications) Articles R. 1223-3 to R. 1223-7, R. 1223-13 (authorization, continuous public service), R. 1223-9 (irradiation), R. 1224-1 to R. 1224-5 (SOTS)	
Other instruments	Guideline on *Preparation* (good practices provided for in Article L. 1223-3 of the CSP) Order of 11 April 2008 on clinical and biological good practices guidelines in medically assisted procreation Decision of the Director-General of the Afssaps of 24 July 2009 on good manufacturing practice *(SD-FFP)* Ministerial orders and decisions of the Director-General of the Afssaps and the ANSM, clarifying and organizing in particular: the transfer price of LBP, the list and characteristics of LBP, determining the content of the application to submit to the Afssaps for the assessment of labile blood products	

CSP: French Public Health Code; LBP: labile blood products; SOTS: plans for the organization of blood transfusion services; Afssaps: French Health Products Safety Agency; SD-FFP: fresh frozen plasma inactivated by solvent/detergent; ANSM: French National Agency for the Safety of Medicines and Health Products.

Donation testing	
Directive European Commission (specific annex)	Directive 2002/98/EC of the European Parliament and of the Council of 27 January 2003 setting standards of quality and safety for the collection, testing, processing, storage and distribution of human blood and blood components and amending Directive 2001/83/EC Directive 98/79/EC (amended) of the European Parliament and of the Council on *in vitro* diagnostic medical devices Commission Decision (amended) of 7 May 2002 on common technical specifications for *in vitro*-diagnostic medical devices
CSP	Articles L. 1221-4, L. 1223-2, L. 6221-13 (accreditation) Articles R. 1221-5, D. 1221-6 to D. 1221-16 (testing) Articles R. 1222-30 to R. 1222-32 (staff qualifications) Articles R. 1223-3 to R. 1223-7 (authorization), R. 1223-11, R. 1223-13 (activity and continuity of service) Articles R. 1224-1 to R. 1224-4-4 (SOTS) Articles R. 5222-3 to R. 5222-18 (reagent vigilance) Articles R. 5232-16 to R. 5232-18 (technological vigilance)
Other instruments	Guideline on donation testing (good practices provided for in Article L. 1223-3 of the CSP) Orders determining special dispensations in the testing and screening of blood donations for urgent therapeutic use, determining the conditions of transferring plasma taken from blood donors by the EFS to the transfusion virology laboratory of the French Institute of Blood Transfusion EFS guidelines determining decision-making algorithms specific to this type of donation testing, the steps to take if the donor's test results are abnormal

CSP: French Public Health Code; SOTS: plans for the organization of blood transfusion services; EFS: French Blood Establishment.

Transfusion medicine: the French model

Patient testing		
Directive European Commission (specific annex)		Directive 98/79/EC (amended) of the European Parliament and of the Council on *in vitro* diagnostic medical devices Commission Decision of 7 May 2002 on common technical specifications for *in vitro*-diagnostic medical devices (Text with EEA relevance) (2002/364/EC) European Federation for Immunogenetics standards (EFI) for EFI accreditation
CSP		Articles L. 1111-2 and L. 1111-4 to L. 1111-7 (information and consent to treatment, access to information), L. 1111-14 (medical records) Articles L. 1223-1 and R. 1223-14 to R. 1223-20 (testing services of ETS) Articles L. 6212-1 et seq (medical testing and organization of laboratories), L. 6213-3 (quality control of tests) Articles L. 1131-1 to L. 1131-7, L. 2131-1, L. 6211-5, R. 2131-1 to R. 2131-9, R. 6122-25 Articles R. 1131-1 and R. 1131-2, R. 1131-6 to R. 1131-20 (genetic testing, prenatal diagnosis) Articles L. 6222-1 to L. 6222-8, R. 6211-1 to R. 6211-25 (conditions for authorization) Articles R. 1222-30 to R. 1222-32, R. 1223-12, R. 1223-14 to R. 1223-20 (IH of recipients) Article R. 4352-13 (laboratory technician) Articles R. 5222-3 to R. 5222-18 (reagent vigilance) Articles R. 5232-16 to R. 5232-18 (technological vigilance)
CSS		In particular, Articles R. 161-46 of CSS et seq, R. 162-17 (inter-laboratory transfer)
Other instruments		Decree 2011-1268 of 10 October 2011 determining the criteria for assessing the activity of an LBM and the maximum percentage of biological samples that can be transferred between LBM Amended Order of 29 May 2009 on the carriage of dangerous goods by road Amended Order of 26 November 1999 on good conduct of medical testing ("GBEA") BS EN ISO 15189 for the accreditation of LBM Orders clarifying the applicable standards and procedures of LBM accreditation, the procedures for transferring biological samples between LBM, the content of the application for authorization to conduct genetic testing Order of 6 August 2008 determining the content of the annual reports of medical testing laboratories authorized to practise cytogenic and biological activities with the aim of providing prenatal cytogenetic diagnoses Order of 16 January 2009 amending the Order of 20 April 1994 on the notification, classification, packaging and labelling of hazardous substances HAS May 2012 guidelines on clinical practice/giving patients information on their health

CSP: French Public Health Code; CSS: French Social Security Code; EEA: European Economic Area; ETS: blood establishment; LBM: medical testing laboratory; IH: immunohaematology; HAS: French National Authority for Health.

Distribution/delivery	
Directive European Commission (specific annex)	Commission Directive 2004/33/EC of 22 March 2004 implementing Directive 2002/98/EC of the European Parliament and of the Council as regards certain technical requirements for blood and blood components
CSP	Articles L. 1221-1 (ethics), L. 1221-4 (testing), L. 1221-8, L. 1221-9 (list and price), L. 1221-10 (banking) and L. 1221-12 (importing) Articles R. 1221-17 to R. 1221-21 (organisation and blood banks), R. 1221-54 (staff qualifications) Articles R. 1222-23 and R. 1222-24 (staff qualifications, transfusion support) Articles R. 1223-3 to R. 1223-7 (authorization), R. 1223-13 (continuity of public service), R. 1224-1 to R. 1224-4 (SOTS) Articles D. 1221-56 to D. 1221-64 (LBP import)
Other instruments	Guideline linked to an *autologous transfusion protocol* and the guideline on *distribution* (good practices provided for in Article L. 1223-3 of the CSP) Orders determining the conditions for training distribution and delivery staff, the technical and qualification conditions of certain blood bank staff members, the content of the agreement between health facilities and the referent ETS on constituting a blood bank, the conditions for storing LBP in the wards of health facilities Afssaps circulars on transfusion safety (quality control prior to transfusion, prescription conditions, steps to take if bacterial incidents are suspected) Amended Decision of 20 October 2010 determining the list and characteristics of LBP Afssaps and HAS guidelines on using LBP

CSP: French Public Health Code; SOTS: plans for the organization of blood transfusion services; LBP: labile blood products; ETS: blood establishment; Afssaps: French Health Products Safety Agency; HAS: French National Authority for Health.

Regulatory references

Transfusion	
CSP	Articles L. 1221-1 (ethics) and L. 1221-10-1 (ANSM role) Articles L. 1111-2 and L. 1111-4 to L. 1111-7 (information and consent to treatment, access to information), L. 1111-14 (medical records) Articles R. 1112-1 to R. 1112-7 (medical records, archiving and data storage), R. 1112-43 (refusal of treatment), R. 1112-45 (anonymity), R. 1125-7, R. 1125-13 (research) Articles R. 1223-13 and R. 1222-24 (transfusion support)
Other instruments	Decision of 6 November 2006 defining the principles of good practices provided for in Article L. 1223-3 of the CSP (guideline on the distribution and guideline linked to an autologous transfusion protocol) Amended Decision of 20 October 2010 determining the list and characteristics of LBP DGS/DHOS/Afssaps circulars on the provision of transfusion care, with guidelines on the steps to take if a transfusion incident involving bacterial contamination is suspected DGS/DH/AFS circular on autologous transfusion in surgery DGS circular on information for patients on the risks of LBP and blood-derived medicinal product, and on the various recall measures for these blood products ANSM/HAS good practice guidelines for the transfusion of plasma, platelets, packed red blood cells and clarifications (TRALI, methylene blue-treated FFP, etc.) on the use of LBP HAS 2006 guidelines on intraoperative blood salvage HAS 2005 professional practice guidelines/Transfusion in anaesthesia-intensive care

CSP: French Public Health Code; ANSM: French National Agency for the Safety of Medicines and Health Products; LBP: labile blood products; DGS: Directorate-General for Health; DHOS: Directorate-General for Hospitalization and Healthcare Organization; Afssaps: French Health Products Safety Agency; DH: Directorate for Hospitals; AFS: French Blood Agency; HAS: French National Authority for Health; TRALI: Transfusion-related acute lung injury; FFP: fresh frozen plasma.

Assessment	
Directive European Commission (specific annex)	Commission Directive 2005/62/EC of 30 September 2005 implementing Directive 2002/98/EC of the European Parliament and of the Council as regards Community standards and specifications relating to a quality system for blood establishments (Text with EEA relevance) Commission Directive 2004/33/EC of 22 March 2004 implementing Directive 2002/98/EC of the European Parliament and of the Council as regards certain technical requirements for blood and blood components (Text with EEA relevance)
CSP	Articles L. 1221-8-2, L. 6213-3, L. 5311-1 (ANSM's role) Articles R. 1222-28 and R. 1222-29, R. 1223-8, R. 1223-9, R. 1125-7, R. 1125-13 (research and quality control)
Other instruments	Amended Decision of 20 October 2010 determining the list and characteristics of LBP Decision of 19 November 2010 determining the content of the application to submit to the Afssaps for the assessment of labile blood products

CSP: French Public Health Code; EEA: European Economic Area; ETS: blood establishments; ANSM: French National Agency for the Safety of Medicines and Health Products; LBP: labile blood products; Afssaps: French Health Products Safety Agency.

Monitoring	
Directive European Commission (specific annex)	Commission Directive 2005/61/EC of 30 September 2005 implementing Directive 2002/98/EC of the European Parliament and of the Council as regards traceability requirements and notification of serious adverse reactions and events
CSP (specific provisions)	Articles L. 1221-13, L. 1222-1 (haemovigilance) Articles R. 1221-22 to R. 1221-52 and R. 1221-54 (haemovigilance), R. 1223-7-1 (ANSM inspection) Articles L. 5212-2 and R. 5212-6, R. 5212-14 to R. 5212-17 (medical devices reporting) Articles L. 5222-3 and R. 5222-3 to R. 5222-15 (reagent vigilance)
Other instruments	Ministerial orders, technical guidance of the AFS, AFS and Afssaps circulars, decisions of the Director-General of the Afssaps, clarifying and organizing in particular: – the roles and responsibilities of healthcare stakeholders in vigilance – the national system for managing adverse reactions or risks pertaining to transfusion services, MD or IVDD (timeframe, paper and electronic materials, recipients of notifications) – the national system of traceability for establishments, persons and blood products (codification of the LBP and ETS, archiving) – the procedures for conducting transfusion investigations

CSP: French Public Health Code; ANSM: French National Agency for the Safety of Medicines and Health Products; AFS: French Blood Agency; Afssaps: French Health Products Safety Agency; MD: medical devices; IVDD: *in vitro* diagnostic medical devices; LBP: labile blood products; ETS: blood establishments.

Annexes

The EFS staff

The workforce in the "core" activities, related activities, research and support services:

9,844 people were working within the French Blood Establishment (EFS) as of 31 December 2012:
– 8,370 private-sector employees;
– 737 civil servants;
– 64 secondments;
– 20 leased public-sector employees;
– 653 temporary workers.

The EFS's "core" activities account for 74% of staff members.

The EFS's workforce has the following statistics:
– women account for three-quarters of the total workforce;
– the average age is 44;
– average length of time that an employee has been employed is 13 years.

640 employees were recruited on a permanent contract (CDI) in 2012:
– 450 clerical workers, technicians and supervisors;
– 131 medical directors;
– 59 non-medical directors.

486 permanent employees left the EFS in 2012:
– 46.7% redundancy;
– 27.8% retirement;
– 25.5% for other reasons (end of probationary period, dismissal, death, etc.).

28.2% of employees are part-time, broken down into the following socio-economic categories:
– 41.7% clerical workers;
– 26.5% technicians and supervisors;
– 8.2% non-medical directors;
– 44.1% medical directors.

Over 60% of the EFS's workforce received training in 2012.

Table showing selling price before tax for labile blood products in France

Product type		Price in euros (ex. tax.)
Whole human blood (adult unit, infant's unit and paediatric unit)		€111.16
Homologous human PRBCs (adult unit, infant's unit and paediatric unit)		€183.84
Homologous human PRBCs, leucocyte-depleted (adult unit, infant's unit and paediatric unit)		€183.84
Granulocyte concentrate by aphaeresis		€583.83
Pool of standard platelet concentrates	Minimum concentration of 1×10^{11} platelets per bag	€75.02
	Then per additional tranche of therapeutic unit of 0.5×10^{11}	€37.51
Aphaeresis platelet concentrate	Minimum concentration of 2×10^{11} platelets per bag	€217.56
	Then per additional tranche of therapeutic unit of 0.5×10^{11}	€54.39
Pool of standard platelet concentrates, amotosalen-inactivated	Minimum concentration of 1×10^{11} platelets per bag	€75.02
	Then per additional tranche of therapeutic unit of 0.5×10^{11}	€37.51
Aphaeresis platelet concentrate, amotosalen-inactivated	Minimum concentration of 2×10^{11} platelets per bag	€217.56
	Then per additional tranche of therapeutic unit of 0.5×10^{11}	€54.39
Fresh frozen plasma	Homologous human, treated for reconstituted blood	€34.50
	Homologous human by aphaeresis, quarantined (adult unit – 200 mL minimum, infant's unit and paediatric unit)	€97.21
	Pathogen reduced by solvent/detergent (at least 200 mL)	€97.21
	Pathogen reduced by amotosalen (at least 200 mL)	€97.21
Flat rate	For autologous PRBCs (adult units SAGM by erythropheresis)	€430.80
	For planned autologous transfusion (including autologous PRBCs and fresh frozen plasma) per collection	€222.82
Surcharge	For "leucocyte-depletion" processing (applicable to autologous PRBCs)	€24.92
	For "cryopreserved" processing	€118.28
	For "RH/K phenotype" determination	€3.23
	For "extended phenotype" determination	€15.00
	For "CMV negative" determination	€10.61
	For "plasma removed" processing	€71.81
	For "irradiated" processing (applicable to each product)	€14.52
	For "volume reduced" processing	€22.14
	For "reconstituted blood for paediatric use" processing	€24.37
	For "cryopreserved PRBCs suspended in SAGM solution after thawing" processing	€166.63

Source: Order of 12 April 2011 published in the *Official Journal* dated 27 April 2011.
SAGM: saline-adenine-glucose-mannitol solution; PRBCs: packed red blood cells; CMV: cytomegalovirus.

Glossary

AABB	American Association of Blood Banks
ABM	French Biomedicine Agency
ACT	Activated cephalin time
AFS	French Blood Agency
Afssaps	French Health Products Safety Agency
ALT	Alanine aminotransferase
ANSM	French National Agency for the Safety of Medicines and Health Products
APC	Aphaeresis platelet concentrate
ARS	French Regional Health Agency
ASIP	French Agency for Shared Health Information Systems
ATMP	Advanced therapy medicinal products
AVIESAN	French National Alliance for Life Sciences and Health
BC	Buffy coat
BDMP	Blood-derived medicinal product
BDN	French National Database
BNSR	French National Rare Blood Bank
CDC	Complement-dependent lymphocytotoxicity
CDS	Health centre
CLIA	Chemiluminescent immunoassay
CHU	University hospital
CHV	Haemovigilance Officer
CIC	Clinical investigation centre
CJD	Creutzfeldt–Jakob disease
CLB	Local Biovigilance Officer
CM	Lymphocyte cross-match
CNRGS	French National Reference Centre for Blood Groups
CNRS	French National Centre for Scientific Research
CNU	French National University Council
Cofrac	French Certification Committee
COP	Objectives and performance contract
CPD	Citrate phosphate dextrose
CREDOC	French Research Centre for the Study and Monitoring of Living Standards
CRH	Regional Haemovigilance Officer
CRPV	Regional Pharmacovigilance Centre
CSP	French Public Health Code
CSTH	Transfusion Safety and Haemovigilance Committee
CTSA	French Armed Forces Blood Transfusion Centre
DES	Specialized qualification
DESC	Advanced specialized qualification
DGOS	Directorate-General for Care Provision
DGS	Directorate-General for Health

DSS	Social Security Directorate
EBMT	European Bone Marrow Transplantation
EBV	Epstein-Barr virus
EFI	European Federation for Immunogenetics
EFS	French Blood Establishment
EID	Adverse reaction in a donor
EIGD	Serious adverse reaction in a donor
EIR	Adverse reaction in a recipient
ELISA	Enzyme-linked immunosorbent assay
EMA	European Medicines Agency
EPST	State-funded science and technology research centres
EQA	External quality assessment
ERA	Test results exchange
ES	Health facilities
ETS	Blood establishment
FACT	Foundation for the Accreditation of Cellular Therapy
FEIGD	Donor serious adverse reaction report
FEIR	Recipient adverse reaction report
FFDSB	French Federation for Voluntary Blood Donation
FFP	Fresh frozen plasma
FIG	Serious incident report
FTE	Full-time equivalent
HAS	French National Authority for Health
Hb	Haemoglobin
HIV	Human immunodeficiency virus
HLA	Human leucocyte antigens
HSCs	Haematopoietic stem cells
Ht	Haematocrit
IAS	Irregular antibody screening
IFI	Indirect immunofluorescence
IG	Serious incident (in the transfusion chain)
IgG	Immunoglobulin G
INSEE	French National Institute for Statistics and Economic Studies
INSERM	French National Institute of Health and Medical Research
InVS	French Institute for Public Health Surveillance
IPD	Post-donation information
IQC	Internal quality control
ISBT	International Society of Blood Transfusion
IUMTC	Transfusion and Cellular Medicine University Institute
IVDD	*in vitro* diagnostic medical devices
JACIE	Joint Accreditation Committee ISCT and EBMT
LBP	Labile blood products
LDL	Low density lipoprotein
LFB	French Fractionation Laboratory
LQL	Limiting quality level
MA	Marketing authorization
MD	Medical device
MEDDEV	Medical devices
MGEN	National health insurance fund for education workers
MNC	Mononuclear cell
NAT	Nucleic acid test
NC	Nonconformity
PBU	Placental blood unit
PC	Platelet concentrate

Glossary

PCC	Prothrombin complex concentrate
PIG	Public interest group
PL	Prothrombin level
PRA	Preliminary risk analysis
PRBCs	Packed red blood cells
PrP (PrPc - PrPres)	Prion protein
P-SD-PC	Pooled standard platelet concentrate
QBD	Donation testing
Q-BS	Quality control by sampling
QC	Quality control
QC-LBP	Quality control of labile blood products
QL	Quality level
SAGM	Saline-adenine-glucose-mannitol solution
SCSTH	Transfusion Safety and Haemovigilance Subcommittee
SOTS	Plans for the organization of blood transfusion services
SP	Sampling plan
STOTS	Area plans for the organization of blood transfusion services
SUD	Single-use device
TRALI	Transfusion-related acute lung injury
TSSE	Transmissible subacute spongiform encephalopathies
UMR	Mixed research unit
UNCAM	French National Union of Health Insurance Funds
UPEC	University Paris-Est Créteil Val-de-Marne
UV	Ultraviolet (rays)
UVA	Ultraviolet A (rays)
VBMD	Voluntary Bone Marrow Donors
vCJD	Variant Creutzfeldt–Jakob disease
WBC	White blood cells
WHO	World Health Organization

IMPRIM'VERT®

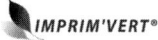

Achevé d'imprimer par Corlet, Imprimeur, S.A.
14110 Condé-sur-Noireau
N° d'Imprimeur : 154262 - Dépôt légal : juin 2013
Imprimé en France